Epigenetics and Epigenomics in Health and Disease

Epigenetics and Epigenomics in Health and Disease

Editor: Kylan Russell

MURPHY & MOORE
www.murphy-moorepublishing.com

www.murphy-moorepublishing.com

MURPHY & MOORE

Cataloging-in-Publication Data

Epigenetics and epigenomics in health and disease / edited by Kylan Russell.
p. cm.
Includes bibliographical references and index.
ISBN 978-1-63987-197-1
1. Epigenetics. 2. Human genome. 3. Medical genetics. 4. Epigenesis. 5. Genomics. I. Russell, Kylan.
QH450 .E65 2022
572.865--dc23

Murphy & Moore Publishing,
1 Rockefeller Plaza,
New York City, NY 10020, USA

ISBN 978-1-63987-197-1 (Hardback)

Contents

Preface

It is often said that books are a boon to mankind. They document every progress and pass on the knowledge from one generation to the other. They play a crucial role in our lives. Thus I was both excited and nervous while editing this book. I was pleased by the thought of being able to make a mark but I was also nervous to do it right because the future of students depends upon it. Hence, I took a few months to research further into the discipline, revise my knowledge and also explore some more aspects. Post this process, I begun with the editing of this book.

Epigenetics is a branch of biology which deals with the study of heritable phenotype changes that are not associated with the alterations in the DNA sequence. It generally involves the alterations which affect gene expression and activity but it may also include any heritable phenotypic change. These effects on cellular and physiological phenotypic characteristics may be a part of normal development or may result from environmental factors. Epigenomics refers to the study of the epigenome which is the complete set of epigenetic modifications taking place in the genetic material of a cell. These epigenetic modifications are reversible in nature. They affect gene expression without altering the DNA sequence. The book studies, analyses and upholds the pillars of epigenetics and epigenomics and their utmost significance in modern times. It consists of contributions made by international experts. As these fields are emerging at a fast pace, this book will help the readers to better understand their concepts.

I thank my publisher with all my heart for considering me worthy of this unparalleled opportunity and for showing unwavering faith in my skills. I would also like to thank the editorial team who worked closely with me at every step and contributed immensely towards the successful completion of this book. Last but not the least, I wish to thank my friends and colleagues for their support.

Editor

1

Genomic Imprinting and Human Reproduction

I.N. Lebedev

1. Introduction

The high frequency of reproductive losses is specific to the human race. The chances of conceiving and giving birth to a healthy child for women between 20 and 30 years old are estimated to be as low as 21-28% per cycle [1]. About 60% of zygotes are eliminated during the pre-implantation or early post-implantation developmental stages and 15-20% of clinically recognized pregnancies are lost during the first trimester [2]. Approximately 50-60% of spontaneously aborted embryos have chromosomal abnormalities which are not compatible with prenatal development [3]. At the same time, the death of another considerable number of embryos with normal karyotypes cannot be explained by existing cytogenetic theories. Considering ontogenesis as a result of the unrolling of the strict developmental program, the epigenetic basis of this process may be of outstanding significance.

According to the classical definition, coined by Conrad Waddington in 1942, epigenetics is a branch of biology which studies "causal mechanisms" by which "the genes of the genotype bring about phenotypic effects" [4]. In its beginning, epigenetics was a synonym for developmental genetics. However, in contrast to classical genetic theories, the subject of epigenetics has a wider diversity of phenomena, which may be unrelated to changes in gene nucleotide sequences [5]. A strong surge of interest in studying the epigenetic basis of human hereditary pathology has been noted over the last several years [6, 7]. New classes of epigenetic diseases, namely chromatin diseases [8] and imprinting disorders [9] have been identified. However, little is known about the features and nature of epigenetic abnormalities, i.e., epimutations, [10] during human prenatal development. In this chapter information on the impact of genomic imprinting abnormalities on embryo development is summarized and discussed.

2. Genomic imprinting and its role in embryogenesis

Genomic imprinting is an epigenetic phenomenon, which is related to differential parent-of-origin gene expression. The term "imprinting" was taken from physiology. It was Konrad Lorenz, an Austrian zoologist, ethologist and ornithologist, who, when working with geese, rediscovered the principle of imprinting (originally described by Douglas Spalding in the 19th century) in the behaviour of nidifugous birds when a young bird acquired several of its behavioural characteristics from one parent.

The term "chromosomal imprinting" was coined in 1960 by Helen Crouse, one of only three PhD students trained by Nobel Laureate Barbara McClintock. Crouse described the selective elimination of paternal chromosomes in the male meiosis in *Sciara* fly [11]. In the first meiotic division of spermatogenesis, a monopolar spindle forms upon which all the maternally derived homologues move to a single pole and all the paternally derived homologues move away from the single pole and are completely eliminated from the cell as a nucleoplasmic bud. Crouse wrote, "the 'imprint' a chromosome bears is unrelated to the genetic construction of the chromosome and is determined only by the sex of the germ line through which the chromosome has been inherited" (cited in [12]). At the time that Crouse first used the term, chromosome imprinting was known to occur in *Sciara* spermatogenesis. This mechanism of selected chromosome segregation remains enigmatic, although much headway has been made in mammalian systems [12].

The first evidence of the parental genome's memory in mammals came from experiments conducted by the Surani, McGrath and Solter groups with pronuclei transplantation in mouse zygotes in 1984 [13, 14]. These studies were aimed at answering the question about the absence of parthenogenesis in mammalian reproduction. It was discovered that diploid androgenic mouse embryos derived from zygotes, which contained two paternal pronuclei and none of the maternal pronuclei, demonstrated an extensive proliferation of extraembryonic tissues but poor development of the embryo *per se*, which usually did not reach a 4-6 somite stage. In contrast, gynogenic zygotes with two maternal pronuclei and an absence of the paternal genome resulted in embryos which developed until the stage of early somites, but then died due to the poor development of supportive extraembryonic tissues. These pioneers' studies established that diploidy alone is not sufficient for embryonic development, but that a balance of maternal and paternal genomes is strongly required for normal embryogenesis. Moreover, the impact of parental genomes on embryo development is different. It seems that the maternal genome is responsible for the development of the embryo body to a greater extent, whereas the paternal one is involved in the support of extraembryonic tissue differentiation.

It is interesting to note that a similar effect of the increasing number of paternal genomes in the zygote is also observed in humans due to an abnormality of fertilization [15]. Fertilization of a diploid oocyte by normal haploid sperm or double fertilization of a normal oocyte by two haploid sperms leads to triploidy in the zygote. In this case, the partial hydatidiform mole (PHM) arises. PHM is characterized by the cystic degeneration of chorionic villi and the presence of a visible embryo in the foetal sac. In the case of the extrusion of the maternal pronucleus from such a triploid zygote, a diploid karyotype is restored through the postzygotic triploid diploidization mechanism [16], but both haploid genomes are paternal in their nature. This bipaternal karyotype is not compatible with the development of an embryo body, but leads to a hyper proliferation of trophoblasts cells and a complete hydatidiform mole (CHM) with an increased risk of chorioepithelioma. The observed effect may be explained by the double increase in the dose of imprinted genes expressed from paternal chromosomes, which promotes proliferative and invasive activity of the trophoblasts cells as well as an absence of activity of the maternal imprinted genes, which, in turn, must suppress trophoblast proliferation.

The parental differences in imprinted genes expression are epigenetic in their nature. They are established during gamete differentiation by sex-dependent epigenetic chromatin modifications, mainly by the differential DNA methylation of promoter regions of imprinted genes or regulatory imprinted centres, which are further stably inherited in the somatic cells of the progeny. These regular and consecutive alterations of chromatin organization are referred to as epigenetic genome reprogramming [17, 18] (Figure 1). This starts in the primordial germ cells when they enter the gonads. Both imprinted and non-imprinted loci become demethylated. This total erasure of epigenetic information is required for the totipontency of future germ cells, imprinting switching and for the prevention of the inheritance of epigenetic defects. The demethylated chromatin's state remains until the duration of the mitotic arrest in male germ cells and the meiotic arrest in female ones. When mitotic divisions of spermogonia are resumed, *de novo* DNA methylation begins, which terminates completely by the time of pachytene of meiosis I. In oocytes, *de novo* DNA methylation starts only at their maturation and ends by metaphase II. In this period, sex-specific methylation of imprinted genes is established. In one imprinting genes, DNA methylation occurs exclusively in oogenesis, whereas in others it occurs during spermatogenesis [19].

The second wave of epigenetic genome reprogramming, which involves somatic cells, begins immediately after fertilization. The paternal chromosomes became decondensed, protamines in the chromatin are replaced by histones and fast demethylation of paternal genome is triggered. The maternal genome undergoes slow passive demethylation. It is believed that demethylation of parental genomes is required to induce pluripotency in embryonic stem cells. Later, during implantation, *de novo* DNA methylation is launched again, which results in specific methylation patterns of particular genomic regions in different cells and tissues. This process, in fact, provides one of the most important mechanisms for committing and regulating tissue specific gene expression during ontogeny. It is significant that imprinted genes avoid this reprogramming wave in somatic cells, preserving their differential methylation pattern inherited from the parents. Genomic imprinting is also regulated through other epigenetic mechanisms, such as histone modifications, antisense transcripts and small non-coding RNA, which have been discussed in detail in some comprehensive reviews [19, 20].

At present, (August 2013), it is reported that there are about 90 imprinted genes in a human genome [21]. Most of them are involved in the regulation of intrauterine foetal development through the control of cell proliferation and the differentiation of placental tissues, regulation of metabolism of some hormones and growth factors [22]. The evolutionary reverse to the haploid expression of a subset of genes in mammalian and flowering plants genomes was a

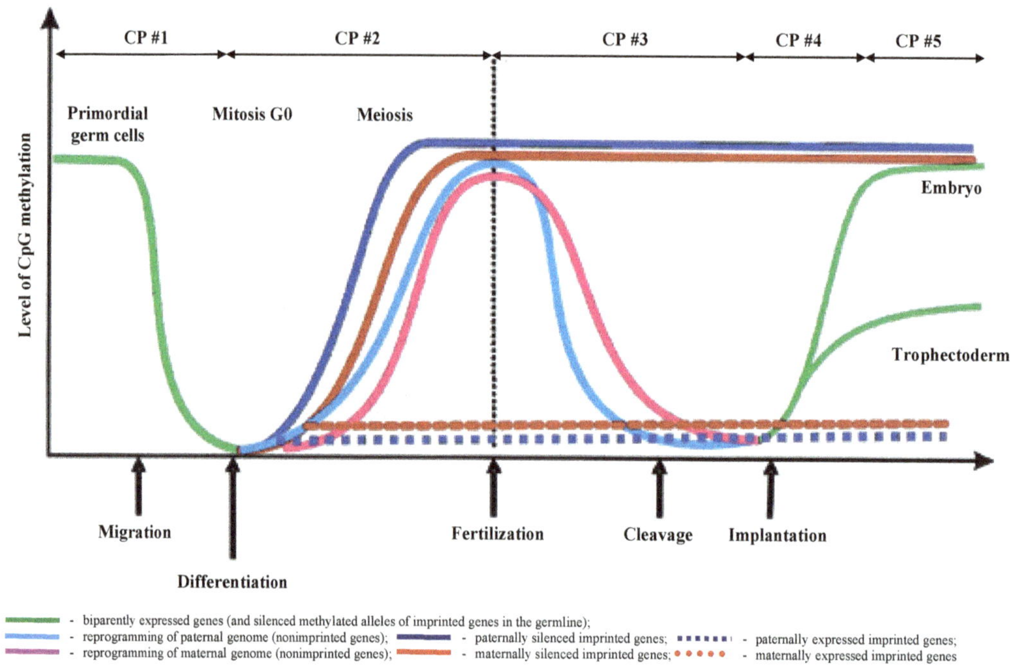

CP – critical periods of reprogramming

Figure 1. Dynamics of epigenetic genome reprogramming

great surprise. Several hypotheses were introduced to explain this intriguing fact, but the "sex conflict" was one the most popular among them [23]. According to this hypothesis, maternal imprinted genes in mammals are responsible for the suppression of foetal growth in order to save maternal resources for subsequent pregnancies. In contrast, paternal imprinted genes are involved in the promotion of foetal growth that provides higher chances of survival for many offspring.

Testing this hypothesis in mouse models, the direct evidence for the significant role of genomic imprinting in mammalian embryo development was obtained. The generation of uniparental disomies (UPD) in progeny of translocation carrier's mice gives nonviable embryos [24]. This fact leads to the idea of searching for UPD in human spontaneous abortions in order to estimate the impact of genomic imprinting abnormalities on prenatal death.

3. UPD in spontaneous abortions

To date, eight studies have been performed to find UPD in spontaneous abortions [25-32] (Table 1). However, the obtained results were modest. Only seven cases of UPD (2.3%) among a total of 305 spontaneous abortions were found and most of them involved chromosomes which did not contain known imprinted genes. Only in three cases segmental UPD (16p/16q (mat), 14q (pat) and 7q (mat)) embryo death can be connected with a disturbance of the dose of imprinted genes localized on these chromosomal regions. Moreover, spontaneous abortions without previous cytogenetic analysis were included in some studies that could have led to overestimation the obtained rate. As a result, the frequency of UPD for chromosomes, which contain known imprinted genes in spontaneous abortions were estimated to be 1% (3/305) or 1.14 per 1,000 occasions of chromosome inheritance from parents to progeny. The latter figure was obtained from the investigation of 6,156 cases of chromosome inheritance by DNA microsatellite analyses and seven cases of UPD were found in the eight cited studies. This figure does not significantly differ from the expected frequency (1.65:1,000), predicted from data about frequencies of chromosome segregation errors in gametogenesis and early embryogenesis, which can lead to uniparental inheritance in humans [33].

Thus, it seems that UPD is a selectively neutral phenomenon in human reproduction. Moreover, UPD for some chromosomes (6, 7, 11, 14 and 15) are compatible with postnatal life leading

Samples	Number of spontaneous abortions	UPD cases	References
Anembryonic pregnancies without cytogenetic analysis	23	UPD(21)mat, UPD(21)mat in combination with trisomies 7 and 9	[25]
Spontaneous abortions: - first trimester, without cytogenetic analysis	18	0	[26]
- with normal karyotype	35	0	[27]
- 6-22 weeks, with normal karyotype	71	UPD(9)mat UPD(21)mat	[28]
- with normal karyotype	24	Maternal segmental heterosomy 16pter-D16S3107 and isodisomy D16S3018-qter	[29]
- with normal karyotype	81	Segmental UPD(14q)pat, UPD(7q)mat	[30]
Missed abortions and anembryonic pregnancies: - with 46,XX karyotype (analysis of X-chromosome inheritance only)	52*	0	[31]*
- with normal karyotype	87*	0	[32]*
Total:	305	7 (2,3%)	

Note: * - samples partially overlap.

Table 1. Results of UPD studies in spontaneous abortions

to a formation of specific genomic imprinting disorders: transient neonatal diabetes mellitus (TNDM), Silver-Russell syndrome (SRS), Beckwith-Wiedemann syndrome (BWS), Wang and Temple syndromes, Prader-Willi syndrome (PWS) and Angelman syndrome (AS), respectively [34]. It became clear that UPD is a rare cytogenetic phenomenon, which cannot explain the mechanisms of imprinted genes disturbances in human pregnancy loss. The only evidence for the pathogenetic role of genomic imprinting abnormalities in human reproduction remains from studies on a hydatidiform mole which originated from the doubling of paternal genome in conception [15]. However, this conclusion does not offer an answer on the possible mechanisms of imprinting disturbances associated with early pregnancy loss.

4. Epimutations of imprinted genes in spontaneous abortions

Taking into account the epigenetic nature of genomic imprinting, we proposed a hypothesis that expected the deleterious effect of abnormal imprinted genes expression to be visible at the epigenetic rather than cytogenetic level [35]. Indeed, UPD formation requires a combination of several subsequent errors in chromosomal segregation during parental meiosis, fertilization and embryo development. For example, the most frequent mechanism of UPD formation is trisomy rescue. It arises from chromosomal nondisjunction in meiosis, trisomy formation in the zygote after fertilization and the loss of additional chromosome in some somatic cells during subsequent mitotic divisions. In a third of the cases of such correction, the situation of inheritance of both homologues from one parent may be observed. If involved chromosome contains an imprinted gene, then the double increase or complete loss of expression of imprinted genes may be detected and it is dependent on the parental origin of expressed allele.

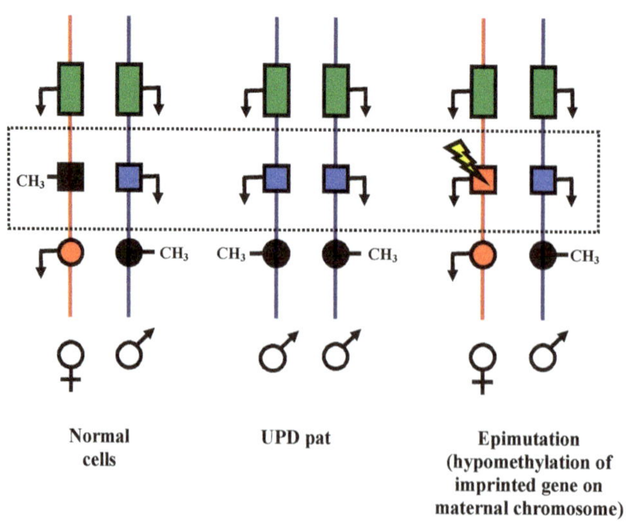

Figure 2. Effects of UPD and epimutations on expression of imprinted genes.

On the other hand, the change of the imprinted gene dose may be achieved by epimutations, i.e., abnormal methylation of the expressed allele or demethylation of the silenced allele. From a functional point of view, epimutations and UPD influences on imprinted genes expression should be similar (Figure 2). It is important that epimutation on a single allele is enough to achieve the imprinted gene dysfunction in a dominant manner.

Before the testing of the hypothesis about the influence of methylation defects in imprinted genes on the aetiology of early pregnancy loss, a classification of epimutations was introduced [36]. They were divided into the following several groups depending on their germinal or somatic origin, hyper- or hypomethylation of active or silenced alleles, and affected parental chromosomes (Table 2):

1. Types of epimutations of imprinted genes by the loci involved:
    - 1.1. Epimutations causing a global disturbance of genomic imprinting at the genome level.
    - 1.2. Epimutations at the imprinting centres causing a disturbance of imprinting of neighbouring genes.
    - 1.3. Epimutations at the imprinted genes.
2. Types of epimutations of imprinted genes by their origin:
    - 2.1. Germinal epimutations
        - 2.1.1. Errors of genomic imprinting erasure in primordial germ cells with retention of methyl groups (Critical Period 1, CP #1, on Figure 1). These errors may lead to transgenerational inheritance of epigenetic defects.
        - 2.1.2. Errors of imprinting establishment during gametogenesis (CP #2 on Figure 1)
            - 2.1.2.1. Absence of methylation of imprinted genes alleles that normally should be methylated in sperm or oocytes.
            - 2.1.2.2. Aberrant methylation of imprinted genes alleles that normally should be unmethylated in sperm or oocytes.
    - 2.2. Somatic epimutations
        - 2.2.1. Abnormal hypomethylation of inactive parental alleles of imprinted genes during epigenetic genome reprogramming (CP #3 on Figure 1).
        - 2.2.2. Abnormal methylation of expressed parental alleles of imprinted genes during de novo DNA methylation upon epigenetic genome reprogramming (CP #4 on Figure 1).
        - 2.2.3. Spontaneous hypomethylation of inactive parental alleles of imprinted genes in somatic cells after epigenetic genome reprogramming (CP #5 on Figure 1).
        - 2.2.4. Spontaneous hypermethylation of expressed parental alleles of imprinted genes in somatic cells after epigenetic genome reprogramming (CP #5 on Figure 1).
3. Types of epimutations of imprinted genes by their functional consequences and affected parental alleles:
    - 3.1. Hypomethylation of the inactive maternal allele of the imprinted gene.
    - 3.2. Hypomethylation of the inactive paternal allele of the imprinted gene.
    - 3.3. Hypermethylation of the expressed maternal allele of the imprinted gene.
    - 3.4. Hypermethylation of the expressed paternal allele of the imprinted gene.

	Type of epimutations	Abnormal hypomethylation of		Abnormal hypermethylation of	
		maternal allele	paternal allele	maternal allele	paternal allele
Germinal epimutations	Errors of genomic imprinting erasure with retention of methyl groups (CP #1)	Not applicable	Not applicable	*IGF2/H19* (BWS)	*SNURF-SNRPN* (PWS); *PEG1/MEST* (SRS)
Germinal epimutations	Absence of imprinted genes alleles methylation (CP #2)	BiCHM; *SNURF-SNRPN* (AS); *KCNQ1OT1* (BWS, TNDM); *PLAGL1* (TNDM, BWS)	*IGF2/H19* (SRS)	Not applicable	Not applicable
Germinal epimutations	Aberrant hypermethylation of imprinted genes alleles (CP #2)	Not applicable	Not applicable	*IGF2/H19* (BWS)	*SNURF-SNRPN* (PWS); *PEG1/MEST* (SRS)
Somatic epimutations	Abnormal hypomethylation of inactive parental alleles of imprinted genes during epigenetic genome reprogramming (CP #3)	*SNURF-SNRPN* (mosaic forms of AS). MHS; mosaic forms of TNDM	Partial hypomethylation of *IGF2/H19* (SRS)	Not applicable	Not applicable
Somatic epimutations	Abnormal hypermethylation of expressed parental alleles of imprinted genes during epigenetic genome reprogramming (CP #4)	Not applicable	Not applicable	*IGF2/H19* (BWS)	*SNURF-SNRPN* (PWS)
Somatic epimutations	Stochastic epimutations (hypo- and hypermethylation) in somatic cells after epigenetic genome reprogramming (CP #5)	*KCNQ1OT1* (oesophagus carcinoma, liver cancer); *PEG3* (choriocarcinoma)	*P73* (renal carcinoma; lung cancer)	*IGF2/H19* (Wilm's tumour); *P73* (acute leukaemia, Burkitt's lymphoma); *DLK1/GTL2* (renal carcinoma)	*SNURF-SNRPN* (mosaic forms of PWS); *PEG3* (cervical and endometrial carcinomas); *PLAGL1* (ovarian cancer)

Table 2. Types of epimutations of imprinted genes in human (according to [36] with modifications)

The first evidence of epimutations in imprinted genes in reproductive losses came from studies of biparental complete hydatidiform mole (BiCHM, MIM #231090). This pathology, as opposed to classical androgenic complete mole, arose in the case of normal biparental karyotype [37] (Figure 3). It was shown that imprinted genes, which are methylated on maternal chromosomes in normal embryos, became hypomethylated in the case of BiCHM both on the paternal and maternal homologues [15]. Functionally, this epigenetic status is the same as an androgenic complete mole. Subsequent studies revealed that BiCHM arose due to germinal epimutations, namely the absence of *de novo* methylation of imprinted genes in oogenesis (type # 2.1.2.1 according to classification) [38]. However, these findings do not offer an answer about the prevalence of imprinting defects in human reproductive losses. The convenient model system for studies became spontaneous abortions.

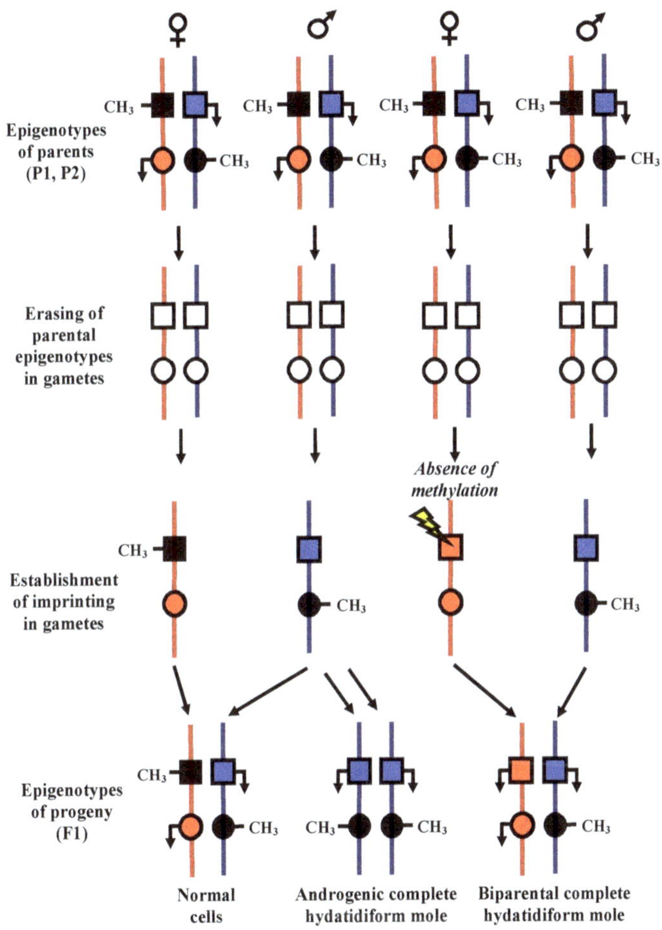

Figure 3. Cytogenetic and epigenetic mechanisms of hydatidiform mole formation.

The first study devoted to the analysis of methylation status of *SNRPN* imprinted gene was published by our group in 2006 [39]. However, it was shown that all investigated spontaneous abortions, as well as the control sample of induced (therapeutic) abortions, had normal differential methylation of parental alleles of this imprinted gene.

Our further studies on imprinted genes *PLAGL1 (ZAC)*, *CDKN1C* and regulatory imprinting centres *IGF2/H19* and *KCNQ1OT1 (LIT1)* in spontaneous abortions revealed that 9.5% and 10.3% of embryos with normal karyotype had hypomethylation of *KCNQ1OT1* and *PLAGL1*, respectively, on maternal chromosomes [35, 40]. It is interesting that in two embryos from the investigated group (2.3%) epimutations were detected in both genes. In both families, the women had not had a successfully delivered pregnancy. In one family, the woman had had four spontaneous abortions, in the other, the woman had had two spontaneous abortions and a stillbirth. It was shown that the frequency of recurrent pregnancy loss (i.e., the loss of three or more consecutive pregnancies) was significantly higher in woman who had had a loss of methylation in *PLAGL1* in spontaneous abortions tissues, in comparison with woman without epimutations in the aborted embryo (33% and 8%, respectively, $p < 0.05$). A similar tendency was observed for *KCNQ1OT1* epimutations, but it does not reach a statistically significant difference.

It was remarkable also that all detected epimutations were confined to one placental tissue (cytotrophoblast or extraembryonic mesoderm) only indicating their somatic origin in post-implantation stages of development after the divergence of embryonic and extraembryonic cell lineages. This observation has an important value for the discussion on the increase of genomic imprinting disorders in children born after the application of assisted reproductive technologies (ART) [20, 41-44]. Indeed, several cases of children with BWS, SRS and AS born after *in vitro* fertilization (IVF) or intracytoplasmic sperm injection (ICSI) have been reported. However, it is more significant that all patients with confirmed molecular diagnosis had hypomethylation of imprinted genes on maternal chromosomes as a cause of disorder among all the other known possible mechanisms which can alter imprinted genes expression – UPD, chromosomal microdeletions or microduplications, point mutations in imprinted genes or regulatory imprinted centres. This fact is supported by results of *in vitro* studies in model organisms [45]. This often leads to a hasty one-sided conclusion that manipulations with gametes and embryos in an artificial medium cannot support correct recording and maintenance of genomic imprinting and they are responsible for an increase of imprinting defects in children after ART. Our, and other, recently published data from spontaneous abortions studies [46] indicates that the same epimutations with relatively high frequency can be observed in embryos from natural cycles also and not only from IVF or ICSI pregnancies. This means that epimutations of imprinted genes arising during human embryo development, and infertile pairs or couples with the history of recurrent pregnancy losses (typical patients of ART clinics), may have increasing chances to produce progeny with epimutations after overcoming the natural reproductive barriers by IVF or ICSI. This conclusion implies that the nature of epimutations involves the interaction of hereditary and environmental factors.

Evidence for epimutations of imprinted genes in spontaneous abortions was also noted in other subsequent studies (See tables 3 and 4). For example, multiple hypermethylation of imprinted genes was detected in 4% (2 out of 55) of spontaneous abortions and 18% (10 out of 57) of stillbirths [47]. In this study, *H19, KCNQ1OT1, PEG3* and *SNRPN* genes with paternal expression and *MEG3* and *NESP55* with maternal expression were investigated. In other studies, the expression level of several imprinted genes was compared between placental tissues from normal pregnancies and pregnancies complicated by intrauterine growth retardation (IUGR) [48]. It was found that *PHLDA2, ILK2, NNAT, CCDC86* and *PEG10* genes had increased expression in IUGR pregnancies, whereas the expression level of *PLAGL1, DHCR24,*

ZNF331, and *CDKAL1* was decreased. In this study, hypomethylation of *DLK1, H19,* and *SNRPN* was demonstrated also in the placental tissues of foetuses with IUGR. In another study, expression levels of four imprinted genes (*IGF2, PEG10, PHLDA2,* and *CDKN1C*) were investigated in embryonic and placental tissues of 38 spontaneous abortions [49]. The increased expression of *PHLDA2* was found both in the embryonic and placental tissues in the first trimester. During the second trimester, elevated expression levels of all four genes were observed in both tissues, however, for the *PHLDA2* gene it was specific to the embryonic tissues only. A decreased expression of *PEG3* was detected in embryonic tissues during the third trimester.

Pathology	Sample size	Tissue	MLMD frequency	*PLAGL1* (6q24)	*PEG10* (7q21)	*DLK1* (14q32)	*PEG3* (19q13.4)	*LIT1* (11p15)	*INS* (11p15)	*SNRPN* (15q11)	*WT1* (11p15)	*KCNQ1* (11p15)	*GABRB3* (15q11)	*HTR2A* (13q14)	*TRPM5* (11p15)	*MEST* (7q32)	*GABRA5* (15q11)	Ref.
SA	55	MT	3.6% (2)	-	-	-	2↑	1↑	-	1↑	-	-	-	-	-	-	-	[47]
SB	57	MT	17.5% (10)	-	-	-	6↑	2↑	-	9↑	-	-	-	-	-	-	-	[47]
SA	87	CC	2.3% (2)	2↓	-	-	-	2↓	-	0	-	-	-	-	-	-	-	[40]
SA	13	CC	100% (13)	1↓	3↓	0	0	0	2↑	2↑	4↓	5↓	3↓	2↓	1↑	0	3↑	[50]
SA	13	EM	100% (13)	2↓	9↓	9↓	0	0	7↑	10↑	10↓	3↓	5↓	6↓	5↑	0	7↑	[50]
SA	165	CC	3.6% (6)	-	-	-	-	6↑	-	7↑	-	-	-	-	-	-	-	[46]
SA	29	CC	10.3% (3)	-	-	-	1↓, 2↑	2↑	-	1↑	-	-	-	-	-	1↑	-	[51]
Total	406		12.1% (49)	5.0% (5/100)	46.2% (12/26)	34.6% (9/26)	7.1% (11/154)	3.2% (13/406)	34.6% (9/26)	7.4% (30/406)	53.8% (14/26)	30.8% (8/26)	30.8% (8/26)	30.8% (8/26)	23.1% (6/26)	1.8% (1/55)	38.5% (10/26)	
				↓ - 16.0% (65/406); ↑ - 18.7% (76/406)														

Notes for tables 3 and 4: SA – spontaneous abortion; SB – stillbirth; MT – muscular tissues of embryo; CC – chorion cytotrophoblast; EM – extraembryonic mesoderm; MLMD – multilocus methylation defects (number of embryos with MLMD is indicated in parentheses); ↓ – hypomethylation; ↑ – hypermethylation.

Table 3. Frequency of epimutations in paternally expressed imprinted genes in spontaneous abortions

Pathology	Sample size	Tissue	MLMD frequency	*GRB10* *(7q21)*	*CPA4* *(7q32)*	*PHLDA2* *(11p15)*	*ZNF215* *(11p15)*	*H19* *(11p15)*	*MEG3* *(14q32)*	*NESP55* *(20q13.3)*	Ref.
SA	55	MT	3.6% (2)	-	-	-	-	0	1↑	0	[47]
SB	57	MT	17.5% (10)	-	-	-	-	4↑	8↑	6↑	[47]
SA	87	CC	2.3% (2)	-	-	-	-	0	0	-	[40]
SA	13	EM	100% (13)	1↓	8↓	2↓	8↓	1↑	0	0	[50]
SA	13	CC	100% (13)	5↓	5↓	9↓	4↓	6↑	0	0	[50]
SA	165	CC	3.6% (6)	-	-	-	-	4↑	-	-	[46]
SA	29	CC	10.3% (3)	-	-	-	-	0	0	0	[51]
Total	406		12.1% (49)	23.1% (6/26)	50.0% (13/26)	42.3% (11/26)	46.2% (12/26)	3.7% (15/406)	3.7% (9/241)	3.9% (6/154)	
				↓ - 10.3% (42/406); ↑ - 7.4% (30/406)							

Table 4. Frequency of epimutations in maternally expressed imprinted genes in spontaneous abortions

It is important to note that all the above mentioned studies were performed by the "candidate gene" approach, i.e., only several interesting genes were tested based on their supposed functions in embryogenesis. A new era in this area of research began with the application of array technologies. They provide comprehensive and unbiased analysis of the human imprintome. Results of the first studies revealed a new, intriguing phenomenon of multilocus methylation defects (MLMD) on imprinted genes. This effect is presented by multiple epimutations (hypo- and/or hypermethylation) affecting several imprinted genes simultaneously in the genome in different combinations. In fact, the first example of MLMD is a BiCHM, which results from errors of imprinting establishment on maternal chromosomes during epigenetic genome reprogramming in oocytes leading to the hypomethylation of maternal alleles of different imprinted genes [38]. MLMD were detected in human reproductive losses [50] as well as in patients with genomic imprinting disorders [52]. Importantly, in one recent study 15 (8%) probands among 194 patients with clinical features of an imprinting disorder but no molecular diagnosis had methylation anomalies, including missed and unexpected molecular diagnosis [53].

Evidence of MLMD in 13 first trimester spontaneous abortions were obtained in our study by DNA methylation array the GoldenGate Methylation Cancer Panel I (Illumina) analysis of 51 imprinted genes [50]. Multiple methylation defects affecting from four to 12 genes in each embryo were found. Epimutations were presented by the hypomethylation of paternal alleles of *GRB10, CPA4, PHLDA2, ZNF215* genes, and maternal alleles of *PEG10, PLAGL1, WT1, HTR2A, DLK1, GABRB3, KCNQ1* genes. Hypermethylation was observed on paternal allele of

H19 and on maternal alleles of *INS, TRPM5, PWCR1, GABRA5* genes. The majority of epimutations (78%) were confined to single placental tissue (extraembryonic mesoderm or cytotrophoblast), indicating postzygotic errors in imprinting maintenance in somatic cells.

Summarizing the published data, it is possible to note that MLMD were observed in 49 of 406 investigated spontaneous abortions (12%) (See tables 3 and 4). It is evident that this value, of a significant magnitude greater than UPD frequency in miscarriages, indicates an appreciable effect of epigenetic defects on imprinted genes in pregnancy losses. The incidence of epimutations for different genes varied from 1.8% (*MEST*) to 53.8% (*WT1*). For genes expressed from maternal chromosomes, the frequency of epimutations was 17.7%, with 10.3 % of these presented by the hypomethylation of respective inactive paternal alleles and 7.4% by the hypermethylation of active maternal alleles. For genes expressed from the paternal allele, the total frequency of epimutations was twice as frequent (34.7%). These epimutations were presented by the hypomethylation of respective inactive maternal alleles (16%) and the hypermethylation of expressed paternal alleles (18.7%).

The results of the studies suggest possible mechanisms of the selective influence of epimutations of imprinted genes on early embryo development. As it was mentioned early, the "sex conflict" hypothesis is the most popular in explaining the imprinted mode of gene expression. From its point of view, the expected suppressive effect of epimutations should emerge from the hypomethylation of paternal alleles, which leads to a loss of imprinting and the biallelic expression of maternal genes responsible for foetal growth suppression, as well as from hypermethylation of paternal alleles, which leads to the absence of products responsible for foetal growth stimulation. The total incidence of such types of epimutations in spontaneous abortions is 29% (10.3 + 18.7). At the same time, the total incidence of epimutations, which can lead to the promotion of foetal growth (hypo- and hypermethylation of maternal alleles), was 23.4% (16 + 17.4). The differences between frequencies of "suppressive" and "promotion" epimutations were not statistically significant ($p = 0.07$). However, this is a relative estimation for several reasons, including complete acceptance of the "sex conflict" hypothesis for each imprinted gene (maternal genes are suppressors, paternal genes are activators) and the idea that there is a strong reverse correlation between gene methylation and its expression. To obtain more precise and weighted estimations, further studies of imprinted gene functions and molecular mechanisms of their expression regulation are encouraged.

Does MLMD arise spontaneously in different loci or is it driven by mutations in a candidate's genes responsible for genomic imprinting establishment and maintenance? To answer this question the evidence of MLMD in patients with imprinting disorders should be discussed.

5. Multiple methylation defects in patients with imprinting disorders

The first evidence of multiple epimutations of imprinted genes was obtained in 2005 in the comparative analysis of methylation status of two genes – *ZAC (PLAGL1)* and *LIT1 (KCNQ1OT1)* in eight patients with BWS and 17 patients with TNDM [54]. The idea for this study was based on the fact that there is partial overlapping of some clinical features in these syndromes. This observation may reflect possible interactions between *PLAGL1* and *P57*^{KIP2} genes. According to the author's suggestion, an overexpression of *PLAGL1* due to the loss of methylation of inactive maternal allele may lead to the suppression or inhibition of cyclin-dependent kinases *P57*^{KIP2} through the hyperactivation of *LIT1 (KCNQ1OT1)*. It was shown that all eight BWS patients had normal *PLAGL1* methylation, whereas in two patients with TNDM hypomethylation at *LIT1* was detected. The first patient had UPD(6)pat. The second one had a normal karyotype, but, typically for TNDM, a loss of methylation at *PLAGL1* on maternal chromosome 6. It is interesting that in the latter patient's situation, clinical signs of TNDM were supplemented with umbilical hernia and macroglassia that are typical for BWS.

In 2006, Mackay and colleagues reported on a study of two patients with TNDM and IUGR who had hypomethylation of *ZAC* and *KCNQ1OT1* on maternal chromosomes 6 and 11 respectively [55]. Significantly, both patients did not have the overgrowth which is typical for BWS in the case of *KCNQ1OT1* hypomethylation. However, they had moderate macroglassia, which is not typical for TNDM, and abdomen wall defects and exomphalos that are frequent in both syndromes.

Later in 2006, Mackay and colleagues described another 12 patients with TNDM and hypomethylation of *ZAC* on maternal chromosome 6q24 [56]. In six patients (50%) additional methylation defects were found in different imprinted genes. It was hypomethylation of *GRB10, PEG1/MEST, KCNQ1OT1,* and *PEG3* on maternal chromosomes in different combinations. All patients with multiple methylation defects had higher birth weight and were more phenotypically diverse than other TNDM patients with different genetic aetiologies, except for *ZAC* hypomethylation, presumably reflecting the influence of dysregulation of multiple imprinted genes. It was proposed the existence of a "maternal hypomethylation syndrome" (MHS), when a patient with the loss of methylation at one maternally-methylated locus may also manifest DNA methylation loss at other loci, potentially complicated or even confounded the clinical presentation [56].

Another specific finding of this study which is also very intriguing, is that the level of mosaicism for the DNA methylation index varied in different investigated tissues (blood, mouth-brushes, fibroblasts) and affected different genes. The presence of mosaicism indicates postzygotyic errors of imprinting maintenance in somatic cells. However, it is more significant that such errors affected only maternally, but not paternally inherited alleles. This type of epigenetic mosaicism may explain another interesting fact that all patients with MHS had a major clinical manifestation of TNDM but no other genomic imprinting disorders that can be expected from the involvement of different imprinted genes. It is reasonable to assume that germinal epimutations at *ZAC*, which in theory must be presented (or at least maintained) in all somatic cells, should lead to TNDM symptoms, whereas somatic epimutations at other different genes can partially modify only a clinical manifestation of the "main" hereditary imprinting syndrome.

Later, MLMD were also reported in other imprinting disorders. However, both maternal and paternal alleles were affected in comparison with MHS. Hypermethylation and hypomethylation of imprinted genes were reported also. For example, in some cases of BWS, loss of methylation at *KCNQ1OT1* was accompanied by hypomethylation at *PLAGL1, PEG/MEST* and

SNURF-SNRPN [57]. In some patients with SRS, hypomethylation at *GRB10* and *IGF2/H19* was observed [58, 59]. Multiple epimutations were observed at *H19, PEG3, NESPAS* and *GNAS* genes in one patient with overlapping clinical symptoms of PWS and BWS [60].

It was mentioned earlier that microarray technologies allow us to obtain comprehensive data sets about the methylation status of imprinted genes over the whole genome. In a recent study, 65 patients with different genomic imprinting disorders (BWS, SRS, PWS, AS, TNDM and pseudohypoparathyroidism (PHP-1B)) were investigated by using "GoldenGate Cancer Panel I" (Illumina) DNA methylation microarray [61]. MLMD were detected in all the diseases except PWS and AS, which demonstrated methylation defects at *SNRPN* only. Multiple epimutations were observed in 33% of BWS patients with *KCNQ1OT1* hypomethylation, 75% of TNDM patients with *PLAGL1* hypomethylation, 50% of PHP-1B patients with *GNASXL/EX1A* hypomethylation, and in 17% of SRS patients with *H19* hypomethylation. MLMD involved an additional one to 16 imprinted genes in each patient.

Thus, examinations of patients with imprinting disorders indicate that the epigenetic basis of these diseases may, in some cases, be supplemented by multiple methylation defects in several other imprinting genes in addition to epimutation at the disease-specific gene, which is responsible for the pathogenesis of major clinical features of a given syndrome. The incidence of MLMD in different imprinting disorders varies from 8.9% (SRS) to 56.3% (TNDM) (Table 5). The incidence of methylation defects at different genes varies also. The *KCNQ1OT1, H19,* and *GNAS/NESPAS* genes are the most frequently involved in MLMD. On the other hand, *SNURF-SNRPN* imprinting centre is a very rare subject in the study of methylation defects in BWS and SRS patients, and scarcely noted in the list of MLMD affected genes in patients with TNDM and MHS.

Is the combination of imprinted genes affected by MLMD in different syndromes and pregnancy losses non-random? Are there any specific features of nucleotide sequences and mechanisms of expression regulation of imprinted genes with different incidence of methylation defects? Does an interaction between imprinted genes that may lead to formation of specific epigenotype and phenotype exist? Further studies are necessary to obtain answers to these questions. However, there is some data which indicates the existence of coordination mechanisms in the regulation of epigenetic status of human imprintome. For example, it was shown that epigenetic changes in the cases of BiCHM and TNDM affected imprinted genes on maternal chromosomes only, whereas other non-imprinted genes were not a subject for epimutations [68, 69]. On the other hand, multiple methylation defects were observed by DNA methylation array analysis both in imprinted and non-imprinted genes in spontaneous abortions [50]. It is also possible that MLMD may have a different molecular nature in comparison with a methylation defect at a single locus. For example, multiple methylation defects in patients with BWS were observed only in the cases of *KCNQ1OT1* hypomethylation, but not in the ones with *H19/IGF2* hypermethylation (Table 5). The possible regulation genetic mechanisms for epigenetic status of imprinted genes are discussed in the last part of the chapter.

Syndrome	Sample size	Disease-specific epimutation	MLMD frequency	*PLAGL1* *(6q24)*	*MEST/* *PEG1* *(7q32)*	*LIT1 (11p15)*	*DLK1/* *GTL2* *(14q32)*	*SNRPN* *(15q11)*	*IGF2R* (6q25)	*GRB10/* *MEG1* *(7p13)*	*H19* *(11p15)*	*GNAS/* *NESPAS* *(20q13)*	Ref.
				Genes with paternal expression					Genes with maternal expression				
TNDM	12	*PLAGL1* hypometh	50% (6)	12↓	5↓	3↓	0	0	n.a.	3↓	0	n.a.	[56]
TNDM	4	*PLAGL1* hypometh	75% (3)	4↓	0	0	0	0	1↓,1↑	1↓	0	0	[61]
Total	**16**	***PLAGL1* hypometh**	***56.3% (9)***	***100%***	***31.4% (5/16)***	***18.8% (3/16)***	***0***	***0***	***12.5% (2/16)***	***25.0% (4/16)***	***0***	***0***	
BWS	40	*LIT1* hypometh	25% (10)	n.a.	3↓	40↓	n.a.	1↓	6↓	n.a.	n.a.	n.a.	[62]
BWS	81	*LIT1* hypometh	21% (17)	7↓	6↓	81↓	0	0	6↓	4↓	0	10↓	[63]
BWS	68	*LIT1* hypometh	23.5% (16)	6↓	6↓	68↓	0	1↓	10↓	n.a.	1↓	n.a.	[64]
BWS	11	*LIT1* hypometh	45.5% (5)	0	1↓	11↓	2↓	n.a.	2↓	2↓	2↓	2↓	[65]
BWS	24	*LIT1* hypometh	25% (6)	2↓	4↓	24↓	0	1↓	n.a.	n.a.	n.a.	n.a.	[57]
BWS	43	*LIT1* hypometh	33% (14)	3↓	3↓	43↓	0	0	3↓	3↓	2↓	3↑	[61]
Total	***267***	***LIT1 hypometh***	***25.5% (68)***	7.9% (18/227)	8.6% (23/267)	***100%***	0.9% (2/227)	1.2% (3/256)	***10.9% (27/243)***	6.7% (9/135)	2.5% (5/203)	11.9% (16/135)	
BWS	20	***H19*** hypermeth	0	0	0	0	0	0	0	0	20↑	0	[63]
SRS	23	***H19*** hypometh	8.2% (2)	0	0	1↓	0	n.a.	1↓, 2↑	1↓	23↓	2↓	[66]
SRS	74	***H19*** hypometh	9.5% (7)	2↓	3↓	3↓	5↓	1↓	2↓	n.a.	74↓	n.a.	[64]
SRS	65	***H19*** hypometh	7.7% (5)	n.a.	1↓	3↓	1↓	n.a.	3↓	0	65↓	n.a.	[67]
SRS	6	***H19*** hypometh	16.6%(1)	0	1↓	0	0	0	0	0	6↓	0	[61]
Total	***168***	***H19 hypometh***	***8.9% (15)***	2.1% (2/103)	2.5% (5/168)	4.3% (7/168)	3.7% (6/168)	1.4% (1/80)	4.9% (8/168)	1.1% (1/94)	***100%***	8.7% (2/29)	
PWS/BWS	1	***SNRPN*** hypometh	–	n.a.	n.a.	1↓	n.a.	1↓	n.a.	n.a.	1↓	1↓	[60]
PHP-1B	10	***GNAS*** hypometh	50% (5)	0	2↓	0	0	0	1↓	0	0	10↓	[61]
Total	***476***		***20.4% (97/476)***	***10.3% (38/370)***	***7.4% (35/475)***	***58.4% (278/476)***	***1.8% (8/435)***	***1.1% (4/377)***	***8.7% (38/439)***	***5.2% (14/269)***	***47.1% (194/412)***	***15.0% (29/193)***	
				↓ – 75.6% (360/476); ↑ – 0.6% (3/476)					↓ – 52.9% (252/476); ↑ – 4.8% (23/476)				

Note: MLMD – multilocus methylation defects (number of patients with MLMD is indicated in parentheses); n.a. – not analysed; ↓ – hypomethylation; ↑ – hypermethylation.

Table 5. Incidence of methylation defects in patients with imprinting disorders

6. Genetic control of epigenetic status of imprinted genes

The story begins again with BiCHM. Recurrent cases of this pathology or classical CHM and PHM in anamnesis, the occurrence of several cases within one pedigree, and the appearance in consanguineous couples provide evidence for an autosomal recessive mode of inheritance of BiCHM by maternal lineage. The first candidate's genes were DNA methyltransferases, however, the sequencing of it in women with a history of BiCHM did not reveal the presence of mutations. Subsequent genome-wide association studies and homozigosity mapping indicated the linkage of BiCHM with chromosomal segment 19q13.42, in which the *NLRP7 (NALP7)* gene was mapped [70]. In this first study, five mutations of *NLRP7* in familial and recurrent cases of hydatidiform mole were reported. Two mutations, IVS3+1G-A and IVS7+1G-, were found in introns 3 and 7, respectively. Three single nucleotide changes were detected in another three families: p.R693W, p.R693P, and p.N913S. All these mutations were absent in the 348 individuals from the control group.

Homozygous c.295G>T (p.Glu99X) and heterozygous c.1970A>T (p.Asp657Val) mutations were observed in a woman with four hydatidiform moles [71]. Her sister with two moles and brother were compound heterozygotes for these mutations. Her father had a homozygous p.Asp657Val mutation. Her mother had a homozygous p.Glu99X mutation, three successful pregnancies and a stillbirth in anamnesis. In another studied family, a brother and his three sisters with recurrent hydatidiform moles (two, three, and five cases in anamnesis, respectively) were homozygous for p.Arg693Pro mutations, but the brother did not have any reproductive problems. The authors of this study made a very important conclusion that mutations of *NLRP7* do not affect the foetal development in the case of paternal inheritance, but lead to recurrent hydatidiform moles when transmitted from the mother.

Several studies combined methylation analysis of imprinted genes and the search for *NLRP7* mutations. For example, homozygous c.2248C>G (p.L750V), c.2471+1G>A missense mutations and heterozygous c.2248C>G (p.Leu750Val), c.2810+2T>G *NLRP7* mutations in women with BiCHM and multiple hypomethylation at the *PEG3, SNRPN, KCNQ1OT1, GNAS* imprinted genes were reported [72]. Studying 11 families with BiCHM, Hayward and colleagues performed methylation analysis of the *ZAC, GNAS-NESP55, LIT1/KCNQ1OT1,* and *SGCE/PEG10* genes in four families. Hypomethylation of maternal alleles at the *ZAC* and *LIT1* as well as hypermethylation of maternal alleles at the *NESP55,* which is unusual for BiCHM, were observed in all four families. The sequencing of *NLRP7* revealed eight not previously described mutations: p.K116X, p.L398R, p.S673X, p.W778X, c.939_952dup14, c.1456dupG, c.2030delT, and c.277+1G>C [73]. Moreover, p.L398R was associated with multiple epimutations of imprinted genes indicating that some mutations in *NLRP7* may be connected with different types of methylation defects, but not restricted by the hypomethylation of maternal alleles only.

A search for *NLRP7* mutations was performed in 40 Tunisian families with sporadic hydatidiform moles [74, 75]. Two sisters in one family had a homozygous mutation p.E570X. Heterozygous mutations were found in 11 patients. There were several new mutations among them: c.544G>A (p.Val182Met), c.1480G>A (p.Ala494Thr), c.1532A>G (p.Lys511Arg) and c.

2156C>T (p.Ala719Val). The authors concluded that the presence of some heterozygous mutations of *NLRP7* in woman may be a risk factor not only for BiCHM, but also for a sporadic mole.

There are current reports on mutations at almost all exons and introns of *NLRP7* gene, which were associated with BiCHM. The product of the gene belongs to CATERPILLER proteins family. These NLRP proteins are implicated in the activation of proinflammatory caspases through multiprotein complexes called inflammasomes. This gene may act as a feedback regulator of caspase-1-dependent interleukin 1-beta secretion, which is pleiotropic cytokine involved in trophoblast invasion in the uterus during implantation [76].

As mentioned previously, *NLRP7* may be a gene with a maternal effect. The products of such genes are necessary for oocytes to support early embryo development before the activation of embryo genome. These genes do not have an influence on ovulation and fertilization, but the absence of their products leads to the termination of early embryo development. This feature may explain the lack of reproductive problems in *NLRP7* mutation's male carriers. It seems that another gene from the NRLP family in mice – *Nalp5,* is a gene with maternal effect also. *Nalp5-/-* females had normal ovaries. Their oocytes fertilized normally, but embryos arrested their development at the 2-cell stage [77].

NLRP7 protein has no DNA-binding motifs in its sequence, which is why it is unclear how it may be involved in imprinting recording during oogenesis. In this situation, an alternative hypothesis is attractive. According to this hypothesis, the involvement of NLRP7 in BiCHM pathogenesis may be related to its participation in inflammation and autoimmune response. It was found that patients with *NLRP7* mutations cannot provide specific responses to different antigens [78]. As a result, in such women androgenic blastocysts, which are in fact are complete allografts, can implant and develop without rejection from the maternal side. It is also possible that androgenic blastocysts arise spontaneously *de novo* with definite frequency due to errors of fertilization or through epigenetic mechanisms independently from *NRLP7* mutations. In women without *NRLP7* mutations and normal immune systems, such androgenic blastocysts die or stop in development. It is interesting that mutations in other members of the CATERPILLER family – *NLRP1* and *NOD2* were also associated with some clinical forms of vitiligo (MIM #606579) and inflammatory bowel disease (MIM #266600) [78]. There were no reports on the association of molar pregnancies with these autoimmune diseases, except for one study [79]. However, the association of Crohn's disease with recurrent pregnancy loss was noted repeatedly [80, 81]. It is possible that this association is based on common pathogenic mechanisms involved in the disturbance of autoimmune response regulation.

Mutations at the *NLRP7* gene have not been found in every case of BiCHM and only 48-60% of patients with recurrent hydatidiform moles indicate a heterogeneous nature of this reproductive pathology. Indeed, in 2011 a type II of BiCHM was described (MIM #614293), which is clinically indistinguishable from the classical variant of the biparental complete mole. It was related to mutations at the *KHDC3L* (*C6orf221*) gene in 6q13. The search for mutations in this gene was performed in 14 pedigrees with BiCHM without *NLRP7* mutations. As a result, homozygous change c.3G>T, deletion c.322_325delGACT and compound heterozygote c. 322_325delGACT were found in three families [82]. This study revealed that *KHDC3L* is mutated in 14% of patients with recurrent a hydatidiform mole who are negative for *NLRP7* mutations.

Sequencing of *KHDC3L* in 97 patients with recurrent moles, reproductive loss and absence of *NLRP7* mutations allows to identify three unrelated patients, each homozygous for one of the two protein-truncating mutations, a novel 4-bp deletion resulting in a frame shift c. 299_302delTCAA (p.Ile100Argfs*2), and a previously described 4-bp deletion c.322_325del-GACT (p.Asp108Ilefs*30), transmitted on a shared haplotype to three patients from different populations [83]. It was also shown that molar tissues from one of the spontaneous abortions were diploid and biparental. In this study, immunofluorescence analysis revealed colocalization of KHDC3L and NLRP7 proteins in lymphoblastoid cell lines from normal subjects. Using cell lines from patients, it was demonstrated that the *KHDC3L* mutations do not change the subcellular localization of protein in haematopoietic cells. This finding highlights the similarities between the two causative genes for recurrent moles, *KHDC3L* and *NLRP7*, in their subcellular localization, the parental contribution to the mole tissues caused by them, and the presence of several founder mutations and variants in different populations in both of them indicating positive selection and adaptation.

It is probable that some patients with imprinting disorders and MLMD also have mutations in two other genes – *NLRP2* (*NALP2*) (19q13.42) and *ZFP57* (6p22.1), which may be involved in imprinting maintenance. The NALP2 is a cytosolic protein of the CATERPILLER's subfamily. It is suggested that NALP2 is a component of inflammosomes, like NLRP7. Mutation c. 1479delAG (p.Arg493SerfsX32) at the *NLRP2* was found in a family with one healthy child and two children with BWS [84]. *KCNQ1OT1* imprinted centres were hypomethylated in both affected children, whereas *PEG1* hypomethylation was observed in only one of them. Homozygous mutation at the *NLRP2* was detected in the mother and the affected child, whereas the father, the healthy child and the other diseased child were heterozygotes. The mutation was absent in the control group. This data is in agreement with the hypothesis that *NLRP2* is a maternal-effect gene, like *NLRP7*. It is interesting that *NLRP2 per se* is imprinted. Its monoallelic expression from the maternal chromosome was detected in decidual tissue, foetal heart and liver [85]. However, there is a single report, which does not support the maternal effect of *NLRP2*. In 2013, a paternally inherited mutation c.2077C>T (p.R693W) was observed in BWS patient with *KCNQ1OT1* hypomethylation [61]. This mutation was absent in individuals from the control group and may be pathogenic according to the "PolyPhen-2" database. However, it seems that this example does not cover multiple methylation defects.

In 2008, mutations at the *ZNF57* were detected for the first time in seven out of twelve families with TNDM and multiple hypomethylation of imprinted genes *PLAGL1, CRB10, PEG3, KCNQ1OT1, PEG1/MEST*, and *NESPAS* [86]. Homozygous mutation p.C241X was found in a brother with hypomethylation at the *KCNQ1OT1, NASPAS* and *PEG1/MEST* and his sister with *KCNQ1OT1* and *PEG1/MEST* hypomethylation. Proband in another family had deletion c.257_258delAG (p.E86VfsX28). His father was a heterozygote for this deletion. Compound heterozygous mutation c.683G>A (p.R228H) was detected in two families, including one patient with hypomethylation of *PEG1/MEST* and *NESPAS*. None of the mutations were found in 200 individuals from the control group.

Two years later, Mackay and Temple reported about *ZFP57* mutations in 10 out of 16 patients with TNDM and hypomethylation at the *PLAGL1, GRB10* and *PEG3* genes [87]. It is interesting that all patients with maternal hypomethylation syndrome, *ZFP57* mutations and *PLAGL1* hypomethylation also had *PEG3* and *GRB10* hypomethylation. However, in the absence of *ZFP57* mutations, *PEG3* and *GRB10* genes were infrequently affected by methylation defects. This observation indicates that *ZFP57* may be involved in imprinting maintenance in somatic cells in contrast to germinal methylation defects, which are associated with mutations at the *NLRP7*.

ZFP57 mutations were also observed in patients with other imprinting disorders, like SRS and BWS. For example, seven mutations at the *ZFP57* were found in 30 patients with SRS and hypomethylation of imprinting centre *H19/IGF2* on chromosome 11 [88]. Other imprinted genes were not tested in this study. Six nucleotide changes were recognized as known polymorphisms, whereas one patient had not previously detected homozygous mutation p.R125Q in the exon 6. This mutation was also found in heterozygous form in two of the 80 (2.5%) healthy individuals.

Twenty-seven BWS patients with *KCNQ1OT1* hypomethylation were tested for the presence of *ZFP57* mutations [89]. As a result, three new nucleotide changes were found. Two twin girls and their father were heterozygous for the c.503C>T (p.Ser168Phe). Two other changes c. 723C>T and c.1026T>C were detected in a diseased child and his father.

ZFP57 mutations were found in a recent study of patients with TNDM, SRS, BWS and methylation defects [61]. New homozygous deletion c.371delC was identified in a patient with TNDM and maternal hypomethylation of five imprinted genes, including *PLAGL1*. Both parents in this family were heterozygous carriers of deletion, whereas it was absent in the 180 individuals from the control group. Two cases of maternal inheritance of the mutation c. 374G>A (p.R125Q) were observed in a SRS patient with *H19/IGF2* hypomethylation and in a BWS patient with a loss of methylation at the *KCNQ1OT1*. This mutation was not found in the control sample. The mother of the SRS patient was a compound heterozygote for p.R125Q and c.559G>A (p.R187C) mutation.

The protein encoded by *ZFP57* is a zinc finger protein containing the Kruppel-associated box repressor (KRAB) domain, which acts as transcription repressor. It is interesting that this domain may be involved in the *de novo* DNA methylation during mouse embryogenesis [90]. It was also shown that *Zfp57* mutations in mice may induce multiple methylation defects of imprinted genes. Partial hypomethylation of maternal and paternal alleles was noted in progeny with *Zfp57-/-* genotype in zygote [Li et al., 2008]. The authors of this study suggested that *Zfp57* is a maternal-zygotic effect gene and its product is required for imprinting maintenance in different genomic loci.

Taking the discussed results together, it is possible to make an unexpected conclusion that some part of imprinting diseases and reproductive disorders associated with abnormal imprinting are related to defects in gene (or genes) involved in the establishment and maintenance of epigenetic organization of imprinted loci. In other words, imprinting diseases, or at least some part of them, that were usually considered epigenetic in nature, have, in fact, a single gene basis sometimes modified by parental-of-origin effects. A similar situation is specific for chromatin diseases (ICF, Rett, Rubinshtein-Taybi, Coffin-Lowry, ATR-X syndromes), which arise due to mutations in genes involved in the control of chromatin organization [8]. From this point of view, the presence of one form of TNDM, a classical imprinting disorder, in the OMIM catalogue (MIM # 601410) as a result of *ZFP57* mutations is not unexpected.

Considering the high incidence of reproductive losses in humans and the elevated level of methylation defects at different imprinted loci in spontaneous abortions, the search for mutations in genes involved in the control of genomic imprinting is a challenge for modern reproductive epigenetics and medicine. In our preliminary study, 11 first trimester missed abortions with MLMD of imprinted genes were tested for the presence of *NLRP7* mutations [92]. Nine genetic variants of *NLRP7* were found. Seven of them were presented in specific databases for women with BiCHM and normal reproductive outcomes. Whereas two new changes, c1405delC and c1444delC, in homozygous form were found in spontaneous abortion with hypomethylation at the *PEG10, KCNQ1, WT1, ZNF215* and hypermethylation at the *INS, PWCR1* and *GABRA5* genes.

7. Conclusion

The reviewed data clearly indicates that epigenetic abnormalities are the leading cause of imprinted gene dysfunction in pregnancy complications and losses. This is not surprising because of the fact that the rate of epimutations is estimated to be one or two orders higher than the incidence of classical gene mutations. It is import to also note that epimutation in one allele is enough to cause the loss of imprinting or the silencing of an imprinted gene due to one of its main inherent features, namely monoallelic expression.

The application of genome wide technologies of DNA methylation analysis revealed the phenomenon of multiple methylation defects at imprinting genes both in spontaneous abortions and in some patients with imprinting disorders. Today we are witnesses of data accumulation about spectrum and the incidence of this type of methylation abnormalities in different diseases. However, cautious estimations should be provided because of a lack of current data about possible benign epipolymorphisms of imprinted genes. However, obtained results change and supplement existent concepts about pathogenesis of imprinting disorders. One of the most intriguing findings is that some part of epigenetic imprinting defects has, in fact, a genetic nature due to mutations in genes, which are responsible for imprinting regulation. This remark may have obvious significance for the likes of molecular genetic diagnosis in the light of the application of high-throughput genomic and post-genomic technologies and for medical genetic counselling. Carriers of mutations in imprinting control genes may have incorrect or instable epigenomes in their gametes or progeny which will be not compatible with fertilization, implantation, normal prenatal development or the delivery of a healthy child. Preimplantation genetic diagnosis for the excluding of embryo transfer with mutations in such genes may be a successful reproductive choice for such couples.

Author details

I.N. Lebedev*

Address all correspondence to: igor.lebedev@medgenetics.ru

Institute of Medical Genetics, Tomsk, Russia

References

[1] Bonde J.P.E., Ernst E., Jensen T.K. et al., Relation between semen quality and fertility: a population based study of 430 first-pregnancy planners. *Lancet* 1998; 352(9135) 1172-1177.

[2] Warburton D., Fraser F.C., Spontaneous abortion risks in man: data from reproductive histories in a medical genetics unit. *American Journal of Human Genetics* 1964; 16(1) 1-24.

[3] Hassold T., Chen N., Funkhouser J. et al., A cytogenetic study of 1000 spontaneous abortions. *Annals of Human Genetics* 1980; 44(2) 151-178.

[4] Waddington C.H. The epigenotype. *Endeavour* 1942; 1 18-20 (See also reprint: Waddington CH. The epigenotype. *International Journal of Epidemiology* 2012; 41 10-13).

[5] Jablonka E., Lamb M., The changing concepts of epigenetics. *Annals New York Academy of Sciences* 2002; 981 82-96.

[6] Horsthemke B., Epimutations in human disease. *Current Topics in Microbiology and Immunology* 2006; 310 45-59.

[7] Feinberg A.P., Genome-scale approaches to the epigenetics of common human disease // *Virchows Archive* 2010; 456(1) 13-21.

[8] Johnson C.A., Chromatin modification and disease. *Journal of Medical Genetics* 2000; 37(12) 905-915.

[9] Falls J.G., Pulford D.J., Wylie A.A., Jirtle R.L., Genomic imprinting: Implications for Human Disease. *American Journal of Pathology* 1999; 154(3) 635-647.

[10] Holliday R., The inheritance of epigenetic defects. *Science* 1987; 238(4824) 163-170.

[11] Crouse H.V., The controlling element in sex chromosome behavior in Sciara. *Genetics* 1960; 45(10) 1429-1443.

[12] Gerbi S.A. Helen Crouse (1914-2006): Imprinting and chromosome behavior. *Genetics* 2007; 175(1) 1-6.

[13] Surani M.A., Barton S.C., Norris M.L., Development of reconstituted mouse eggs suggests imprinting of the genome during gametogenesis. *Nature* 1984; 308(5959) 548-550.

[14] McGrath J., Solter D. Completion of mouse embryogenesis requires both maternal and paternal genomes. *Cell* 1984; 37(1) 179-183.

[15] Devriendt K., Hydatidiform mole and triploidy: the role of genomic imprinting in placental development. *Human Reproduction Update* 2005; 11(2) 137-142.

[16] Golubovsky M.D., Postzygotic diploidzation of triploids as a source of unusual cases of mosaicism, chimerism and twinning. *Human Reproduction* 2003; 18(2) 236-242.

[17] Reik W., Fean W., Walter J. Epigenetic reprogramming in mammalian development. *Science* 2001; 293(5532) 1089-1093.

[18] Li E., Chromatin modification and epigenetic reprogramming in mammalian development. *Nature Reviews Genetics* 2002; 3(9) 662-673.

[19] Reik W., Walter J., Genomic imprinting: parental influence on the genome. *Nature Reviews Genetics* 2001; 2(1) 21-32.

[20] Arnaud P., Feil R., Epigenetic deregulation of genomic imprinting in human disorders and following assisted reproduction. *Birth Defects Research (Part C)* 2005; 75(2) 81-97.

[21] Geneimprint. Imprinted genes database: http://www.geneimprint.com/site/genes-by-species.Homo+sapiens.imprinted-All (Accessed 29 August 2013).

[22] Tycko B., Morison I.M., Physiological functions of imprinted genes. *Journal of Cell Physiology* 2002; 192(3) 245-258.

[23] Haig D., Graham C., Genomic imprinting and the strange case of the insulin-like growth factor II receptor. *Cell* 1991; 64(6) 1045-1046.

[24] Cattanach B.M., Jones J., Genetic imprinting in the mouse: Implications for gene regulation. *Journal of Inherited Metabolic Disease* 1994; 17(4) 403-421.

[25] Henderson D.J., Sherman L.S., Loughna S.C. et al., Early embryonic failure associated with uniparental disomy for human chromosome 21. *Human Molecular Genetics* 1994; 3(8) 1373-1376.

[26] Shaffer L.G., McCaskill C., Adkins K., Hassold T.J., Systematic search for uniparental disomy in early fetal losses: the results and a review of the literature. *American Journal of Medical Genetics* 1998. V. 79(5) 366-372.

[27] Smith M., Creasy M.R., Clarke A., Upadhyaya M., Sex ratio and absence of uniparental disomy in spontaneous abortions with a normal karyotype. *Clinical Genetics* 1998; 53(4) 258-261.

[28] Fritz B., Aslan M., Kalscheuer V. et al., Low incidence of UPD in spontaneous abortions beyond the 5th gestational week. *European Journal of Human Genetics* 2001; 9(12) 910-916.

[29] Kondo Y., Tsukishiro S., Tanemura M. et al., Maternal uniparental disomy of chromosome 16 in a case of spontaneous abortion. *Journal of Human Genetics* 2004; 49(4) 177-181.

[30] Tsukishiro S., Li Q.Y., Tanemura M. et al., Paternal uniparental disomy of chromosome 14 and unique exchange of chromosome 7 in cases of spontaneous abortion. *Human Genetics* 2005; 50(3) 112-117.

[31] Evdokimova V.N., Nazarenko S.A., The absence of uniparental X-chromosome inheritance in spontaneous abortions with normal karyotype. *Russian Journal of Developmental Biology* 2000; 31(3) 201-204.

[32] Nikitina T.V., Sazhenova E.A., Sukhanova N.N. et al., Evaluation of the role of uniparental disomy in early embryolethality of man. *Russian Journal of Developmental Biology* 2004; 35(4) 297-306.

[33] Engel E., DeLozier-Blanchet C.D., Uniparental disomy, isodisomy, and imprinting: probable effects in man and strategies for their detections. *American Journal of Human Genetics* 1991; 40(4) 432-439.

[34] Online Mendelian Inheritance in Man. An Online Catalog of Human Genes and Genetic Disorders: http://omim.org (Accessed 29 August 2013).

[35] Sazhenova E.A., Lebedev I.N., Epimutations of the *KCNQ1OT1* imprinting centre of chromosome 11 in early human embryo lethality. *Russian Journal of Genetics* 2008; 44(12) 1609-1616.

[36] Lebedev I.N., Sazhenova E.A., Epimutations of imprinted genes in the human genome: classification, causes, association with hereditary pathology. *Russian Journal of Genetics* 2008; 44(10) 1176-1190.

[37] Judson H., Hayward B.E., Sheridan E., Bonthron D.T., A global disorder of imprinting in the human female germ line. *Nature* 2002; 416(6880) 539-542.

[38] Van den Veyver I.B., Al-Hussaini T.K.. Biparental hydatidiform moles: a maternal effect mutation affecting imprinting in the offspring. *Human Reproduction Update* 2006; 12(3) 233-242.

[39] Kashevarova A.A., Sazhenova E.A., Lebedev I.N., Nazarenko S.A., Methylation status of *SNRPN* imprinted genes in early embryonic death in human. *Bulletin of Siberian Branch of Russian Academy of Medical Sciences* (Rus) 2006; 119(1) 101-105.

[40] Sazhenova E.A., Lebedev I.N., Epimutation of the imprinted gene *PLAGL1* in recurrent pregnancy losses. *Medical Genetics* (Rus) 2010; 9(11) 34-38.

[41] Horsthemke B., Ludwig M., Assisted reproduction: the epigenetic perspective. *Human Reproduction Update* 2005; 11(5) 473-482.

[42] Lebedev I.N., Puzyrev V.P., Epigenetic perspectives of safety in assisted reproductive technologies. *Russian Journal of Genetics* 2007; 43(9) 961-972.

[43] Amor D.J., Halliday J., A review of known imprinting syndromes and their association with assisted reproductive technologies. *Human Reproduction* 2008; 23(12) 2826-2834.

[44] Owen C.M., Segars J.H., Imprinting disorders and assisted reproductive technology. *Seminars in Reproductive Medicine* 2009; 27(5) 417-428.

[45] Khosla S., Dean W., Reik W., Feil R., Epigenetic and experimental modifications in early mammalian development: Part II. Culture of preimplantation embryos and its long-term effects on gene expression and phenotype. *Human Reproduction Update* 2001; 7(4) 419-427.

[46] Zheng H.Y., Tang Y., Niu J. et al., Aberrant DNA methylation of imprinted loci in human spontaneous abortions after assisted reproduction techniques and natural conception. *Human Reproduction* 2013; 28(1) 265-273.

[47] Pliushch G., Schneider E., Weise D. et al., Extreme methylation values of imprinted genes in human abortions and stillbirths. *American Journal of Pathology* 2010; 176(3) 1084-1090.

[48] Diplas A.I., Lambertini L., Lee M.J. et al., Differential expression of imprinted genes in normal and IUGR human placentas. *Epigenomics* 2009; 4(4) 235-240.

[49] Dória S., Sousa M., Fernandes S. et al., Gene expression pattern of *IGF2, PHLDA2, PEG10* and *CDKN1C* imprinted genes in spontaneous miscarriages or fetal death. *Epigenetics* 2010; 5(5) 444-450.

[50] Sazhenova E.A., Skryabin N.A., Sukhanova N.N., Lebedev I.N., Multilocus epimutations of imprintome in the pathology of embryo development. *Molecular Biology* 2012; 46(2) 183-191.

[51] Zechner U., Pliushch G., Schneider E. et al., Quantitative methylation analysis of developmentally important genes in human pregnancy losses after ART and spontaneous conception. *Molecular Human Reproduction* 2010; 16(9) 704-713.

[52] Eggermann T., Leisten I., Binder G. et al., Disturb methylation of multiple imprinted loci: an increasing observation in imprinting disorders. *Epigenomics* 2011; 3(5) 625-637.

[53] Poole R.L., Docherty L.E., Al Sayegh A. et al., Targeted methylation testing of a patient cohort broadens the epigenetic and clinical description of imprinting disorders. *American Journal of Medical Genetics Part A* 2013; 161(9) 2174-2182.

[54] Arima T., Kamikihara T., Hayashida T. et al., ZAC, LIT1 (KCNQ1OT1) and p57KIP2 (CDKN1C) are in an imprinted gene network that may play a role in Beckwith-Wiedemann syndrome. *Nucleic Acids Research* 2005; 33(8) 2650–2660.

[55] Mackay D.J.G., Hahnemann J.M., Boonen S.E. et al., Epimutation of the TNDM locus and the Beckwith-Wiedemann syndrome centromeric locus in individuals with transient neonatal diabetes mellitus. *Human Genet*ics 2006; 119(1-2) 179–184.

[56] Mackay D.J.G., Boonen S.E., Clayton-Smith J. et al., A maternal hypomethylation syndrome presenting as transient neonatal diabetes mellitus. *Human Genetics* 2006; 120(2) 262–269.

[57] Lim D., Bowdin S., Tee L. et al., Clinical and molecular genetic features of Beckwith-Wiedemann syndrome associated with assisted reproductive technologies. *Human Reproduction* 2009; 24(3) 741-747.

[58] Yamazawa K., Kagami M., Nagai T. et al., Molecular and clinical findings and their correlations in Silver-Russell syndrome: implications for a positive role of *IGF2* in growth determination and differential imprinting regulation of the IGF2-H19 domain in bodies and placentas. *Journal of Molecular Medicine* 2008; 86(10) 1171-1181.

[59] Bartholdi D., Krajewska-Walasek M., Ounap K. et al., Epigenetic mutations of the imprinted IGF2-H19 domain in Silver-Russell syndrome (SRS): results from a large cohort of patients with SRS and SRS-like phenotypes. *Journal of Medical Genetics* 2009; 46(3) 192-197.

[60] Baple E.L., Poole R.L., Mansour S et al., An atypical case of hypomethylation at multiple imprinted loci. *European Journal of Human Genetics* 2011; 19(3) 360-362.

[61] Court F., Martin-Trujillo A., Romanelli V. et al., Genome-wide allelic mathylation analysis reveals disease-specific susceptibility to multiple methylation defects in imprinting syndromes. *Human Mutation* 2013; 34(4) 595-602.

[62] Rossignol S., Steunou V., Chalas C. et al., The epigenetic imprinting defect of patients with Beckwith–Wiedemann syndrome born after assisted reproductive technology is not restricted to the 11p15 region. *Journal of Medical Genetics* 2006; 43(12) 902-907.

[63] Bliek J., Verde G., Callaway J. et al., Hypomethylation at multiple maternally methylated imprinted regions including PLAGL1 and GNAS loci in Beckwith–Wiedemann syndrome. *European Journal of Human Genetics* 2009; 17(5) 611-619.

[64] Azzi S., Rossignol S., Steunou V. et al., Multilocus methylation analysis in a large cohort of 11p15-related foetal growth disorders (Russell Silver and Beckwith Wiedemann syndromes) reveals simultaneous loss of methylation at paternal and maternal imprinted loci. *Human Molecular Genetics* 2009; 18(24) 4724-4733.

[65] Bliek J., Alders M., Maas S.M. et al., Lessons from BWS twins: complex maternal and paternal hypomethylation and a common source of haematopoietic stem cells. *European Journal of Human Genetics* 2009; 17(12) 1625-1634.

[66] Turner C.L., Mackay D.M., Callaway J.L. et al., Methylation analysis of 79 patients with growth restriction reveals novel patterns of methylation change at imprinted loci. *European Journal of Human Genetics* 2010; 18(6) 648–655.

[67] Begemann M., Spengler S., Kanber D. et al., Silver–Russell patients showing a broad range of ICR1 and ICR2 hypomethylation in different tissues. *Clinical Genetics* 2011; 80(1) 83-88.

[68] Djuric U., El-Maarri O., Lamb B. et al., Familial molar tissues due to mutations in the inflammatory gene, NALP7, have normal postzygotic DNA methylation. *Human Genetics* 2006; 120(3) 390-395.

[69] Martin-Subero J., Bibikova M., Mackay D. et al., Microarray-based DNA methylation analysis of imprinted loci in a patient with transient neonatal diabetes mellitus. *American Journal of Medical Genetics Part A* 2008; 146(24) 3227-3229.

[70] Murdoch S., Djuric U., Mazhar B. et al., Mutations in *NALP7* cause recurrent hydatidiform moles and reproductive wastage in humans. *Nature Genetics* 2006; 38(3) 300-302.

[71] Qian J.H., Deveault C., Bagga R. et al., Woman heterozygous for NALP7/NLRP7 mutations are risk for reproductive wastage: report of two novel mutations. *Human Mutation* 2007; 28(7) 741.

[72] Kou Y.C., Shao L., Peng H.H. et al., A recurrent intragenic genomic duplication, other novel mutations in *NLRP7* and imprinting defects in recurrent biparental hydatidiform moles. *Molecular Human Reproduction* 2008; 14(1) 33-40.

[73] Hayward B.E., De Vos M., Talati N. et al., Genetic and epigenetic analysis of recurrent hydatidiform mole. *Human Mutation* 2009; 30(5) E629-639.

[74] Landolsi H., Rittore C., Philibert L. et al., Screening for *NLRP7* mutations in familial and sporadic recurrent hydatidiform moles: report of 2 Tunisian families. *International Journal of Gynecologic Pathology* 2011; 30(4) 348-353.

[75] Landolsi H., Rittore C., Philibert L. et al., *NLRP7* mutation analysis in sporadic hydatidiform moles in Tunisian patients: *NLRP7* and sporadic mole // *Archives of Pathology and Laboratory Medicine* 2012; 136(6) 646-651.

[76] Kinoshita T., Wang Y., Hasegawa M. et al., PYPAF3, a PYRIN-containing APAF-1-like protein, is a feedback regulator of caspase-1-dependent interleukin-1beta secretion. *Journal of Biological Chemistry* 2005; 10(23) 21720-21725.

[77] Tong Z.B., Gold L., Pfeifer K.E. et al., Mater, a maternal effect gene required for early embryonic development in mice. *Nature Genetics* 2000; 26(3) 267-268.

[78] Deveault C., Qian J.H., Chebaro W.A. et al., NLRP7 mutations in women with diploid androgenetic and triploid moles: a proposed mechanism for mole formation. *Human Molecular Genetics* 2009; 18(5) 888-897.

[79] Hovdenak N., Ulcerative colitis, vitiligo and hydatidiform mole. *Tidsskrift for Den Norske Legeforening* 1979; 20(23) 1089-1090.

[80] Gasbarrini A., Torre E.S., Trivellini C. et al., Recurrent spontaneous abortion and intrauterine fetal growth retardation as symptoms of coeliac disease. *Lancet* 2000; 356(9227) 399-400.

[81] Lejeune V. Early recurrent spontaneous abortion: How to take care in 2006? //*Gynécologie Obstétrique & Fertilite* 2006;34(10) 927-937.

[82] Parry D.A., Logan C.V., Hayward B.E. et al., Mutations causing familial biparental hydatidiform mole implicate *c6orf221* as a possible regulator of genomic imprinting in the human oocyte. *American Journal of Human Genetics* 2011; 89(3) 451-458.

[83] Reddy R., Akoury E., Nguyen N.M.P. et al., Report of four new patients with protein-truncating mutations in *C6orf221/KHDC3L* and colocolization with *NLRP7*. *European Journal of Human Genetics* 2013; 21(9) 957-964.

[84] Meyer E., Lim D., Pasha S. et al., Germline mutation in *NLRP2* (*NALP2*) in a familial imprinting disorder (Beckwith-Wiedemann syndrome). *PloS Genetics* 2009; 5(3) e1000423 doi: 10.1371/journal.pgen.1000423.

[85] Bjornsson H.T., Albert T.J., Ladd-Acosta C.M. et al., SNP-specific array-based allele-specific expression analysis. *Genome Research* 2008; 18(5) 771-779.

[86] Mackay D.J., Callaway J.L., Marks S.M. et al., Hypomethylation of multiple imprinted loci in individuals with transient neonatal diabetes is associated with mutations in *ZFP57*. *Nature Genetics* 2008; 40(8) 949-951.

[87] Mackay D.J., Temple I.K.. Transient neonatal diabetes mellitus type 1. *American Journal of Medical Genetics Part C Seminars in Medical Genetics* 2010; 154(3) 335-342.

[88] Spengler S., Gogiel M., Schönherr N. et al., Screening for genomic variants in ZFP57 in Silver-Russell syndrome patients with 11p15 epimutations. *European Journal of Medical Genetics* 2009; 52(6) 415-416.

[89] Boonen S.E., Hahnemann J.M., Mackay D.J. et al., No evidence for pathogenic variants or maternal effect of ZFP57 as the cause of Beckwith-Wiedemann Syndrome. *European Journal of Human Genetics* 2012; 20(1) 119-121.

[90] Wiznerowicz M., Jakobsson J., Szulc J. et al., The Kruppel-associated box repressor domain can trigger *de novo* promoter methylation during mouse early embryogenesis. *Journal of Biological Chemistry* 2007; 282(47) 34535-34541.

[91] Li X., Ito M., Zhou F. et al., A maternal-zygotic effect gene, *Zfp57*, maintains both maternal and paternal imprints. *Developmental Cell* 2008; 15(4) 547-557.

[92] Lepshin M.V., Sazhenova E.A., Lebedev I.N.. Search for NLRP7 mutations in first trimester missed abortions with multiple methylation changes in imprinted genes. *European Journal of Human Genetics* 2013; 21(Supplement 2) 588.

2

Epigenetic Mechanisms in Autism Spectrum Disorders

Tafari Mbadiwe and Richard M. Millis

1. Introduction

Autism spectrum disorders (ASDs) are neurodevelopmental diseases characterized by repetitive, stereotyped behavior and maldevelopment of social and language skills. Classical autism, Asperger syndrome and pervasive development disorder-not otherwise specified (PDD-NOS) are the most commonly diagnosed ASDs. There are also a significant number of cases that are considered idiopathic because the etiology is unclear (Gillis and Rouleau, 2011). The incidence of ASDs has increased substantially in the past twenty years, growing by as much as 5-10 fold; although, the approximate 4:1 ratio of affected males to females has been relatively constant (Kadesjö et al., 1999). Some of this increase has likely been driven by shifting diagnostic criteria, heightened awareness and improved diagnostic techniques (Levy et al., 2007). However, some of this increase could be attributable to an authentic increase in the frequency of ASDs. The factors fueling this increase remain unclear and the precise causes of ASDs remain unknown (Stoltenberg et al., 2010). Although its basis is thought to be multifactorial, ASDs are known to have a heritable component (Hu et al., 2006). The inheritance patterns can to some extent be explained by typical genetic processes but, especially in light of studies noting discordance among monozygotic twins, this is unlikely to be the whole story (Ptak and Petronis, 2010). Substantial scientific evidence is emerging suggesting that epigenetic influences may be partly responsible for the development of ASDs.

2. Epigenetic protein-DNA interactions: proteins mediating epigenetic signaling

2.1. Mecp2 and the frontal cortex

Methyl CpG binding protein 2 (Mecp2) is an epigenetic regulator required for development of neuronal synaptic contacts (Luikenhuis et al., 2004) that is thought to function mainly as a gene silencing molecule (Chahrour et al., 2008). The Mecp2 gene is located on the q arm of the

X chromosome and is subject to X-inactivation (Cohen et al., 2008). The Mecp2 mechanism involves binding to methylated DNA (Yasui et al., 2007) and, after binding, complexing with histone deacetylase-1 (HDAC1). HDAC1 is responsible for removing acetyl groups from histones; this removal causes the chromatin to condense and this suppresses gene transcription at the gene promoter site. Mecp2 is also purported to be an activator of some genes (Mehler, 2008) and, although it is not clear whether the role of Mecp2 in ASDs is dependent on its role as a gene silencer or promoter, there appear to be strong associations between decreased expression of Mecp2 and ASDs.

Decreased expression of Mecp2 in frontal cortex and fusiform gyrus (Nagarajan et al., 2006) - the latter associated with neural processing of face recognition (LaSalle et al., 2001; Pelphrey et al., 2004) - has been reported. The Mecp2 gene on the X chromosome and all males actively express one X chromosome. Hence, aberrant methylation patterns of autistic males (the predominant sex affected by ASDs) cannot be counteracted by a second X chromosome, as occurs in females. Aberrant methylation of the 5' portion of the Mecp2 regulatory region has been reported for brain samples from males affected by ASDs and, as expected, there is an inverse correlation between promoter region methylation and Mecp2 expression. There is a well-established relationship between a missense mutation of Mecp2 and Rett syndrome, a pervasive developmental disorder of females exhibiting ASD-like behaviors (O'Conner et al., 2009).

3. Epigenetic DNA-protein interactions

3.1. Protein kinase c beta and the temporal lobe

Downregulation of the gene for protein kinase C beta (PRKCB1) in the temporal lobe is reported to be correlated with ASDs (Lintas et al., 2009). Phosphorylation of histone H3 at threonine 6 (H3T6) by PRKCB1 appears to prevent lysine-specific demethylase-1 (LSD1) from demethylating H3K4 during androgen receptor-dependent gene activation (Metzger et al., 2010). Consequently, downregulation of PRKCB1 could play a role in the predominance of male ASD patients. Further, this downregulation may impact deep temporal lobe (limbic system) synaptogenesis and consequently preferentially sensitize males (who are generally exposed to higher fetal androgen concentrations than females) to the environmental stressors thought to be involved in the development of ASDs.

3.2. The oxytocin receptor and hypermethylation

Generally, females lack androgen-facilitated arousal inputs to the amygdala and might, therefore, be protected from the development of ASDs by high fetal levels of estrogens and oxytocin (Pfaff et al., 2011). A role for an oxytocin receptor polymorphism in ASDs is reported (Wu et al., 2005; Liu et al., 2010) and aberrant DNA methylation in the promoter region of the oxytocin receptor gene has been observed after acute psychosocial stress (Unternaehrer et al., 2012). Epigenetic dysregulation of the oxytocin receptor gene (OXTR) has been implicated in the etiology of ASDs (Jacob et al., 2007) and oxytocin, together with vasopressin, has also been shown to have socialization functions (Gouin et al., 2010). A link between oxytocin and ASDs in humans (Insel, 1992) and in knockout mice is also suggested by the decreased memory and face recognition abilities which are commonly found among ASD patients (Ferguson et al., 2000; Takayanagi et al., 2005) and also adversely impact socialization. It is noteworthy that OXTR-knockout decrements in social interactions appear to be sex-specific (Sun et al., 2008).

These findings suggest that any defect of the oxytocin pathway, including a deficiency of oxytocin receptors, has the potential to contribute to the development of ASDs. A diminished number of oxytocin receptors can have a variety of causes, including both genomic and epigenetic. A study involving a family in which the mother had a hemizygous deletion of the OXTR gene, noted that the mother passed down the deletion to one of her sons, but not the other; however, both sons were diagnosed with autism and it turned out that the promoter region of the OXTR gene of the affected sibling without the deletion was hypermethylated (Gregory et al., 2009). Prior studies had identified two CpG island regions of the OXTR gene that, as a consequence of variable methylation, seem to be associated with differential OXTR expression in liver and myometrium (Kimura et al., 2003). The first CpG island overlaps with exons 1, 2 and 3 of the OXTR gene and the second CpG island was localized to the third intron. The second CpG island, within intron 3, was found to be heavily methylated in all three family members studied. The other CpG island -- overlapping exons 1,2 and 3 -- was found to be methylated differently in each of the family members; specifically, the affected sibling without the deletion showed significantly more methylation than his brother or mother at three sites within the intron. This hypermethylation occurred at locations that have previously been shown to impact OXTR expression. Since both siblings were autistic in spite of the fact that one had a genomic deletion and the other displayed hypermethylated promoter regions, this study demonstrates that epigenetic and genetic mechanisms can have equivalent effects on phenotype. Furthermore, this study showed that five differentially methylated CpG islands which were examined in a group of 20 autistic and 20 phenotypically normal individuals exhibited significantly greater methylation at several of the examined loci. These observations were made in both blood and cerebral cortex samples. Additionally, low levels of OXTR expression were found to be associated with increased methylation at a statistically significant level. This finding strengthens the idea that promoter region methylation causes gene silencing. Moreover, when the data were stratified by sex, two of the loci showed significant differences in methylation for males only, implying that the different frequencies of autism in males and females might be driven by epigenetic mechanisms.

3.3. Bcl-2 and apoptosis

Bcl-2 (B-cell lymphoma 2) is a protein regulator of apoptosis (Tsujimo et al., 1984) and it s gene has been linked to ASDs (Glantz et al., 2006). Decreased expression of Bcl-2 has been shown in cerebellum and frontal cortex of subjects diagnosed with ASDs (Fatemi et al., 2001; Fatemi and Halt, 2001), and lymphoblastoid cell lines from sets of monozygotic twins discordant for ASDs.

3.4. RORA and oxidative stress

A novel hypothesis suggests that ASDs may develop from epigenetic dysregulation of the retinoic acid-related orphan receptor alpha (RORA), a regulator of circadian rhythm and neuroprotection from oxidative stress and inflammation, is reported (Akashi and Takumi, 2005; Boukhtouche et al., 2006). The Bcl-2 and RORA hypotheses are similar in that both depend on the idea that oxidative stress plays a key role in some instances of apoptosis. The RORA hypothesis is supported by reports that oxidative stress and inflammation are increased in patients diagnosed with ASDs (Pardo et al., 2005; Chauhan and Chauhan, 2006). Differences in RORA gene promoter region methylation and protein product expression is reported for some subjects diagnosed with ASDs and their (non-twin) unaffected siblings (Nguyen et al., 2010). Furthermore, decreased RORA expression was found only in the ASD subjects with severe language impairment.

3.5. Beta-catenin, estradiol and lithium

Estrogens are important for sex-related differentiation of the brain and it is likely that brain estrogen levels are increased in subjects diagnosed with ASDs (MacLusky et al., 1987). Estrogens, being steroid hormones, and their receptors - including estrogen receptor alpha (ERα) - are located in the nucleus and in the cytosol of target cells. One of the targets of cytosolic ERα is GSK3B, which is known to complex with β-catenin in the degradation of β-catenin. ERα activation by estradiol is reported to release β-catenin from this complex, thereby increasing β-catenin availability (Cardona-Gomez et al., 2004). An increase in the cytosolic concentration of estrogens is thought to result in increases in cytosolic and nuclear β-catenin during critical periods of prenatal and neonatal development during which β-catenin binding to the LEC/TCF promoter has positive effects on Wnt pathway gene transcription. Such increased transcription in the Wnt pathway is strongly associated with the development of ASDs. The effect of ERα is to cause the dissociation of β-catenin from a complex whose integral members include the proteins GSK3β, axin and adenomatous polyposis coli tumor suppressor (APC). GSK3β, axin and APC are negative regulators of the Wnt signaling pathway and the complex requires all of these constituents to initiate the destruction of β-catenin. The absence or downregulation of any of these components may increase the availability of cytosolic β-catenin, and consequently the various knock-in effects discussed previously - increased nuclear β-catenin with greater Wnt pathway transcription. Lithium, used mostly as a mood stabilizing drug, exerts an inhibitory effect on GSK3β both directly and indirectly, by interrupting the dephosphorylation of phospo-GSK3β (Jope, 2003). In either case, the effect is the same, and also the same as that of increased estrogen levels; i.e., the complex responsible for initiating the degradation of β-catenin is made nonfunctional, and the concentration of cytosolic β-catenin increases.

3.6. SHANK3 and the neurexin-neuroligin pathway

SHANK3 is a scaffolding protein in the neurexin-neuroligin pathway that interacts with synaptic proteins. Recent research suggests that copy number variations or mutations of either of these proteins may be associated with the development of ASDs (Liu et al., 2013). It appears that epigenetic mechanisms are used to control the expression of this gene. Five CpG islands in the SHANK3 gene (the post-translational methylation of which determines gene expression) and one specific locus - CpG island 2 - appear to particularly impact tissue SHANK expression (Beri et al., 2007). The SHANK3 gene is well conserved between humans and rodents and neonatal expression of certain SHANK3 transcripts in mice is known to temporarily decrease methylation of CpG island 2 after birth (Uchino and Waga, 2013). These findings suggest that the expression of SHANK3 (and thus its effect on the development of ASDs) is regulated by epigenetic mechanisms, though this connection has yet to be directly established in humans. Additionally, two genes responsible for the production of cell adhesion molecules in this pathway, NLGN3 and NLGN4, have also been associated with the development of ASDs (Liu et al., 2013). However, epigenetic regulation of these genes are, at this time, unproven (Yasuda et al., 2011).

3.7. IGF-2 and the cerebellum

Disruption of cerebellum cytoarchitecture with loss of Purkinje cells, effects that could have a negative impact on cerebellum development and postmortem cerebellum weight, has been described in subjects diagnosed with ASDs (Whitney et al., 2009). Insulin like growth factor-2 (IGF-2) is the product of a paternally imprinted gene, the allele-specific expression of which is regulated by DNA methylation. DNA methylation at a key transcriptional repressor (CTCF2) is shown to be correlated with cerebellum weight. Paradoxically, DNA methylation at CTCF3 of the maternally-inherited allele also appears to be associated with an increase in cerebellum weight (Pidsley et al., 2012).

3.8. Neurotrophins

Contemporary thinking has seized upon neurotrophins (proteins tasked with promoting the development, and, later, survival of neurons) as potentially important factors in the later development of ASDs. Neutrophins are growth factors whose prenatal presence (or absence) might affect neurogenesis in such a way as to make the later development more or less likely. In particular, a recent investigation focused on the role of three neurotrophic factors -- brain derived neurotrophic factor (BDNF), neurotophin-4 (NT4) and the immunosuppressive cytokine transforming growth factor beta (TGF-β) - in the development of ASDs (Nickl-Jockschat and Michel, 2011). The results, which were based on analysis of dried blood spot samples of neonates later diagnosed with ASDs and frequency-matched controls, suggest a role for each of studied neurotrophins: neonates with BDNF and TGF-β concentrations in the bottom decile were more likely to be diagnosed with ASDs, and eventual ASD neonates were less likely to have a NT4 concentration in the top decile (Abdallah et al., 2013). In spite of the authors' conspicuously cautious concluding remarks, their finding may have far reaching implications (Pareja-Galeano et al., 2013). BDNF has also been implicated in the etiology of a variety of neurological and psychiatric conditions - such as Alzheimer's and Huntington - that are posited to be involved in dysfunctional CNS synapse development. The results of the neurotrophin study are in line with this idea. The BDNF gene has been linked to early life stressors and their concomitant brain responses and behavioral outcomes, which suggests than an aberrant BDNF gene - or aberrant epigenetic regulation of that gene - might compromise the brain's advanced paternal capacity to mount a robust response to early life stressors, including those that were linked to ASDs in our earlier discussion. Furthermore, BDNF has been proposed as a link mediating interactions between genes, environmental conditions, synaptic plasticity and apoptosis and some research suggests that environmental and social conditions early in life may affect the epigenetic regulation of BDNF (Balaratnasingam and Janca, 2012). This points to a (somewhat speculative) mechanism for the development of ASDs: Adverse perinatal conditions alter the epigenetic regulation of BDNF which in turn limits the young brain's ability to properly respond to its adverse environment which then makes the development of ASDs more likely. These ideas may also be the first steps towards a strategy to reduce the ASD frequency. Since the higher concentrations of BDNF (as well as NT4 and TGF-β) are associated with decreased frequency of ASDs, promoting the upregulation of those proteins may be protective. Mouse models have shown that music exposure can increase the brain BDNF concentration in mice, however this finding is yet to be extended to the perinatal human context (Angelucci et al., 2007). Similarly, controlled physical exercise demonstrably increases BDNF concentrations in rats (Lee et al., 2013). Either, or both, of these approaches may be useful in encouraging a perinatal environment that minimizes the eventual development of ASDs.

3.9. The locus coeruleus-noradrenergic system and fever

The study of epigenetics encompasses more than differential methylation and acetylation of gene promoter regions. Indeed, any mechanism that affects gene expression, without altering the genetic code, may be considered an epigenetic mechanism. This broader view of epigenetics can help explain a curious, but common, observation: Autistic children consistently exhibit diminished ASD symptoms when febrile (Curran et al., 2007). This effect of fever appears to have nothing to do with methylation, gene silencing or promotion. Furthermore, there is no reason to suspect that the appearance of fever would result in the addition of methyl groups to particular portions of the genome. However, one hypothesis argues that febrile episodes temporarily modify the functional integrity of the locus coeruleus-norandrenergic (LC-NA) system, the dysregulation of which has been implicated as a proximate cause of ASD symptoms (Mehler and Purpura, 2009). This hypothesis is plausible, particularly in view of the functions of the LC-NA system. LC is in the pontine tegmentum and is notable for containing the most widely spread efferent projections of any nucleus in the brain (Foote et al., 1983). Most of the norepinephrine in the brain is transported by these neurons. This property of the LC-NA system is significant because distributed neural networks - those that are associated with the ability to make behavioral adaptations to environmental changes and that tend to be disrupted in ASD patients - are modulated by the LC-NA system. Indeed, the LC-NA system is also implicated in several other neurodegenerative and psychiatric disorders. The key point is that autism is frequently associated with dysregulation of the LC-NA system and fever also affects the LC-NA system. Moreover, febrile symptoms are typically induced by bacterial lipopolysaccharide and symptoms in the brain are, in turn, mediated by norepinephrine (Linthorst et al., 1995). Because most of the brain's norepinephrine is released from LC neurons, it is reasonable to think that the LC-NA system is somehow altered in the febrile state, especially since LC neurons are known to exhibit extremely synchronized activity. Consequently, fever may induce a change in LC-NA system functions that diminishes ASD symptoms. The discovery of this relationship between ASD symptoms and LC-NA functions implies that the neural networks of autistic patients are not irreparably damaged but, rather, are functionally intact. Theoretically, these findings suggest that fever-related changes in the brain might provide a useful experimental model for the development of drugs and other targeted therapies for ASDs. Moreover, the existence of this relationship between fever and LC-NA system functions points to a broader view of the concept of epigenetic mechanisms. Indeed, epigenetic effects may be thought of as relatively static, such as in the case of DNA methylation, or dynamic such as in the case represented by the connection between fever and the LC-NA system. This difference is roughly analogous to that between chronic and acute symptoms of a disease. A fully effective treatment of ASDs might require targeting both of the aforementioned types of epigenetic causative mechanisms.

4. Role of maternal hypomethylation

Development of the LC-NA system seems to be strongly impacted by prenatal events, reflecting the importance of environment-gene interactions. Maternal hypomethylation is an epigenetic mechanism that has effects on the intrauterine environment and which, in turn, may predispose fetuses to developing ASDs. Greater prevalence of ASDs is reported in children whose mothers were exposed to hurricanes or tropical storms during gestation (Beversdorf et al., 2005) and if the accompanying stress causes dysregulation in a distributed neural network such as the LC-NA system, it could result in a predilection for ASDs. Thus, epigenetic influences on the maternal genome could alter the intrauterine environment such that the probability of the offspring developing ASDs is increased or decreased. DNA hypomethylation linked to variants in the maternal folate pathway have been linked to aberrant fetal development (Foote et al., 1983; Linthorst et al., 1995). Because folate is the primary one carbon donor in methylation reactions, epigenetic dysregulation of the folate pathway should provide insight into the availability of methylation precursors and also the extent of genomic methylation in mothers of unaffected children compared to mothers of children diagnosed with ASDs.

Indeed, mothers of children diagnosed with ASDs often exhibit aberrant DNA methylation (James et al., 2008). Moreover, mothers of children diagnosed with ASDs also exhibit significantly lower levels of methylfolate and methionine - essential precursors for DNA methylation - than their non-ASD counterparts. In addition, levels of the methylation-inhibiting proteins S-adenosylmethoinine, adenosine and homocysteine were all elevated in autism mothers. S-adenosylmethonine (SAM) is the primary methyl donor for the DNA methyltransferase reaction, which produces S-adenosylhomocysteine (SAH) and methylated DNA. Because SAM and SAH are linked by the transferase reaction the SAM/SAH ratio is generally considered to be a good indicator of DNA methylation potential. Mothers of children diagnosed with ASDs often exhibit lower SAM/SAH ratios than control groups, indicative of a diminished capacity for methylation. Furthermore, the DNA of the mothers of children diagnosed with ASDs appears to be less methylated than that of mothers of unaffected children; the ratio of 5-methylcytosine to total cytosine - a measure of overall genomic methylation - was significantly lower in the mothers of autistic children (James et al., 2008). Taken together, this evidence strongly suggests that hypomethylation of maternal DNA may be linked to ASDs. However, the significance of these findings about the influences of epigenetics on the development of autism is not entirely clear.

5. Role of advanced paternal age in autism

Advanced paternal age is strongly associated with a variety of childhood conditions (Goriely et al., 2013). The relationship between advanced paternal age and autism is especially well-established. Large-scale studies have shown that advanced paternal age may increase the offspring's risk of developing an ASDs by as many as six fold. Despite such a striking effect, the specific mechanism underlying the relationship between older fathers and autistic children is not precisely clear. It seems likely that the link is at least partly explained by the effect of paternal age on germ cell integrity; a greater number of sperm divisions (and therefore opportunities for duplication errors) occur as paternal age increases, and the disparity between paternal and maternal germ line divisions widens. Of course, advanced paternal age may covary with a number other factors that may exert an effect on ASD frequency, not the least of which is maternal age. It's worth noting that none of these proposed mechanisms are mutually exclusive; in fact, it is entirely possible that the observed effects are the consequence of combination of a number of factors.

Some of these factors may have an epigenetic nexus. Rat model studies have demonstrated the germ cells of older rats tended to have changes in chromatin packaging, and consequently decreased gene integrity. In one notable study, sensitivity to oxidative treatment was used as a proxy for resilience and integrity of chromosomal packaging. Four-month-old and 21-month-old Brown Norway rats were systematically exposed to L-buthionine-[S,R]-sulphoximine (BSO) (a drug with well-known glutathione depleting properties) and hydrogen peroxide. The chromatin from spermatozoa of the younger rats demonstrated less nuclear chromomycin A3 penetration, decreased thiol oxidation, fewer DNA breaks and reduced tendency to dissociate from acridine orange - all indications of more fragile genetic material (Zubkova and Robaire, 2006). Researchers have also conducted systematic searches for age-related global and gene-specific methylation patterns. Using restriction landmark genomic scanning to determine methylation patterns of CpG islands, one study detected a ribosomal DNA locus the methylation of which is correlated with age; interestingly, the methylation of all studied single copy CpG island sequences were independent of age (Oakes et al., 2003). Together, these results suggest the presence of a direct effect of paternal age on the epigenome.

The science underlying the effect paternal age on genetic integrity is well-known and relatively straightforward; the hundreds of replications that spermatogonial undergo allow for greater numbers of point mutations, chromosomal breakages and copy number alterations than are typically observed in maternal cell lines (Perrin et al., 2007). However, the pervasive nature of the *genetic* effects of advanced paternal age somewhat complicates the evaluation of its *epigenetic* impacts. Consequently, separating the genetic and epigenetic effects can be delicate work. The evidence required to make such a determination must be biochemical; merely noting an association between increased paternal age and frequency of ASDs is insufficient to account for possibly confounding genetic effects. On the other hand, we know that dysregulation of imprinted genes, which as noted earlier often occur in clusters that are regulated by imprinting centers, is associated with altered brain development, and, notably, neurocognitive conditions such as autism. Recent studies have bridged this gap by demonstrating that advanced paternal age may increase the likelihood of the epigenetic dysregulation of the imprinting centers. Specifically, mouse models have indicated that the epigenetic loss of suppression of particular genes occurs more frequently in older mice than younger mice. Two examples of specific genes are illustrative (Bennett-Baker et al., 2003). The first, copper-transporting ATPase 1 (Atp7a), is located on the X chromosome and is consequently subject to X-linked inactivation. Quantitative comparison of RNA transcripts from young and old mice (2 and 24 months of age, respectively) have shown significantly less consistent X-inactivation among the transcripts from the older mice. This, in turn, suggests that, to some extent, the Atp7a gene of the older mice is hypomethylated as compared to the younger cohort. When we recall that the methylation resulting in gene inactivation is heritable, it follows that the offspring of older mice are more likely to inherit hypomethylated, and thus not inactivated, paternal alleles. A similar epigenetic mechanism has been demonstrated for the insulin growth factor 2 gene (Igf2). Unlike Atp7a, Igf2 is subject to genomic imprinting. As we've noted previously, epigenetic effects may manifest through manipulation of the imprinting process. It has also been demonstrated that older mice cohorts produce RNA transcripts from silenced alleles more frequently than their younger counterparts. Here again, this alteration of the imprinting process - mediated through changes in methylation patterns - is a heritable epigenetic change that results as a consequence of advanced paternal age. Further, we're beginning to see similar results in studies of human subjects. Most notably, a study of the cord blood of a group of Chinese Han newborns (approximately 20% of whom had non-imprinted Igf2 genes) found that although no measured maternal factor was statistically correlated with loss of imprinting, this epigenetic alteration was associated with increased paternal age (Dai et al., 2007). These studies comprise fairly compelling evidence of the effect exerted by advanced paternal age on the epigenome. It follows closely that these mechanisms have the potential to result in the passing of genetic material to ASD-susceptible offspring.

6. Nutritional factors

The ultimate effect of nutritional imbalances depends greatly on the developmental period during which the imbalance occurs. Different organs have critical developmental stages, and the time point at which they are compromised will predispose individuals to specific diseases. Also, depending on the function of the gene, epigenetic modifications that occur during development may not be expressed until later in life. While the majority of studies implicate prenatal and perinatal periods as critical time windows, some research has shown that nutritional intake during adulthood can also affect the epigenome.

Genetic polymorphisms of cytochrome P450 enzymes have been linked to ASDs, specifically the cytochrome P450 family 27 subfamily B gene (CYP27B1), which is essential for proper vitamin D metabolism. Epigenetic regulation of cytochrome P450 genes for hydroxylation and activation of vitamin D in has been shown in prostate cancer cells (Luo et al., 2010). Vitamin D is important for neuronal growth and neurodevelopment, and defects in its metabolism or deficiency have also been implicated in ASDs (Currenti, 2010). Mutations of Mecp2 associated with impaired methylation are known to be associated with autism and a related neurological disorder, Rett syndrome. One component of Rett syndrome is abnormal bone formation caused by abnormal vitamin D metabolism, which is associated with epigenetic dysregulation of cytochrome P450 genes (O'Connor et al., 2009) which could be a conceptual model for epigenetic interactions between Mecp2, vitamin D and cytochrome P450 genes (Currenti et al., 2010). As noted earlier, abnormal folic acid metabolism may play a role in the decreased capacity for methylation and DNA hypomethylation associated with significantly higher-than-normal levels of plasma homocysteine, adenosine, and SAH in mothers of subjects diagnosed with ASDs (James et al., 2010). Indeed, nutritional factors such as folic acid appear to be protectors against the epigenetic dysregulation associated with ASDs. DNA methylation, the most established epigenetic gene regulation, is a one-carbon transfer dependent mechanism requiring folate, choline, betaine and other B vitamins (Anderson et al., 2012) and it is, therefore, not surprising that folic acid supplementation in pregnancy appears to be protective against the development of ASDs (Surén et al., 2013). Changes in autism-related behaviors are reported to be strongly associated with vitamin-supplementation associated changes in plasma levels of biotin and vitamin K (Adams et al., 2011). Although biotin is a known cofactor in bioavailability of methyl groups for DNA methylation, a vitamin K-related epigenetic mechanism has not been described.

7. Toxic factors

7.1. Exposure to valproic acid

Valproic acid (VPA) is a therapeutic anticonvulsant and mood stabilizing drug that gained attention in the 1980s as a potential teratogen. VPA exposure is highly correlated with autism; as many as 60% of infants who exhibit the suite of symptoms associated with VPA teratogenicity also display two or more autistic characteristics (Moore et al., 2000). Autism has also been shown to occur in 9% of cases of prenatal exposure to VPA (Rasalam et. al., 2005). The mechanisms underlying the pharmacological actions of VPA are also suggestive of a correlation between VPA and ASDs (Shimshoni et al., 2007). VPA is responsible for inhibiting two enzymes: myo-inositol-1-phosphate (MIP) synthase and the class 1 and 2 histone deacetylase

(HDAC). HDAC1 is an important inhibitor of DNA transcription that works by associating with the LEC/TCF transcription factor. When HDAC1 is removed from the LEC/TCF complex, it leaves behind a primed (but inactive) promoter of gene transcription. The primed promoter then forms a complex with β-catenin, thus activating the promoter, and increasing transcription rates of a variety of genes in the wingless-type, mouse mammary tumor virus (MMTV) integration site family, in the type 1 (Wnt) signaling pathway including cyclin D1, as well as in those required for the transition from the G1 to S phases of mitosis. Additionally, the removal of HDAC1 causes the an increase in the transcription rate of MYC, which is a transcription enhancer for many genes throughout the genome (Billin et al., 2000). Accordingly, the consequence of VPA-mediated inhibition of HDAC1 is to upregulate the transcription of Wnt pathway genes. In addition, VPA increases cellular levels of β-catenin, presumably in response to the increased availability of primed LEC/TCF promoters (Wang et al., 2010). The effect of VPA on Wnt gene transcription is well understood but fails to explain the connection between VPA and autism. In order to complete this link, it is necessary to note that an increase in the number of neocortical minicolumns is highly correlated with autism (Williams and Casanova, 2010). This observation is supported by fMRI studies that report differences in how autism brains coordinate the processing of information (Minshew and Williams, 2007). It is reasonable to assume that processes which upregulate genes of the Wnt signaling pathway - such as prenatal exposure to VPA - may result in poorly regulated mitosis and cellular proliferation, one manifestation of which could be an increase in the number of neocortical minicolumns and macrocephaly. This mechanism has been observed at work in a slightly different context. Recall that Mecp2 inactivates genes by forming complexes with a variety of different molecules. One of these molecules is HDAC1 (Nan et al., 1998) and in the absence of HDAC1, or even when HDAC1 has merely been downregulated, the gene inactivating properties of Mecp2 will be expected to have a diminished effect. One of the promoters on which Mecp2 typically exerts its regulatory effect is the LEC/TCF promoter, which, as mentioned previously, ultimately regulates the transcription rates of the Wnt signaling pathway. Although Mecp2 has effects on gene methylation, the function of HDAC1 concerns acetylation of histones. However, in order for a gene to be transcriptionally deactivated, they must often be both methylated and deacetylated. Thus, VPA-induced inhibition of HDAC1 interferes with the functionality of Mecp2 which appears to increase the risk of developing ASD.

7.2. Exposure to sex steroids and antidepressants

Endocrine disruption early in pregnancy during sex-related differentiation of the brain suggests several mechanisms for the development of ASD. Sex steroids are known to be potent inhibitors of 3(17) alpha-hydroxysteroid dehydrogenase (AKR1C1), a bifunctional enzyme that catalyzes the oxidoreduction of the 2- and 17-hydroxy/keto groups of sex steroid hormones, the main metabolite of which is epitestosterone. Epitestosterone is a sex steroid produced in the mammalian brain, including that of humans. Epitestosterone is also shown to occur in higher concentrations in females than in males and could be an important central nervous system epigenetic regulator of gene expression that might help explain some of the male predominance of ASDs. Epitestosterone metabolism may also be linked to the features of ASDs associated with prenatal exposure to citrapolam, estradiol and valproic acid (Sanders,

2012). Several in vitro studies show that sex steroids can also alter serotonin homeostasis and mice expressing the common serotonin reuptake transporter (SERT) polymorphism, SERT Ala56 – which is associated with increased serotonin clearance rates and plasma serotonin concentrations and found in children with ASDs, (Dufour-Rainfray et al., 2010; Simpson et al., 2011; Veenstra-Vanderweele et al., 2012). The serotonin reuptake inhibitor citrapolam (Celexa), which increases plasma serotonin levels, is also implicated in heightened risk of ASDs in the children born to mothers who were prescribed the drug in the early stages of their pregnancies (Rai et al., 2013). These connections between sex steroids and serotonin homeostasis appear to be complex, as evidenced by the finding that citrapolam exposure modulates both cerebral cortical and noradrenergic locus coeruleus functions (previously discussed in relation to ASDs) as well as produces autistic-like behaviors in male rats (Darling et al., 2011).

7.3. Prenatal exposure to organic environmental pollutants

ASDs have also been linked to perinatal exposure to a flame retardant chemical, pentabromodiphenyl ether, BDE-47 (Woods et al., 2012). BDE-47 is one of a group of chemicals whose industrial production is required to be halted under the Stockholm Convention, a treaty intended to protect against environment exposures to persistent organic pollutants. Exposure to BDE-47 is known to negatively impact Mecp-2. Mecp2 has been discussed previously in terms of the X chromosome-linked mutation that produces Rett syndrome, a pervasive autistic-like neurodevelopmental disorder in females. Mecp2(308/+) mice are knock-in animal models shown to exhibit global hypomethylation of adult brain DNA, specifically in female offspring following perinatal exposure to BDE-47. This hypomethylation is associated with decreased social interactions and decreased expression of DNMT3a, a DNA methyltransferase required for learning and memory in hippocampus, specifically in BDE-47-exposed Mecp2(308/+) offspring (Woods et al., 2012). Collectively, these results demonstrate that some chemical environment-gene interactions relevant to social and cognitive behaviors exhibit sexual dimorphism and epigenetic dysregulation that are likely relevant to the pathogenesis ASDs.

8. Other ASD-like diseases

8.1. Angelman syndrome

Epigenetic effects may also manifest through aberrant methylation patterns of imprinted genes. The expression of imprinted genes, which are mostly found in clusters on chromosomes 6, 7, 11, 14 and 15, is controlled by a series of DNA methylations and histone modifications. Imprinting defects may be primary or secondary. Primary imprinting defects cause changes in observed methylation patterns, but leaves the DNA sequence unaltered, and thus may be classified as an epigenetic mechanism (Gos, 2013). Angelman syndrome, which is caused by an absence of active maternal genes in the 15q11-1q13 region, may result from a primary imprinting defect, although the syndrome is more commonly caused by a deletion on the maternal chromosome or a paternal uniparental disomy. There is some basis to suspect a link between Angelman syndrome and autism. For instance, in one particular study, though the frequency of Angelman syndrome was only found to be 4 out of approximately 49,000, each of those four children were found to demonstrate autistic behaviors. (Steffenburg et al., 1996). However, other studies place the rate of co-occurrence of autism and Angelman syndrome at a rate of as low as 2%. It seems reasonable to assert that, to the extent that Angelman syndrome and autism are linked, the condition of some percentage of these patients will be related to an epigenetic primary imprinting defect. However, the available evidence does not establish whether the epigenetic defect causing Angelman syndrome leads directly to autistic symptoms or whether the relationship between Angelman syndrome and autism are merely correlative, and not causative.

8.2. Prader-Willi syndrome

On the other hand, secondary imprinting defects occur when a gene mutation results in improper epigenetic regulation. Such a defect may occur in Prader-Willi syndrome, which is characterized by the lack of a paternal contribution at the 15q11-q13 locus. The specific mutation most commonly responsible for secondary imprinting in Prader-Willi syndrome is a cis-acting defect of the imprinting regulatory center of the Prader-Willi syndrome gene (Dykens, and Shah, 2003). Prader-Willi patients present with autistic behavior more frequently than Angelman syndrome patients; studies suggest the frequency of autism co-occurrence with Prader-Willi syndrome is between 18% and 38% (Veltman et al., 2004), though the causative nature of this relationship has not been established.

8.3. Fragile X syndrome

Fragile X syndrome is the leading single-gene cause of autism accounting for as many at 5% of all cases (McLennan et al., 2011). As with Prader-Willi and Angelman syndromes, epigenetic mechanisms can contribute to the development of the Fragile X, which is characterized by the presence of 200 or more CGG repeats in the 5' untranslated region of the FMR1 gene (Willemsen et al., 2011). The resulting increased concentration of cytosine and guanine nucleotides causes the global methylation of not only the CGG-repeat region but also adjacent regions, which happen to include FMR1 promoter elements.

8.4. Rett syndrome

A missense mutation of the protein Mecp2 is known to produce Rett syndrome, a disease formerly termed cerebral atrophic hyperammonemia, the signs and symptoms of which are often confused with Angelman syndrome. Interestingly, hyperammonemia can also be produced by urea cycle disorders and exposure to valproic acid (the latter being a known risk factor for ASDs). Damage to the locus coeruleus-noradrenergic and midbrain dopaminergic systems have been demonstrated and the etiology of Rett syndrome appears to be confirmed by a study demonstrating that restoration of Mecp2 activity may be achieved by an IGF-1 treatment (Tropea et al., 2009).

9. Role of epigenetic drift in autism

Earlier, we discussed investigations involving identical twins to elucidate the effects of the intrauterine environment on the epigenome. As it happens, twin studies are also valuable because they allow us to explore the concept of epigenetic drift. The idea of epigenetic drift closely parallels the more familiar notion of genetic drift: Beginning with identical starting conditions, epigenetic drift is the divergence of two formerly identical epigenomes in response to external pressures. An investigation of global histone H3 and H4 acetylation, 5 methyl cytosine methylation and X chromosome inactivation concluded that despite very few differences between the epigenomes of monozygotic twins at birth, significant differences between the epigenomes develop as the twins age (Fraga et al., 2005). Some studies have indicated that epigenomic drift may occur on a scale two orders of magnitude more substantial than genetic drift (Martin, 2012). Clearly, any number of factors - smoking, diet and physical activity among them - may be responsible for these different changes. But it might also be the case that an intermittent failure to properly transfer epigenetic information during the gene replication process may play a role as well. In any event, regardless of the specific etiology of the epigenomic changes, these are the sorts of heritable changes in methylation and acetylation that we've previously seen to be linked to the development of ASDs in offspring.

10. Summary and conclusions

Figure 1 summarizes the main epigenetic mechanisms that appear to play roles in ASDs include low activity of Mecp2 at CpG islands in genes of frontal cortex is shown to reduce the capacity for inhibiting HDAC1 and chromatin condensation for gene silencing. HDAC1 inhibition by valproic acid and GSK3β inhibition by lithium are shown to upregulate the Wnt signaling pathway, which in turn causes accumulation of β-catenin in the cytoplasm and its translocation to the nucleus. In the nucleus β-catenin can act as an activator of transcription and cause macrocephaly and the attendant increase in the number of cerebral cortical columns. DNMT is shown to methylate the oxytocin receptor gene and silence it, resulting in the low oxytocin and estrogen activity necessary for androgen receptor mediation of high arousal inputs to the amygdyla. This defect is associated with antisocial behaviors after exposure to environmental stressors. Histone H3 phosphorylation by protein kinase C beta is shown to activate the LSD1, an HMT that prevents demethylation of H3K4, which is also necessary for androgen receptor mediation of high arousal inputs to the amygdyla. Hypomethylation by decreased availability of S-adenosyl methionine (SAM) is shown to occur in mothers of autistic children. Environmental and nutritional conditions acting as pro- or anti-autism factors by epigenetic mechanisms suggest strategies for decreasing the prevalence of ASDs. This knowledge of putative epigenetic targets should motivate clinical practitioners and educators to develop novel treatment strategies based on the environment-gene interactions which could contribute to the core symptoms of ASDs.

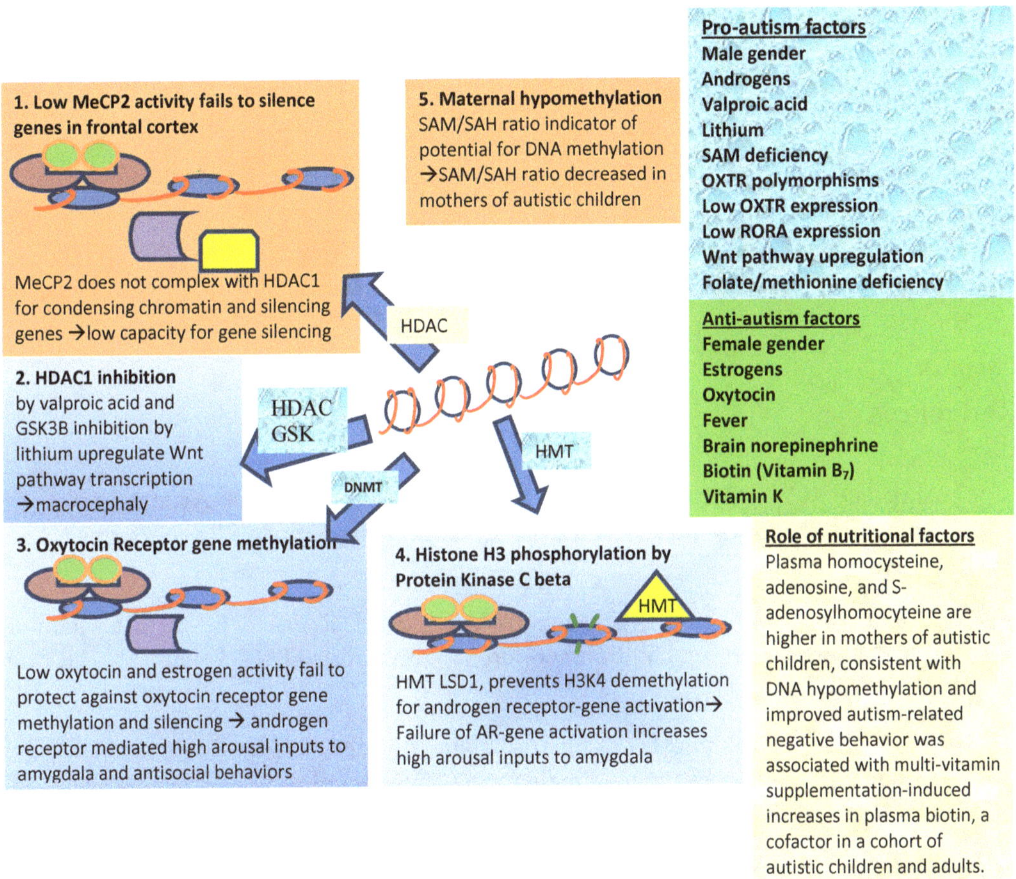

Figure 1. Main mechanisms of epigenetic alterations in autism. Each alteration involves many enzymes but the main players to cause methylation or acetylation are shown by arrows. These are not separate mechanisms and the enzymes do not act alone. Several enzymes act at a promoter simultaneously. 1. Low methyl CpG binding protein-2 (Mecp2) at CpG islands of frontal cortex reduces capacity for complexing with histone deacetylase 1 (HDAC1) for gene silencing. 2. HDAC1 inhibition by valproic acid exposure and glycogen synthetase kinase-3B (GSK3B) inhibition by lithium upregulate Wnt signaling pathway, activates transcription, associated with macrocephaly with increased number of cerebral cortical column. 3. DNA methyltransferase (DNMT) methylates oxytocin receptor gene produces low oxytocin and estrogen activity necessary for androgen receptor mediated high-arousal inputs to amygdala. 4. Histone H3 phosphorylation by protein kinase c beta activates the histone methyltransferase (HMT) lysine demethylase 1 (LSD1) which prevents demethylation of lysine-4 site of histone-3 (H3K4) also necessary for androgen receptor (AR) mediation of high arousal inputs to amygdala. 5. Maternal hypomethylation by dietary folic acid deficiency decreases availability of S-adenosyl methionine (SAM), associated with abnormal intrauterine growth.

Acknowledgements

This research supported in part by NIH/NCRR/RCMI Grant 2G12RR003048 to Howard University.

Author details

Tafari Mbadiwe and Richard M. Millis

Department of Physiology & Biophysics Howard University College of Medicine Washington, DC, USA

The authors have no conflicts of interest, financial or otherwise, to disclose.

References

[1] Abdallah, M.W., Mortensen, E.L., Greaves-Lord. K. et al (2013). Neonatal levels of neurotrophic factors and risk of autism spectrum disorders. *Acta Psychiatr Scand*. 128, 61-69.

[2] Adams, J.B., Audhya, T., McDonough-Means, S., et al (2011). Effect of a vitamin/mineral supplement on children and adults with autism. *BMC Pediatr*. 11, 111, doi: 10.1186/1471-2431-11-111.

[3] Akashi, M. and Takumi, T. (2005). The orphan nuclear receptor RORα regulates circadian transcription of the mammalian core-clock Bmal1. *Nature Struct Mol Biol*. 12, 441-448.

[4] Anderson, O.S., Sant, K.E. and Dolinoy, D.C (2012). Nutrition and epigenetics: an interplay of dietary methyl donors, one-carbon metabolism and DNA methylation. *J Nutr Biochem*. 23, 853-859.

[5] Angelucci, F., Ricci, E., Padua, L. et al (2007). Music exposure differentially alters the levels of brain-derived neurotrophic factor and nerve growth factor in the mouse hypothalamus. *Neurosci Lett*. 429, 152-155.

[6] Perrin, M.C., Brown, A.S. and Malaspina, D (2007). Aberrant epigenetic regulation could explain the relationship of paternal age to schizophrenia. *Schizophr Bull*. 33, 1270-1273.

[7] Balaratnasingam, S. and Janca, A (2012). Brain derived neurotrophic factor: a novel neurotrophin involved in psychiatric and neurological disorders. *Pharmacol Ther*. 134, 116-124.

[8] Beri, S., Tonna, N., Menozzi, G., et al (2007). DNA methylation regulates tissue-specific expression of Shank3. *J Neurochem*. 101, 1380-1391.

[9] Beversdorf, D.Q., Manning, S.E., Hillier, A., et al (2005). Timing of prenatal stressors and autism. *J Autism Dev Dis*. 35, 471-478.

[10] Billin, A.N., Thirlwell, H. and Ayer, D.E (2000). Beta-catenin-histone deacetylase interactions regulate the transition of LEF1 from a transcriptional repressor to an activator. *Mol Cell Biol.* 20, 6882-6890.

[11] Boukhtouche, F., Vodjdani, G., Jarvis, C.I., et al (2006). Human retinoic acid receptor-related orphan receptor $\alpha 1$ overexpression protects neurones against oxidative stress-induced apoptosis. *J Neurochem.* 96, 1778-1789.

[12] Cardona-Gomez, P., Perez, M., Avila, J., et al (2004). Estradiol inhibits GSK3 and regulates interaction of estrogen receptors, GSK3, and beta-catenin in the hippocampus. *Mol Cell Neurosci.* 25, 363-373.

[13] Chahrour, M., Jung, S.Y., Shaw, C., et al (2008). MeCP2, a key contributor to neurological disease, activates and represses transcription. *Science.* 320, 1224-1229.

[14] Chauhan, A. and Chauhan, V (2006). Oxidative stress in autism. *Pathophysiology* 13, 171-181.

[15] Cohen, S., Zhou, Z. and Greenberg, M.E (2008). Medicine. Activating a repressor *Science.* 320, 1172–1173.

[16] Curran, L.K., Newschaffer, L.C., Lee, S.O., et al (2007). Behaviors associated with fever in children with autism spectrum disorders. *Pediatrics.* 120, 1386-1392.

[17] Currenti, S.A (2010). Understanding and determining the etiology of autism. *Cell Mol Neurobiol.* 30, 161-171.

[18] Dai, Y.M., Hu, Y.L., Wang, Z.Q. et al (2007). Loss of imprinting of IGF2 in cord blood of newborns of Chinese Han population. *Zhonghua Yi Xue Yi Chuan Xue Za Zhi.* 24, 10-14.

[19] Darling, R.D., Alzghoul, L., Zhang, J., et al (2011). Perinatal citalopram exposure selectively increases locus ceruleus circuit function in male rats. *J Neurosci.* 31, 16709-16715.

[20] Dufour-Rainfray, D., Vourc'h, P., Le Guisquet, A.M., et al (2010). Behavior and serotonergic disorders in rats exposed prenatally to valproate: a model for autism. *Neurosci Lett.* 470, 55–59.

[21] Dykens, E. and Shah, B (2003). Psychiatric disorders in Prader-Willi syndrome: epidemiology and management. *CNS Drugs.* 17, 167-178.

[22] Ebert, D.H., Gabel, H.W., Robinson, N.D., et al (2013). Activity-dependent phosphorylation of MeCP2 threonine 308 regulates interaction with NCoR. *Nature.* 499, 341-345.

[23] Fatemi, S.H. and Halt, A.R (2001). Altered levels of Bcl2 and p53 proteins in parietal cortex reflect deranged apoptotic regulation in autism. *Synapse.* 42, 281-284.

[24] Fatemi, S.H., Stary, J.M., Halt, A.R., et al (2001). Dysregulation of reelin and bcl-2 proteins in autistic cerebellum. *J Autism Dev Dis* 31, 529-535.

[25] Ferguson, J.N., Young, L.J., Hearn, E.F., et al (2000). Social amnesia in mice lacking the oxytocin gene. *Nature Gen.* 25, 284-288.

[26] Foldi, C.J., Eyles, D.W., Flatscher-Bader, T. et al (2011). New perspectives on rodent models of advanced paternal age: relevance to autism. *Front Behav Neurosci.* 5, 32. doi: 10.3389/fnbeh.2011.00032.

[27] Foote, S.L., Bloom, F.E. and Aston-Jones, G (1983). Nucleus locus ceruleus: new evidence of anatomical and physiological specificity. *Physiol Rev.* 63, 844-914.

[28] Fraga, M.F., Ballestar, E., Paz, M.F. et al (2005). Epigenetic differences arise during the lifetime of monozygotic twins. *Proc Natl Acad Sci U S A.* 102, 10604-10609.

[29] Gillis, R.F. and Rouleau, G.A (2011). The ongoing dissection of the genetic architecture of autistic spectrum disorder. *Mol Autism.* 2, 12. doi: 10.1186/2040-2392-2-12.

[30] Glantz, L.A., Gilmore, J.H., Lieberman, J.A., et al (2006). Apoptotic mechanisms and the synaptic pathology of schizophrenia. *Schiz Res.* 81, 47–63.

[31] Goriely, A., McGrath, J.J., Hultman, C.M. et al (2013). Selfish spermatogonial selection: a novel mechanism for the association between advanced paternal age and neurodevelopmental disorders. *Am J Psychiatry.* 170, 599-608.

[32] Gos, M (2013). Epigenetic mechanisms of gene expression regulation in neurological diseases. *Acta Neurobiol Exp (Warsaw).* 73, 19-37.

[33] Gouin, J.P., Carter, C.S., Pournajafi-Nazarloo, H., et al (2010). Marital behavior, oxytocin, vasopressin, and wound healing. *Psychoneuroendocrinology.* 35, 1082-1090.

[34] Gregory, S.G., Connelly, J.J., Towers, A.J., et al (2009). Genomic and epigenetic evidence for oxytocin receptor deficiency in autism. *BMC Med.* 7, 62, doi: 10.1186/1741-7015-7-62.

[35] Hu, V.W., Frank, B.C., Heine, S. et al (2006). Gene expression profiling of lymphoblastoid cell lines from monozygotic twins discordant in severity of autism reveals differential regulation of neurologically relevant genes. *BMC Genomics.* 7, 118.

[36] Insel, T.R (1992). Oxytocin--a neuropeptide for affiliation: evidence from behavioral, receptor autoradiographic, and comparative studies. *Psychoneuroendocrinology.* 17, 3-35.

[37] Jacob, S., Brune, C.W., Carter, C.S., et al (2007). Association of the oxytocin receptor gene (OXTR) in Caucasian children and adolescents with autism. *Neurosci Lett.* 417, 6-9.

[38] James, S.J., Melnyk, S., Jernigan, S., et al (2008). Abnormal transmethylation/transsulfuration metabolism and DNA hypomethylation among parents of children with autism. *J Autism Dev Dis.* 38, 1966-1975.

[39] James, S.J., Melnyk, S., Jernigan, S., et al (2010). A functional polymorphism in the reduced folate carrier gene and DNA hypomethylation in mothers of children with autism. *Am J Med Gen B Neuropsychiat Gen.* 153B, 1209-1220.

[40] Jope, R.S (2003). Lithium and GSK-3: one inhibitor, two inhibitory actions, multiple outcomes. *Trends Pharmacol Sci.* 24, 441-443..

[41] Kadesjö, B., Gillberg, C. and Hagberg, B (1999). Brief report: autism and Asperger syndrome in seven-year-old children: a total population study. *J Autism Dev Dis.* 29, 327-331.

[42] Kimura, T., Saji, F., Nishimori, K., et al (2003). Molecular regulation of the oxytocin receptor in peripheral organs. *J Mol Endocrinol.* 30, 109-115.

[43] LaSalle, J.M., Goldstine, J., Balmer, D., et al (2001). Quantitative localization of heterogeneous methyl-CpG-binding protein 2 (MeCP2) expression phenotypes in normal and Rett syndrome brain by laser scanning cytometry. *Hum Mol Gen.* 10, 1729-1740.

[44] Lee, M.H., Amin, N.D., Venkatesan, A. et al (2013). Impaired neurogenesis and neurite outgrowth in an HIV-gp120 transgenic model is reversed by exercise via BDNF production and Cdk5 regulation. *Neurovirol.* 19, 418-431.

[45] Levy, S.E., Mandell, D.S. and Schultz, R.T (2007). Autism. *Lancet.* 374, 1627-1638.

[46] Lintas, C., Sacco, R., Garbett, K., et al (2009). Involvement of the PRKCB1 gene in autistic disorder: significant genetic association and reduced neocortical gene expression. *Mol Psychiat.* 14, 705-718.

[47] Linthorst, A.C., Flachskamm, C., Holsboer, F., et al (1995). Intraperitoneal administration of bacterial endotoxin enhances noradrenergic neurotransmission in the rat preoptic area: relationship with body temperature and hypothalamic--pituitary--adrenocortical axis activity. *Eur J Neurosci.* 7, 2418-2430.

[48] Liu, X., Kawamura, Y., Shimada, T., et al (2010). Association of the oxytocin receptor (OXTR) gene polymorphisms with autism spectrum disorder (ASD) in the Japanese population. *J Hum Gen.* 55, 137-141.

[49] Liu, Y., Du, Y., Liu, W., et al (2013). Lack of association between NLGN3, NLGN4, SHANK2 and SHANK3 gene variants and autism spectrum disorder in a Chinese population. *PLoS One.* 8, e56639, doi: 10.1371/journal.pone.0056639.

[50] Luikenhuis, S., Giacometti, E., Beard, C.F., et al (2004). Expression of MeCP2 in post-mitotic neurons rescues Rett syndrome in mice. *Proc Natl Acad Sci USA.* 101, 6033–6038.

[51] Luo, W., Karpf, A.R., Deeb, K.K., et al (2010). Epigenetic regulation of vitamin D 24-hydroxylase/CYP24A1 in human prostate cancer. *Cancer Res.* 70, 5953-5962.

[52] MacLusky, N.J., Clark, A.S., Naftolin, F., et al (1987). Estrogen formation in the mammalian brain: possible role of aromatase in sexual differentiation of the hippocampus and neocortex. *Steroids.* 50, 459-474.

[53] Martin, G.M (2012). Stochastic modulations of the pace and patterns of ageing: impacts on quasi-stochastic distributions of multiple geriatric pathologies. *Mech Ageing Dev.* 133, 107-111.

[54] McLennan, Y., Polussa, J., Tassone, F et al (2011). Fragile x syndrome. *Curr Genom.* 12, 216-224.

[55] Mehler, M.F (2008). Epigenetic principles and mechanisms underlying nervous system functions in health and disease. *Prog Neurobiol.* 86, 305-341.

[56] Mehler, M.F. and Purpura, D.P (2009). Autism, fever, epigenetics and the locus coeruleus. *Brain Res Rev.* 59, 388-392.

[57] Metzger, E., Imhof, A., Patel, D., et al (2010). Phosphorylation of histone H3T6 by PKCbeta(I) controls demethylation at histone H3K4. *Nature.* 464, 792-796.

[58] Minshew, N.J. and Williams, D.L (2007). The new neurobiology of autism: cortex, connectivity, and neuronal organization. *Arch Neurol.* 64, 945-950.

[59] Moore, S.J., Turnpenny, P., Quinn, A., et al (2000). A clinical study of 57 children with fetal anticonvulsant syndromes. *J Med Gen.* 37, 489-497.

[60] Nagarajan, R.P., Hogart, A.R., Gwye, Y., et al (2006). Reduced MeCP2 expression is frequent in autism frontal cortex and correlates with aberrant MeCP2 promoter methylation. *Epigenetics.* 1, 31-e11.

[61] Nan, X., Ng, H.H., Johnson, C.A., et al (1998). Transcriptional repression by the methyl-CpG-binding protein MeCP2 involves a histone deacetylase complex. *Nature.* 393, 386-389.

[62] Nguyen, A., Rauch, T.A., Pfeifer, G.P., et al (2010). Global methylation profiling of lymphoblastoid cell lines reveals epigenetic contributions to autism spectrum disorders and a novel autism candidate gene, RORA, whose protein product is reduced in autistic brain. *FASEB J.* 24, 3036-3051.

[63] Nickl-Jockschat, T. and Michel, T.M (2011). The role of neurotrophic factors in autism. *Mol Psychiatry.* 16, 478-490.

[64] Oakes, C.C., Smiraglia, D.J., Plass, C. et al (2003). Aging results in hypermethylation of ribosomal DNA in sperm and liver of male rats. *Proc Natl Acad Sci U S A.* 100, 1775-1780.

[65] O'Connor, R.D., Zayzafoon, M., Farach-Carson, M.C., et al (2009). Mecp2 deficiency decreases bone formation and reduces bone volume in a rodent model of Rett syndrome. *Bone.* 45, 346-356.

[66] Pardo, C.A., Vargas, D.L. and Zimmerman, A.W (2005). Immunity, neuroglia and neuroinflammation in autism. *Int Rev Psychiat.* 17, 485-495.

[67] Pareja-Galeano, H., Sanchis-Gomar, F. and Mayero, S (2013). Autism spectrum disorders: possible implications of BDNF modulation through epigenetics. *Acta Psychiatr Scand.* 128, 97. doi: 10.1111/acps.12071.

[68] Pelphrey, K., Adolphs, R. and Morris, J.P (2004). Neuroanatomical substrates of social cognition dysfunction in autism. *Ment Retard Dev Dis Res Rev.* 10, 259-271.

[69] Perrin, M.C., Brown, A.S. and Malaspina, D (2007). Aberrant epigenetic regulation could explain the relationship of paternal age to schizophrenia. *Schizophr Bull.* 33, 1270-1273.

[70] Pfaff, D.W., Rapin, I. and Goldman, S (2011). Male predominance in autism: neuroendocrine influences on arousal and social anxiety. *Autism Res.* 4, 163-176.

[71] Pidsley, R., Dempster, E., Troakes, C., et al (2012). Epigenetic and genetic variation at the IGF2/H19 imprinting control region on 11p15.5 is associated with cerebellum weight. *Epigenetics.* 7, 155-163.

[72] Ptak, C. and Petronis, A (2010). Epigenetic approaches to psychiatric disorders. *Dialog Clin Neurosci.* 12, 25-35.

[73] Rai, D., Lee, B.K., Dalman, C., et al (2013). Parental depression, maternal antidepressant use during pregnancy, and risk of autism spectrum disorders: population based case-control study. *BMJ.* 346, f2059, doi: 10.1136/bmj.f2059.

[74] Rasalam, A.D., Hailey, H., Williams, J.H., et al (2005). Characteristics of fetal anticonvulsant syndrome associated autistic disorder. *Dev Med Child Neurol.* 47, 551-555.

[75] Sanders, B.K (2012). Flowers for Algernon: steroid dysgenesis, epigenetics and brain disorders. *Pharmacol Rep.* 64, 1285-1290.

[76] Scholl, T.O. and Johnson, W.G (2000). Folic acid: influence on the outcome of pregnancy. *Am J Clin Nutr.* 71, 1295S-1303S.

[77] Shimshoni, J.A., Dalton, E.C., Jenkins, A., et al (2007). The effects of central nervous system-active valproic acid constitutional isomers, cyclopropyl analogs, and amide derivatives on neuronal growth cone behavior. *Mol Pharmacol.* 71, 884-892.

[78] Simpson, K.L., Weaver, K.J., de Villers-Sidani, E., et al (2011). Perinatal antidepressant exposure alters cortical network function in rodents. *Proc Natl Acad Sci USA.* 108, 18465–18470.

[79] Steffenburg, S., Gillberg, C.L., Steffenburg, U., et al (1996). Autism in Angelman syndrome: a population-based study. *Pediatr Neurol.* 14, 131-136.

[80] Stoltenberg, C., Schjølberg, S., Bresnahan, M. et al (2010). ABC Study Group. The Autism Birth Cohort: A paradigm for gene-environment-timing research. *Mol Psychiat.* 15, 676-680.

[81] Sun, L., Huang, L., Nguyen, P., et al (2008). DNA methyltransferase 1 and 3B activate BAG-1 expression via recruitment of CTCFL/BORIS and modulation of promoter histone methylation. *Can Res.* 68, 2726-2735.

[82] Surén, P., Roth, C., Bresnahan, M., et al (2013). Association between maternal use of folic acid supplements and risk of autism spectrum disorders in children. *JAMA.* 309, 570-577.

[83] Takayanagi, Y., Yoshida M., Bielsky, I.F., et al (2005). Pervasive social deficits, but normal parturition, in oxytocin receptor-deficient mice. *Proc. Natl Acad Sci USA.* 102, 16096-16101.

[84] Tropea, D., Giacometti, E., Wilson, N.R., et al (2009). Partial reversal of Rett syndrome-like symptoms in MeCP2 mutant mice. *Proc Natl Acad Sci USA.* 106, 2029-2034.

[85] Tsujimoto, Y., Finger, L.R., Yunis, J., et al (1984). Cloning of the chromosome breakpoint of neoplastic B cells with the t(14;18) chromosome translocation. *Science.* 226, 1097-1099.

[86] Uchino, S. and Waga, C (2013). SHANK3 as an autism spectrum disorder-associated gene. *Brain Dev.* 35, 106-110.

[87] Unternaehrer, E., Luers, P., Mill, J., et al (2012). Dynamic changes in DNA methylation of stress-associated genes (OXTR, BDNF) after acute psychosocial stress. *Translat Psychiat.* 2, e150, doi: 10.1038/tp.2012.77.

[88] Veenstra-Vanderweele, J., Muller, C.L., Iwamoto, H., et al (2012). Autism gene variant causes hyperserotonemia, serotonin receptor hypersensitivity, social impairment and repetitive behavior. *Proc Natl Acad Sci USA.* 109, 5469–5474.

[89] Veltman, M.W., Thompson, R.J., Roberts, S.E., et al (2004). Prader-Willi syndrome--a study comparing deletion and uniparental disomy cases with reference to autism spectrum disorders. *Eur Child Adol Psychiat.* 13, 42-50.

[90] Wang, Z., Xu, L., Zhu, X., et al (2010). Demethylation of specific Wnt/β-catenin pathway genes and its upregulation in rat brain induced by prenatal valproate exposure. *Anat Rec (Hoboken).* 293, 1947-1953.

[91] Whitney, E.R., Kemper, T.L., Rosene, D.L., et al (2009). Density of cerebellar basket and stellate cells in autism: evidence for a late developmental loss of Purkinje cells. *J Neurosci Res.* 87, 2245-2254.

[92] Willemsen, R., Levenga, J. and Oostra, B.A (2011). CGG repeat in the FMR1 gene: size matters. *Clin Gen.* 80, 214-225.

[93] Williams, E.L. and Casanova, M.F (2010). Autism or autisms? Finding the lowest common denominator. *Boletin de la Asociacion Medica de Puerto Rico.* 102, 17-24.

[94] Woods, R., Vallero, R.O., Golub, M.S., et al (2012). Long-lived epigenetic interactions between perinatal PBDE exposure and Mecp2308 mutation. *Hum Mol Genet.* 21, 2399-2411.

[95] Wu, S., Jia, M., Ruan, Y., et al (2005). Positive association of the oxytocin receptor gene (OXTR) with autism in the Chinese Han population. *Biol Psychiat.* 58, 74-77.

[96] Yasuda, Y., Hashimoto, R., Yamamori, H., et al (2011). Gene expression analysis in lymphoblasts derived from patients with autism spectrum disorder. *Mol Autism.* 2, 9, doi:10.1186/2040-2392-2-9.

[97] Yasui, D.H., Peddada, S., Bieda, M.C., et al (2007). Integrated epigenomic analyses of neuronal MeCP2 reveal a role for long-range interaction with active genes. *Proc Natl Acad Sci USA.* 104, 19416-19421.

[98] Zubkova, E.V. and Robaire, B (2006). Effects of ageing on spermatozoal chromatin and its sensitivity to in vivo and in vitro oxidative challenge in the Brown Norway rat. *Hum Reprod.* 21, 2901-2910.

3

Epigenetic Mechanisms of the Vascular Endothelium

Alexandra A. Majerski, Anthony C. Quinton and Philip A. Marsden

1. Introduction

In the same way that Watson and Crick's breakthrough in identifying the molecular structure of the DNA double helix revolutionized the last sixty years of molecular biology, the field of epigenetics is set to do the same for the next sixty (or more) years! An alphabet of four letters, and strict guidelines dictating their arrangement, comprise the genome of all known living organisms. This same system has allowed us to unravel many of the secrets to human health and to comprehend a great number of once-elusive conditions and diseases. Nevertheless, a vast number of puzzles remain to be solved, and the genetic code is but one tool used to make sense of them.

Our understanding of our genetics has grown enormously over the last several decades and the iconic image of the DNA double helix has become a cornerstone for the field. Most certainly, the information contained within this static DNA code is but a starting point. Yet, a number of seemingly straightforward questions cannot be answered without going beyond the highly conserved script. Undoubtedly, many ask: Why and how is an endothelial cell different from a brain cell when the static DNA genome is identical? To answer this and many other complex and fascinating phenomena, we must, instead, go over or above (epi-) genetics because the DNA blueprint is identical in each of the abovementioned somatic cells. A term coined in the 1940s by Conrad Waddington, epigenetics refers to chromatin-based mechanisms important in the regulation of gene expression that do not involve changes to the DNA sequence per se. Epigenetic principles, in eukaryotic organisms, are linked by an important common thread: DNA does not exist in a "naked" state. Figure 1 provides a visual representation of the added layer of chemical species, as well as proteins which themselves can be modified – all of which contribute to a layer of chemical complexity and significant implications that epigenetics strives to classify and understand.

Division and differentiation are fundamental processes for sending cells of common origin to different destinations. Logically, the timing and regulation of these processes must be dependent on more than an identical code contained in all body cells. Thus, the epigenome comprises the ever-expanding repertoire of chemical alterations that regulate the expression of genes and, hence, dictate the function of cells and the role of proteins. A number of genetic determinants, as well as lineage-specific markings, and environmental responses are used to construct the epigenome [1]. The existence of an epigenetic code is a highly contested topic [2] and one which will be explored throughout this chapter. Indeed, it is not only mistakes in the genetic code, but also deviations in the epigenome that may provide clues to understanding the onset of detrimental conditions and diseases.

2. Three mechanisms of epigenetics

2.1. Posttranslational histone modifications

Compaction of the entire 6 billion base pair genome, 3 billion in each copy of the haploid genome, into each one of 50 trillion human body cells is a truly breathtaking achievement! In each cell, 2 meters of DNA are condensed by at least 10, 000 fold in order to fit into the roughly 6 μm diameter of the nucleus. In accomplishing this monumental feat, intricate folding and wrapping are the first steps in organizing the DNA. Covalent and non-covalent interactions further alter the three-dimensional arrangement of the chromatin. Chromatin refers to the state of DNA when it is spooled around the fundamental repeat unit: the nucleosome [3]. Each nucleosome consists of an octamer containing four different core histone units: histones H2A, H2B, H3 and H4. Two of each core histone unit are present within one nucleosome such that a tetramer of H3 and H4 joins two dimers of H2A and H2B [3]. At least one fifth of the amino acids in each core protein are lysine or arginine – those with highly basic side chains [4]. Approximately 147 base pairs of DNA wrap around each nucleosome. Linker histones, especially H1, interconnect each nucleosome. Structurally, each of the canonical histone core proteins has a characteristic N-terminal tail of amino acids extending out from the core, which is highly susceptible to modifications [3].

Contrary to what biologists believed for many years, kinetic experiments have shown that DNA wrapping around a nucleosome is surprisingly dynamic. Open exposure for 10 to 50 milliseconds – the length of time between rapid winding and unwinding – means that DNA is available for binding other proteins [5]. The formation of nucleosomes converts a DNA molecule into thread-like chromatin approximately one-third of its initial length [4].

Since the initial work in histone acetylation and methylation by Allfrey and colleagues [6], many other modifications have been documented, with the most frequently found to be, at steady state, lysine acetylation, mono-, di-, and tri-methylation of lysines, and the phosphorylation of serines [7]. Concomitantly, a particular collection of enzymes is responsible for each of these additions: histone acetyl transferases (HATs) and histone methyl transferases (HMTs). Importantly, each of these modifications are reversible, the opposite reactions catalyzed by a group of histone deacetylases (HDACs) and histone demethylases (HDMTs). Most often, the

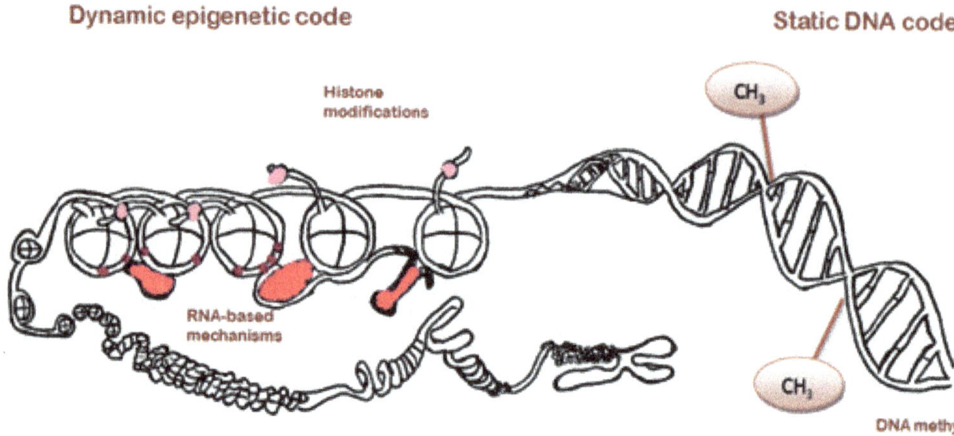

Figure 1. Three defining epigenetic mechanisms: DNA methylation, posttranslational histone modifications, and RNA-based mechanisms. The four-lettered (**a**denine, **c**ytosine, **g**uanine, **t**hymine) code that constitutes an individual's genetic makeup is identical in all cell types and is highly conserved during mitotic and meiotic divisions, whereas the three epigenetic modifications differ amongst cell types and are only partly conserved during mitosis and meiosis. In the "Nurture vs. Nature" debate, genetics characterizes the latter with strong evolutionary convergence while epigenetics is influenced by the former, such that the dynamic patterns that classify it diverge rapidly through evolution.

binding of DNA gene regulatory proteins, or transcription factors, is a pre-requisite for the recruitment action of any of these enzymes. Such events occur at different times in the developmental history of a cell and groups of nucleosomes may be modified in a multitude of ways based on the status of the cell [4].

The mechanism by which histone posttranslational modifications (PTMs) occur can be broadly categorized into 3 groups: a) altering chromatin structure with small (acetylation, phosphorylation, methylation) or large (ubiquitylation, sumoylation) chemical groups, b) inhibiting binding factors to the chromatin, and c) attracting a particular set of proteins to the newly modified regions. In the following, we will highlight the notable features of the well-studied mechanisms and allude to the implications of them throughout the remainder of this chapter.

First, acetylation is a posttranslational histone mark that is known to be correlated with transcriptional activation. Broadly speaking, chromatin structure is loosened by the acetylation of lysine (denoted by K) residues. This modification allows for DNA binding sites to be made more accessible, at the same time that a new collection of proteins are recruited to this region of modified chromatin [8]. Positive charges at highly basic histone tails are neutralized with lysine acetylation, which reduces the binding of the amino acid to the negatively charged DNA [9]. An actual change of the physical properties of the histone tails, such as neutralization, is an example of a *cis*-effect. In this instance, a segmental expansion of the chromatin allows for easier access to transcriptional regulators. When other proteins are actively recruited to the chromatin and read snippets of it, a *trans*-effect is said to occur. The example HPTM recruiting new proteins was observed with histone tail acetylation. Bromodomain are specialized protein domains, found in HATs such as Gcn5 and CBP/p300. [10, 11].

Histone methylation has proven to be more perplexing than histone acetylation due to the fact that lysine can be mono-, di-, or tri-methylated and arginine can be mono-or di-methylated. Knowing that there are 24 sites of lysine and arginine methylation on the four histone core proteins, means that a tremendous number of methylated/unmethylated states are possible [12-15]. Astonishingly, lysine methylation can result in either the activation or silencing of gene expression. Generally, the methylation of lysines 4, 36, and 79 on histone H3 (H3K4me, H3K36me, H3K79me, respectively) are correlated with transcriptional activation, while the remainder have repressive activity [15]. Two of these marks, namely methylation on lysine 79 of histone H3 and 20 on histone H4, also play a vital role in DNA repair [15]. Arginine methylation is similar, in that the process has been correlated with both negative and positive transcriptional regulation in numerous contexts [16-19].

In contrast to the addition of small chemical species, other larger modifications of histones are described (acetyl, phosphate, and methyl). Ubiquitylation and sumoylation, the addition of ubiquitin (Ub) and small ubiquitin-like modifier (SUMO), respectively, increases the size of the histone by up to two-thirds [20]. Depending on the site of ubiquitylation, this process can result in either transcriptionally active or inactive segments of chromatin [21]. Currently, there are no known ubiquitin chromatin binding proteins, but it is hypothesized that ubiquitin protein is again likely involved in a more diverse array of interactions than are the smaller chemical additions. Although much less well studied, SUMO is thought to recruit deacetylases and/or block lysine substrates that could be acetylated. Both mechanisms are consistent with results that have shown sumoylation to be correlated with transcriptional repression [20].

As a final note on PTMs, chromatin remodelling complexes that rely on the hydrolysis of ATP are known to temporarily alter the structure of nucleosomes by reducing the attraction between DNA and its neighbouring histone. This is commonly referred to as "nucleosome sliding" and the action briefly makes the DNA more susceptible to the effects of other proteins [4]. This sequence of events likely allows for a greater range of interactions of which we are not yet fully aware. It is important to stress that chromatin structure is highly regulated by nucleosome eviction and alternative histone core protein usage. This is a new area of study.

2.2. DNA methylation

The second major epigenetic pathway is DNA methylation - the addition of a methyl group (-CH_3) to the five position of the nitrogenous base, cytosine (Figure 1). Often referred to as the "fifth base pair," the product of this reaction, 5-methylcytosine (5mC), is the most common mutagenic base in the mammalian genome. Mutation of methyl CpG to uracil pG then TpG results in CpG depletion and TpG enrichment in the mammalian genome. DNA methylation is predominantly observed at CpG sites in the mammalian genome, with the methyl modification at non-CpG dinucleotides unusual, except perhaps in stem cells and mature neurons. Not to be confused with cytosine complementarily binding with guanine *across* the DNA double helix, CpG sites refer to locations where cytosine and guanine are separated by a phosphodiester bond, adjacent to one another. The vast majority, approximately 70-80%, of all CpG sites in the mammalian genome are, indeed, methylated [22]. Distribution of methylation across the genome shows enrichment at centromeric heterochromatin, repetitive element (transposon), and non-coding regions [23].

Unlike the great variability of histone modifications, DNA methylation is well known to be a mark of transcriptional repression [24]. Having been the first epigenetic mechanism identified, DNA methylation has been studied for the longest time and its consequences are well entrenched in a variety of essential biochemical processes, abnormal conditions, and diseases. X chromosome inactivation and imprinting are two such phenomena where normal DNA methylation in early development plays a vital role in setting the stage for monoallelic expression from chromosones during cellular maturation [25]. Deregulation of the methylation mechanism can lead to Immunodeficiency Centromeric instability, and Facial abnormalities syndrome (ICF) as well as being a contributing factor to cancer progression [26].

There are two main hypothesized mechanisms by which DNA methylation is proposed to repress gene expression. The first of these is a physical interference with the binding of regular transcription factors. The methyl group itself may physically project into the major groove of the DNA double helix, whereby it interferes with the sequence-specific recruitment of DNA proteins [27]. In support of this, a number of transcription factors have been found to recognize GC rich regions of the genome – the very same regions that are most susceptible to CpG methylation. Subsequently, these factors are unable to bind when methylcytosine takes the place of cytosine. The second proposed mechanism is in opposition to the first, as proteins are not repelled by the presence of 5mC, but are instead attracted to it. After the purification and cloning of an individual methyl-CpG binding protein, MeCP2 [28], four more similar proteins were identified and are now referred to as methyl-CpG binding domain proteins (MBDs). The attraction of these MBDs has been shown to block the binding of activating transcription factors and to actually recruit to the chromatin, histone-modifying enzymes, chromatin remodelers, and RNA molecules [29-31]. Several such conglomerates have been proposed to co-operatively silence gene expression [32].

2.2.1. DNA methyltransferases

The reaction that yields 5mC as its product is catalyzed by a family of three DNA methyltransferases (DNMTs): DNMT1, DNMT3A and DNMT3B [33]. DNMT1, the first of three family members, is a maintenance methyltransferase as it is responsible for transmitting methylation patterns from one cellular generation to the next. Replication of DNA demands that the two strands first be unwound, and it is during this time that DNMT1 is recruited to the replication fork. Binding of proliferating cell nuclear antigen (PCNA) to both strands and UHRF1 (ubiquitin-like with PHD and RING finger domains 1) protein via its characteristic SET-and RING-associated (SRA) domain, are pre-requisites for the recruitment of DNMT1 [34-36]. This enzyme exhibits methylation preference for hemi-methylated DNA, that is, double stranded DNA where only one strand exhibits methylation [37, 38]. Following replication, the parent strand displays the necessary methylation patterns and is subsequently used as a template for the DNMT1-mediated methyl addition to the nascent, naked strand of DNA. Such sites are accurately methylated due to the palindromic nature of the CpG sequences and the fact that methylation patterns between the two strands are symmetrical. Two other DNMTs include

DNMT3A and DNMT3B, both of which have been shown to function as *de novo* methyltransferases, displaying preferential methyl addition to unmethylated DNA [39]. These DNMTs play a crucial role in embryonic development, during which time the methylation patterns to be propagated in somatic cells are established [40].

The catalytic domain of the DNA methyltransferases is conserved amongst all of the DNMTs. Despite this, very little similarity is seen at their N-terminal domain. The regulatory domain of DNMT1 is composed of at least five motifs that are not present on the other enzymes, whereas DNMT3A and 3B exhibit two unique motifs. DNMT1 motifs include: a PCNA-interacting domain, a nuclear localization signal, a replication foci-targeting domain, a DNA-binding CXXC region, and a protein-protein interaction motif called the bromo-adjacent homology domain [26]. Those of DNMT3A and 3B include a motif essential for heterochromatin association, PWWP [41, 42] or "pro-trp-trp-pro," as well as a motif for protein-protein interactions: the ATRX-related cysteine-rich region containing a zinc finger and an atypical PHD domain [26].

2.2.2. CpG Islands

The fact that 5mC is the most common mutagenic base of the mammalian genome can be explained by methylcytosine's susceptibility to deamination [43, 44]. Upon deamination, the modified nitrogenous base is replaced by thymine and a T:G mismatch is generated. Rather than the rapid repair mechanism activated by cytosine deamination to uracil, T:G mismatches tend to accumulate and are not readily removed. Consequently, the genome becomes CpG depleted and TpG enriched. As indicated in Table 1, CpG islands (CGIs) are regions of the genome that have been spared this phenomenon; the number of CpG sites observed (O) is equivalent to the number that would be expected (E) based on C or G nucleotide abundance. As a result, the ideal situation would be an O/E of 1.

The definition of a CpG island has undergone a great deal of revision since the earliest studies dealing with these genomic regions [45] and are now rather arbitrarily defined as being > 500 bp [46], but averaging around 1000 bp. The O/E range determines the strength of a CpG island with the strongest having O/E > 0.75, a weak one with an O/E between 0.45 and 0.75, and a poor CGI having an O/E < 0.45. These regions are characterized by their elevated C+G content with the %C+G content > 55% [46]. These segments are especially fascinating due to their unusually low levels of DNA methylation marks. In essence, these regions are very often observed to be unmethylated. Due to the lack of repressive flags, genes that are downstream of CGI containing promoters are often in an active state of expression. It has been speculated that practically all CGIs are transcription start sites (TSS), largely of housekeeping and developmentally important genes [47, 48]. Approximately 70% of all gene promoters are CGIs [49].

The relationship between structure and function is seen most vividly in many of the compositional characteristics of CGIs. For instance, a recent study found that the CGI at the promoters of a particular group of genes was relatively nucleosome-deficient [50]. That is, the underlying DNA was highly accessible to activating transcription factors because less of it was spun around nucleosomes. Evidence from additional studies has shown that this nucleosome deficiency is a feature of CGI promoters, in general [51-53]. It is not yet known whether this phenomenon is a result of intrinsic chromatin instability or nucleosome exclusion due to the presence of the transcription initiation complex. Interestingly, it was found early in the study of CpG islands that, when found at promoter regions, these segments lack the canonical TATA box that so many eukaryotic promoters possess [54, 55]. Constitutive binding of RNA polymerase II is a frequently documented feature of CGIs. Presence of RNA polymerase II would evidently be associated with transcriptional activation as it is the major player involved in regular transcription.

Several histone chromatin features are also known to typify CpG islands, one of which is the depletion of histone 3 lysine residue 36 dimethylation, H3K36me2 [56]. Even though no conclusion has been reached as to why it is the absence of this dimethylation that characterizes most CpG islands, the modification has been reported, in yeast, to inhibit transcriptional initiation via histone deacetylase attraction. [57-59]. This absence makes way for the transcriptionally permissive state of CGIs. Furthermore, CGIs are marked by activating histone acetylation; both H3 and H4 acetylation are frequently observed [51, 60]. Notably, Cfp1 (CXXC finger protein 1) is a well characterized and fundamental component of the Setd1 H3K4 methyltransferase complex [61] and is drawn towards the overwhelming majority of CGIs in the mouse genome [62]. In the context of CpG islands, this protein directs H3K4 trimethylation, the activity of which has been shown to prevent DNA methylation of the underlying code [63, 64]. Hence, the DNA is maintained in a potentially active transcriptional state.

2.2.3. 5-hydroxymethylcytosine: the 6th base pair

The long-standing study of DNA methylation took a significant turn in 2009 with the rediscovery of what is now commonly referred to as the "6th base pair:" 5-hydroxymethylcytosine (5hmC) [65]. This base is the product of an enzymatic reaction that adds a hydroxyl (-OH) group to the methyl of 5-methylcytosine as shown in Figure 2. 5hmC was initially detected in 1972 in mammalian DNA [66], but has since been found primarily, and abundantly, in Purkinje neurons [67], the central nervous system (in the brainstem, spinal cord, and especially the cerebellum [67] and cerebral cortex) [68], and in embryonic stem (ES) cells [65, 69]. The highest tissue levels of 5hmC have been consistently found in the brain [69-71]. The striking abundance of 5hmC in ES cells and PGCs has led scientists to delve into the possibility that 5hmC is linked with the removal of 5mC in such settings, *in vivo*. There is evidence to suggest that, unlike 5mC, 5hmC may be correlated with transcriptional activation, after having been found at euchromatic regions in mice [72, 73]. In essence, while 5mC is known to be a mark of transcriptional repression, 5hmC may be associated with turning genes back on. Since 2009, a large quantity of research has been generated, dedicated to studying the potential role of 5hmC in gene expression regulation. Despite this, we have only just scratched the surface of discovery as the role of 5hmC in the genome continues to remain highly elusive.

A vital question regarding 5hmC is whether it functions as an intermediate in enzymatic reactions or as a stable entity unto itself. In this chapter, considerable space will be dedicated to discussing the possible demethylation pathways in which 5hmC is speculated to be involved. In this and many contexts, demethylation is defined to be the removal of 5mC and

Distinguished by	Unusually high levels of CpG sites, within a GC rich region, in comparison to the rest of the genome
GC percentage	% C + G > 55%
Length	Arbitrarily defined as > 500 bp
	Average 1000 bp
Location	Most often associated with transcription start sites (TSSs)
	Roughly 70% of mammalian gene promoters contain CGIs
Classification of CGI	Strong CGI O/E > 0.75
	Weak CGI 0.45 < O/E < 0.75
	Poor CGI O/E < 0.45
Epigenetic Patterns	Generally unmethylated
	H3K36me2 depletion
	Nucleosome deficiency
	Histone acetylation (H3/H4 Ac)
	H3K4me3 enrichment
	Cfp1 binding
	Constitutive binding of RNA polymerase II

CpG islands are regions of the genome that have remained CpG, rather than TpG rich, the latter being the product of CpG deamination that has taken place over evolutionary time. O/E indicates the ratio of observed CpG sites: expected number of CpG sites. Strong CGIs tend to have a high O/E meaning that the number of observed CpG sites is approaching the expected number of CpG sites, making for a maximum O/E of 1. Often unmethylated, these regions of the genome are associated with transcription start sites. A number of epigenetic patterns have been found to characterize CGIs (H3K36me2=dimethylation of lysine 36 on histone H3 and H3K4me3=trimethylation of lysine 4 on histone H3).

Table 1. Characteristics of CpG Islands (CGIs)

(eventual) replacement by cytosine. In the majority of these pathways where 5hmC is required, it is often thought to act as an intermediate, rapidly replaced by another chemical species. Levels of 5hmC are substantially lower than 5mC in the genome, at approximately 10% of 5mC and 0.4% of all cytosines [74]. These minute levels are thought to be consistent with the short-lived species hypothesis as elevated levels would indicate a longer duration. If 5hmC generation is merely a pre-requisite for subsequent demethylation pathways regardless of what form they take, then 5hmC would be considered a transient species.

Evidence is also emerging which supports the notion of 5hmC as an entirely new landmark in the epigenetic gene regulatory landscape. In fact, the modified nitrogenous base may even be responsible for attracting a unique panel of chromatin and transcriptional modifiers. Numerous mechanisms have been proposed based on preliminary observations. Methyl-CpG binding domain protein 1 (MBD1) specifically recognizes methylated DNA and attracts histone deacetylases and H3 lysine 9 methyltransferases (also repressive in action) [75-79]. 5hmC has been shown to greatly inhibit the binding of these MBDs to DNA [80-82]. On the same note, DNMT1 is also well known to recruit H3K9 methyltransferases, but the enzyme is blocked by the very presence of 5hmC, so the likelihood of H3K9 methyltransferase binding is also reduced. Methylation has also been implicated in nucleosome compaction, making DNA less accessible to transcription factors [83]. Conversely, the effect of 5hmC on nucleosome compaction has yet to be determined, but the nuclei of Purkinje neurons have been reported to exhibit marked decondensation [84].

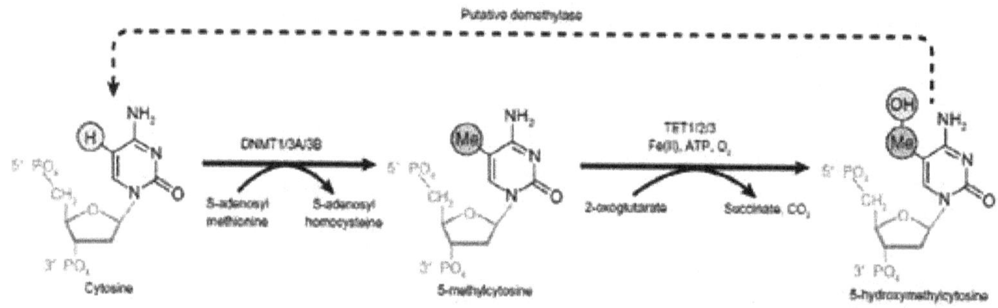

This figure is adapted from Matouk CC, Turgeon PJ, Marsden PA. Epigenetics and stroke risk-beyond the static DNA code. Advances in Genomics and Genetics. 2012;2012:2:67-84.

Figure 2. Methyl modification to cytosine and hydroxyl addition to 5-methylcytosine. The addition of a methyl group at the 5-position of cytosine is mediated by the DNA methyltransferase (DNMT) family, where S-adenosylmethionine serves as the methyl donor. Notes: The ten-eleven translocation (TET) family of enzymes is able to oxidize 5-methylcytosine to 5-hydroxymethylcytosine in an oxygen-dependent reaction requiring adenosine triphosphate and 2-oxoglutarate. Cytosine can then be generated from the action of putative demethylases on 5-hydroxymethylcytosine, but has not yet been fully described.

2.2.4. Ten eleven-translocation (TET) enzymes

The 2009 seminal paper by Tahiliani *et al.* identified the TET (ten-eleven translocation) enzymes as being those responsible for the generation of 5hmC by the hydroxylation of 5mC [65]. Adding yet another layer of complexity to uncovering the role of 5hmC in the genome, TET enzymes are also responsible for the further oxidation of 5hmC into new products: 5-formylcytosine (5fC) and 5-carboxycytosine (5caC) (70, 85, 86). TET enzymes are present throughout the Metazoa and the three forms, TET1, TET2, and TET3, are thought to have arisen as a result of a triplication event that occurred in jawed vertebrates [87]. All three murine forms have been seen to oxidize 5mC to 5hmC *in vitro* and *in vivo* [88, 89]. Moreover, the presence of 5mC consistently appears to be a pre-requisite for the generation of 5hmC *in vivo* [69, 72], suggesting that TET-mediated oxidation is the only means of formation. All of the TET proteins are Fe^{+2} and 2-oxoglutarate dependent dioxygenases (65, 88, 90). The term, *dioxygenase*, refers to an enzyme that catalyzes the addition of both oxygen atoms from molecular oxygen to another organic substrate. The iron ion is utilized as a co-factor, whereas 2-oxoglutarate is a co-substrate.

The mammalian TET enzymes all exhibit a high degree of homology amongst their C terminal domains. It is the Cys-rich and double stranded-helix DSBH region (CD domain) [87] belonging to the Cupin-like dioxygenase superfamily, that contains the catalytic domain for 2-oxoglutarate and iron (II) activity [65, 88]. Further oxidation of 5hmC into 5fC and 5caC also takes place at this same active site [85]. This CD domain also contains the largest identifiable portion of the enzyme: the spacer region. For the most part, the function of this region is unknown, although some leads for future research do exist. For instance, Upabhyay *et al.* noted remarkable sequence overlap between the spacer region of TET1 and the C-terminal domain of RNA polymerase II of *S. cerevisiae* [91]. Likely of most significance are the conserved residues that are key sites for posttranslational modifications such as histone methylation and phosphorylation [92]. Located on the N terminus (~60 amino acids) of TET1 and TET3 (not TET2) enzymes is the CXXC zinc finger domain [65, 87]. Even though its function has not been conclusively determined, the CXXC domain in TET1 has been shown to bind to unmodified cytosine, as well as 5mC and 5hmC [93, 94]. Speculation has tended towards this domain serving as the functional unit responsible for directing the enzymes to particular genomic regions, almost always CpG sites, so they can execute their oxidative action [92]. A similar CXXC domain on DNMT1, the enzyme on which it was first discovered, possesses comparable DNA binding properties [95], initially having suggested an equivalent role for the domain in TETs.

2.3. Long non-coding RNA

Contrary to the central dogma of biology, in which RNA plays a passive role in transmitting genetic information to be translated into proteins, recent advances have shown RNA to play a much more active role in cellular regulation. Long non-coding RNAs (lncRNAs) are the most recent and least well characterized of functional "non-coding" RNAs. The distinction between lncRNAs and miRNAs is arbitrary, but has been defined as greater than 200 nucleotides for an lncRNA [96]. Unlike miRNAs, however, which seem to function through similar pathways, lncRNAs have been shown to play a diverse assortment of regulatory roles, including posttranscriptional repression, RNA splicing, and RNA degradation [97]. Despite this variety, perhaps the most interesting and well-studied mechanism is the ability of many lncRNAs to act as epigenetic modulators, interacting with chromatin remodeling complexes and other epigenetic machinery [98].

Xist was one of the first lncRNAs to be discovered [99] and, consequently, is the most well described. The *Xist* gene is found in the X chromosome inactivating center (XIC) where it plays a major role in the inactivation of one of the two X chromosomes in females [100], a process which equalizes X chromosome dosage to that of a male karyotype. *Xist* acts in *cis* to repress the transcription of the chromosome on which it is transcribed [101]. *Xist*'s function as an epigenetic regulator was confirmed with the discovery of an interacting factor, the polycomb repressive complex 2 (PRC2) [102], a complex that mediates the repressive histone trimethylation mark H3K27me3. PRC2 is recruited to the inactive X chromosome (*Xi*) by a short repetitive sequence, Repeat A (*RepA*), conserved on the *Xist* transcript [102]. Tethering of *Xist* to the chromosome from which it was transcribed allows for allele specific recruitment of the PRC2 complex and subsequent inactivation [101].

Another important lncRNA in X chromosome inactivation is the *Xist* antisense RNA, Tsix. Tsix is expressed on the active chromosome and blocks *Xist* expression, thereby preventing its inactivation [103]. The action of Tsix illustrates another mechanism of epigenetic regulation in which lncRNA can take part: DNA methylation. Recently, evidence has suggested that Tsix mediates DNA methylation at the *Xist* promoter, silencing the *Xist* gene [104]. Tsix may activate DNA methyltransferase 3A (DNMT3A), one of the *de novo* methyltransferases, and guide it to the *Xist* promoter where it is involved in maintaining the silencing of the *Xist* gene after initial repression.

X chromosome inactivation is not the only cellular process in which lncRNA is involved, and there are numerous other examples of lncRNAs as epigenetic regulators. For example, HOTAIR is an lncRNA located in the homeobox C (HOXC) cluster of genes [105]. The *HOX* genes are a family of genes that serve as developmental cues in the embryo [106]. The expression pattern of different *HOX* genes corresponds to specific tissue development and ensures the correct relative positions of body parts. The 39 *HOX* genes are present in 4 gene clusters, HOXA-D, each present on a separate chromosome [107]. HOTAIR is expressed in the HOXC cluster where it acts in *trans* to suppress expression on the HOXD cluster. In this way, HOTAIR is required to maintain the specific expression pattern of *HOX* genes throughout embryonic development. Like the *Xist* RNA, HOTAIR achieves this repression through the recruitment of the PRC2 complex, which then catalyzes the repressive H3K27 trimethylation mark. Indeed, knockdown of HOTAIR has shown loss of H3K27 trimethylation in the HOXD gene cluster, as well as an absence of the PRC2 complex. This suggests that ncRNA may be a global requirement for activation of PRC2 H3K27me3.

3. DNA methylation and development

Most methylation patterns are stably inherited, remaining static throughout the lifetime of an organism. Specific cellular processes as well as cell-lineage specificity require activation or elimination of these patterns. Fluctuations in 5mC and 5hmC levels are most vividly seen in the cases of pre-implantation development and primordial germ cell formation (Figure 3). In order to understand the significance of the rapid changes in modified cytosine levels, a number of recent and vital observations must be taken into account.

a. Pre-implantation embryo

Throughout the duration of development, especially cellular differentiation, somatic-cell lineages acquire specialized DNA methylation and histone modification patterns. Even in the earliest stages, both sperm and oocyte are known to contain appreciable levels of DNA methylation. Many of the methylated regions are shared between oocyte and sperm, such as intracisternal A particles (IAPs) [108], although there are differentially methylated regions (DMRs) which is oocyte-or sperm-specific. Active and repressive histone modifications are present in the oocyte at this time [109], and it is maternally inherited proteins that will direct the events of early cleavage divisions. On the other hand, sperm arrive with temporary histone substitutes, protamines, which play a similarly functional role in packaging [110].

Upon fertilization, the sperm genome is the earliest to undergo major modifications, the first of which is protamine removal and substitution with histones [111]. Prior to the fusion of the maternal and paternal pronuclei, a vast genome-wide demethylation event occurs in the paternal pronucleus [112-115], whereby its methylation patterns are erased almost in their entirety. This event can occur in as few as six hours following fertilization [112, 113, 116]. This demethylation has been assessed repeatedly via immunostaining with antibodies specific for 5mC [112, 113, 116] as well as bisulfite sequencing which has clearly shown that one of two genomes becomes demethylated. A recently discovered and intriguing fact is that this genome-wide demethylation is actually a mass oxidation event [117-119]. 5mC specific antibodies do not recognize 5hmC or any other oxidized cytosine, yet it has been repeatedly and conclusively demonstrated that the male pronucleus does exhibit a marked increase in 5hmC levels at this time [117-119]. Complimentary antibody staining has taken place in order to deduce this. Regions unaffected by this event include paternal DMRs in imprinted genes [120, 121] and IAPs [108]. It is now well known that it is the maternal TET3 enzyme that executes the oxidative action on the paternal pronucleus [119]. In contrast to the other TET enzymes, TET3 knock-down has been demonstrated to result in the near deficit of 5hmC.

The presence of histone modifications unique to the maternal pronucleus is linked to its spared erasure at this time of otherwise mass oxidation. Developmental pluripotency-associated 3 protein (DPPA3, also known as stella), has been identified as the key protector of the maternal pronucleus as well as that of a few paternally imprinted genes [122]. As a matter of fact, the protection offered by this protein is almost indisputable, as experiments have shown that an absence of DPPA3 results in the hydroxymethylation of both paternal and maternal genomes [117, 122]. This protein was originally identified as a result of the upregulation of its encoding gene during initial PGC development [123]. Dimethylation of H3 histone at lysine 9, a mark that is restricted to these sites [122], has been reported to be responsible for the attraction of DPPA3 to these regions.

As indicated in Figure 3, the 2-16 cell stage exhibits a substantial decrease in both maternally dominant 5mC and paternally specific 5hmC levels. It is a well known fact that the maternal genome also loses all methylation marks during early embryogenesis. This, however, has not been attributed to a mass oxidation event, hence, no generation of 5hmC takes place at this time. The cytoplasmic localization of DNMT1o, a splice variant of DNMT1, is attributed to the passive replication-dependent dilution of all oxidized cytosines, [112, 116, 124] accounting also for maternal genome methylation erasure. That is, with each division, 50% of the genomic methylation and hydroxymethylation patterns are lost due to the absence of maintenance methylation [125], until virtually no modified cytosines remain by the sixteen cell stage [112, 116].

Another generally accepted fact is that a wave of *de novo* methylation takes place at approximately the time when the blastula implants into the uterus [116, 120]. This activity occurs very rapidly and 5mC levels plateau once all of the necessary methylation patterns have been instilled (Figure 3). That is, no more demethylation is known to take place because patterns placed onto the genome at this stage are the same as those that will be found in somatic cells of later development and maturation. This *de novo* methylation is now known to be catalyzed by the *de novo* methyltransferases 3A and 3B [116]. In fact, inactivation of both DNMT3A and 3B has been shown to result in early embryonic lethality while mutations in the encoding genes have also resulted in postnatal or embryonic lethality [126, 127]. Establishing the patterns of the genome at this stage allows for the predictable mitotic transmission of methylation marks throughout the lifetime of an organism [40].

As opposed to the undoubtedly critical role of TET3 following fertilization in mice, TET1 and TET2 are thought to have modulatory, yet not essential roles in development, ES cell endurance, and pluripotency [84]. At the blastula stage, the function of TET1 and TET2 proteins in the inner cell mass is likely to repress lineage-specific genes, counteracting the effect of methylation, so as to permit activation of certain genes later in development [128, 129]. Consequently, they are thought to be fine tuning methylation patterns at this point [84].

Consistent experimental results indicate that there is, however, much still to be confirmed about the relative role of TET proteins in development. As a point of discrepancy, TET1 deficient mouse ES cells have been seen to maintain their self-renewal capabilities *in vitro* and develop ordinarily *in vivo* [130]. Furthermore, numerous groups have demonstrated that the knockout of both TET1 and TET2 results in the normal development and healthy adulthood of fertile mice [130-134]. It is hypothesized that such discrepancies may be a result of the alternate TET proteins compensating for the depletion of one another [92]. Although the biological roles of TET1 and TET2 in zygotic development are still highly disputable, that of TET3 appears to be more comprehensive. One study, in particular, highlighted the importance of this particular enzyme in embryogenesis by introducing a homozygous mutation in the TET3 encoding gene, subsequently observing neonatal lethality [119]. The same study came to the conclusion that failure to demethylate the male pronucleus is a direct result of TET3 depletion.

Evidently, epigenetic modifications play an unquestionably enormous role in early development. Despite remaining relatively constant in the mitotic transmission of later development, methylation patterns undergo rapid, yet precisely timed fluctuations in zygotic development. 5hmC abundance points to a vital role of the TET enzymes, as no other pathway has been conclusively verified for the generation of hydroxymethylcytosine from methylcytosine. In light of the recent re-discovery of 5hmC and already substantial amount of scientific inquiry that has gone into deciphering its role in development, we can hope for a great deal more to come in the near future!

b. Primordial Germ Cells

Primordial germ cells (PGCs) are the cells that ultimately give rise to the germ line, the oocyte and sperm. Similar to what has been observed in zygotic development, mouse PGCs, derived from epiblast cells, are known to experience a correspondingly fast decline in 5mC levels [135] between embryonic day (E) 9.5 and 13.5 [124, 136, 137]. Very recently, Hackett *et al.* decisively demonstrated that the demethylation that takes place in PGCs is conceptually equivalent to

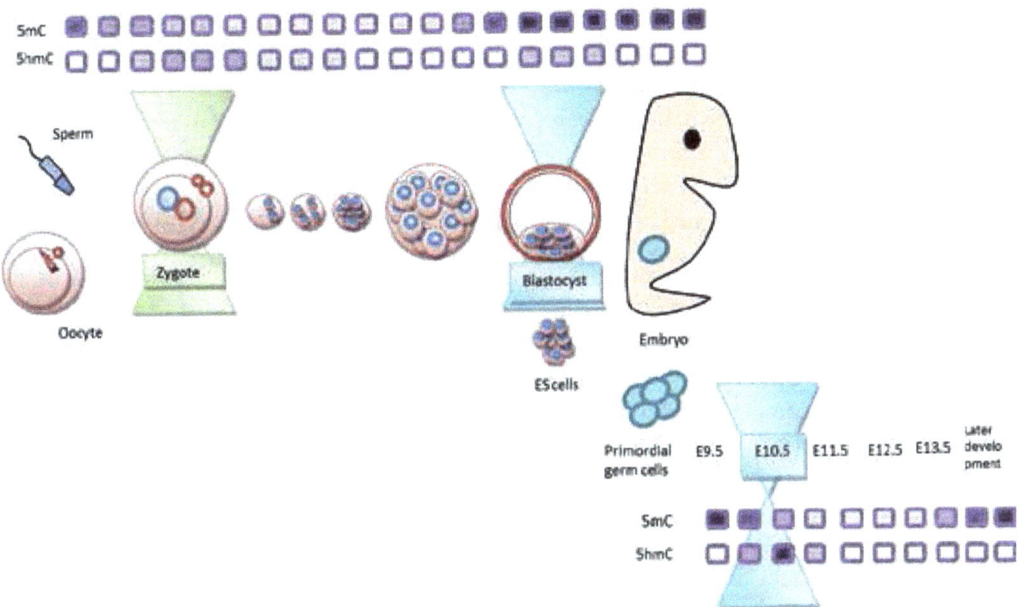

Figure 3. Dynamic nature of 5mC, 5hmC, and TET enzyme levels in the pre-implantation embryo and primordial germ cell development. Intensity of purple shading indicates the relative level of modified cytosine at that stage in development. Green shading indicates high levels of TET3 activity, while blue shading shows elevated levels of TET1 and TET2 at these stages in development. Sperm and oocyte begin with high levels of 5mC. Paternal methylation patterns are erased just after fertilization and a mass oxidation event takes place with increasing levels of 5hmC by the zygotic stage. 5mC and 5hmC (from the paternal genome) levels diminish by means of a passive-replication dependent manner whereby both the maternal and paternal genomes are practically devoid of either modified cytosine by the 16 cell stage. Upon implantation in the uterus, mass *denovo* methylation takes place whereby somatic cell methylation patterns are established. Primordial germ cells are also subject to demethylation between E9.5 and E13.5, accompanied by increasing 5hmC levels until approximately E 11. Paternal re-methylation takes place beginning at about E15 and, in females, after birth.

the mass oxidation event that has been observed during embryonic development. In this case, TET1 and TET2 are responsible for the generation of 5hmC [124, 138].

Thus far, the acquisition of 5hmC appears to take place between E9.5 and E11.5 [124], but seems to be lost at a rate that is typical of replication-dependent pattern dilution [124]. Such circumstances closely parallel those seen in zygotic development. In the same way that the DNMT1o splice variant has been seen to be excluded from the nucleus in zygotic development, UHRF1 consistently appears to be down-regulated in PGC formation [84]. Such a situation prevents DNMT1 from performing its prescribed action. Evidence indicates that TET-mediated oxidation in PGCs is likely made possible by passive, rather than active demethylation [124]. This observation is further substantiated by the absence of both 5fC and 5caC following PGC demethylation, as shown in immunocytochemistry studies [124], whereas their presence in zygotic development indicates an increased likelihood for an active demethylation mechanism at work.

By definition, methylation patterns at CpG islands will never be erased during normal development. Yet, CpG island methylation in the DMR of imprinted genes must undergo erasure so as to ensure that gender-specific methylation associated with imprinting can be put into place during the remainder of germ cell development [123]. Demethylation at this time has also been proposed to be responsible for reinstating the pluripotent state in PGCs. Clearly, those regions whose expression had been repressed are now turned on, allowing for the germ cell lineage acquisition of pluripotent characteristics, perhaps a pre-requisite to achievement of totipotency. Similar to the spared erasure of paternally imprinted genes in zygotic development, certain transposons such as IAPs remain moderately methylated at this time [34].

In contrast to zygotic development, the demethylation of imprinted regions is absolutely critical because germ cells possess imprints that are uniquely exclusive to the gender of the organism. As indicated in the bottom half of Figure 3, an analogous round of *de novo* methylation also takes place later in oogenesis and spermatogenesis. Re-methylation along with the re-installation of imprints starts at approximately E15 in males and, in females, after birth [139].

3.1. DNA demethylation pathways

As illustrated above, it is a well ingrained fact that epigenetic reprogramming does take place in zygotic development and PGC formation. More recently, TET protein activity has been observed in relation to the timing of particular developmental events. Consequently, levels of 5hmC have been monitored and correlated with the activity of TET proteins at each stage of interest. Truly novel is the fact that this reprogramming involves a mass oxidation event, that is, the generation of 5hmC. The function of 5hmC in these stages is a highly debated and controversial area of research. We have already addressed the first disputed issue regarding the stability of this oxidized base, but we will now draw our attention to the second debate: What are the possible demethylation pathways by which reprogramming takes place? We will define demethylation as the eventual replacement of 5mC with unmodified cytosine. Possible mechanisms for this can be broadly grouped into passive and active pathways. In analyzing the possibilities, it is important to note that absolutely no consensus exists as to which mechanism predominates and that there is experimental evidence to both confirm and rebuke nearly all pathways.

3.1.1. Passive demethylation

Passive demethylation is fairly well established as one of perhaps several operating processes. As mentioned above, the maintenance DNMT places methylation patterns on a progeny strand using the parental strand as a template, similar to the synthesis of a new strand of DNA whereby DNA polymerase utilizes the parent strand as a template for construction of a complementarily base-paired DNA strand. Like the DNA double helix, the maintenance of methylation patterns also occurs through a semi-conservative pathway. This particular setup yields a hemi-methylated (partly methylated) pattern on the DNA. UHRF1 binding and PCNA recruitment are the first steps in the faithful copying of methylation patterns from one strand to another, thereby ensuring the transmission of methylation patterns through mitotic division. From the perspective of demethylation pathways, if this faithful re-installation of methylation patterns is disturbed, every generation will subsequently exhibit 50% less methylation. Eventually, such patterns will undergo what is called passive replication-dependent dilution.

As mentioned, this appears to be the way in which the methylation patterns of the zygotic maternal genome are erased. Thus, the plausibility of this mechanism is not debated. Paternal genome erasure prior to replication is significant evidence that defies the notion of passive demethylation as the *only* demethylation pathway.

As far as active or replication-independent pathways go, the central tenets of a variety of these pathways will be discussed in the following. A common thread that runs beneath a number of these is the coupling of TET protein activity with a well known DNA repair pathway, base excision repair (BER), whereby a nitrogenous base is excised by a glycosylase enzyme and replaced with a new one. Some sort of replacement mechanism is practically inevitable given that an unmodified cytosine must take the place of a previous base in order to complete demethylation.

3.1.2. Pathways in which 5fC and 5caC are involved

The first of these proposed pathways involves the other two oxidized bases, 5-formylcytosine (5fC) and 5-carboxylcytosine (5caC) that can be generated by further oxidation of 5hmC by TET enzymes [70, 85, 86]. Their presence at very low quantities in the genome (5fC: 0.03% of 5mC in mouse ES cells; 5caC: 0.01% of 5mC in mouse ES cells) [70, 85, 86], has been attributed to the preference of TET enzymes towards 5mC, not 5hmC, as a substrate, as well as an exceedingly fast removal of the oxidized bases [85, 140]. Thymine DNA glycosylases (TDGs) are capable of excising both bases once they are produced. Kinetic studies by Maiti & Drohat clearly demonstrated that TDG excises 5fC and 5caC, but not 5hmC [141]. Neither when left for a longer time nor performed at a lower temperature (for enzyme stability maintenance) was there any significant 5hmC excision [141]. Excision of the oxidized bases opens the door for base excision repair (BER) action that completes the guanine base on the opposite strand with a brand new cytosine, hence, completing the demethylation pathway. Several labs have confirmed that the proposed is a highly plausible mechanism [85, 141, 142].

Interestingly, a number of studies have shown that TDG exhibits strong specificity in its action: it excises bases which are complementarily base paired with G and/or those which are also followed by guanine [143-146]. Such an observation is entirely consistent with the proposed role of TDG and CpG sites [147] whereby the cytosine has undergone a further modification, yet still fulfills the remainder of the criteria. More research must be undertaken to confirm whether TDG action on modified cytosines, followed by BER, is a plausible demethylation mechanism *in vivo*. Whether such a pathway is of sufficient speed to play a role in demethylation is one concern which must be addressed. Another comes about when we consider the exceedingly minute quantities of both of the bases in the genome: How prevalent can this pathway realistically be? Is it enough to account for mass demethylation in both zygotic and PGC development?

There is limited evidence that supports a decarboxylation pathway of 5caC, mediated by proteins present in lysates of ES cells [148]. Although the factors that catalyze this reaction have yet to be concisely identified, Schiesser *et al.* utilized isotope tracing to detect the direct conversion of 5caC to cytosine without interference from BER [148]. The existence of a deformylation pathway involved in the direct conversion of 5fC to cytosine has also been postulated.

3.1.3. Direct removal of 5-methylcytosine

What about a simple removal of the 5mC base followed by TDG action? Scientists have noted that, due to the strength of the carbon-carbon bond needed to be broken, an enzyme with unwieldy catalytic power would be needed to achieve such a feat [140]. Methyl-CpG binding domain protein 2 (MBD2) was first and foremost reported to catalyze just such a reaction. By its very nature, MBD2 is known to *bind* to methylated cytosine, so it was often questioned how it could be responsible for mediating such an active reaction if it first must attach itself [28, 75]. Numerous other downfalls of this theory emerged and no lab was apparently able to replicate the results, so the theory of MBD2-mediated direct removal of the methyl group of 5mC fell out of favour. Hence, the inevitability of some sort of TDG/BER activity is further substantiated [149].

A model plant used in genetics and epigenetics studies, *Arabidopsis thaliana,* is the only source that has thus far provided evidence for such a direct removal of 5mC (reviewed in [150]). The existence of ROS1, DME, DML2, and DML7-a family of four 5mC DNA glycosylases has been acknowledged in this plant [150]. Their preference for acting on 5mC in double stranded DNA, has led researchers to claim that these enzymes are indeed necessary for active demethylation of particular genes. The function of these glycosylases is similar to that of BER, in that a nick created leaves an abasic site which is rapidly repaired. Yet, the enzymes and mechanisms in mammals appear to be quite distinct from those that have been identified in the plant [151].

3.1.4. AID/APOBEC activity

The second well investigated, yet still highly debated active replication-independent demethylation pathway is one which also utilizes a DNA repair pathway. AID (activation-induced cytidine deaminase) and APOBEC (apolipoprotein B mRNA editing enzymes, catalytic polypeptide) family members are primarily known for their ability to deaminate cytosine to uracil [152]. *In vitro* studies have demonstrated the further ability of AID/APOBEC to deaminate 5mC in DNA, to thymine, resulting in a T:G mismatch [149]. The excision conducted by a TDG glycosylase would subsequently result in an abasic site (apurinic and apyrimidinic [AP] site) which would then be subject to repair by BER. The final product of such a chain reaction would be the regeneration of cytosine in place of the modified base [149].

There are a number of variations and caveats of this and related processes. For instance, AID and APOBEC have frequently been seen to function in a single-stranded DNA environment [149]. Deamination in single-stranded DNA has been experimentally observed *in vitro* and in an *E. coli* assay [149]. Despite this, AID and APOBEC are both present at appreciable levels in oocytes as well as PGCs, so their potential role in developmental demethylation has not been dismissed [149].

An alternate pathway through which AID/APOBEC are thought to function involves the deamination of 5hmC to 5-hydroxymethyluracil (5hmU) and its subsequent removal by a TDG glycosylase or BER pathway [153]. This process would result in the eventual replacement by cytosine. The over-expression of TET1 and AID have been observed to lead to a global accumulation of 5hmU [153]. Two potential pathways may compete with one another because both TDG as well as selective monofunctional uracil-DNA glycosylase 1 (SMUG1) have strong affinity towards the mismatch that would be generated upon deamination: G:hmU [153, 154]. Hence, one of these mechanisms is thought to play a vital role in mediating the downstream commencement of BER following 5mC hydroxylation. Such observations substantiate what many studies propose: that TDG plays an absolutely essential role in active demethylation, regardless of what mechanism succeeds it.

Perhaps what could be considered the downfall of the AID/APOBEC pathway was elucidated in a series of experiments and simulations conducted by Nabel *et al.* [152]. Insisting that the role of this deamination-based mechanism is limited, the researchers examined the plausibility of this pathway by investigating the biochemistry of natural and non-natural modified cytosines. The series of substrates represented a 150 fold difference in reactivity, with the size of the substituent being an integral determinant of susceptibility to deamination. At one end of the scale was unmodified cytosine, the behavior of which as a deaminase substrate was unequivocally superior to all other larger natural and unnatural substrates. The bulky 5hmC not only sterically hindered the activity of AID/APOBEC, but its poor hydrophobic character was also implicated in substantially decreasing its reactivity, in comparison to all other bases. The researchers consolidated their results and firmly stated that AID/APOBEC family members preferentially deaminate unmodified cytosine, yet strongly discriminate against any and all 5-substituted cytosine substrates [152]. Clearly, this result contradicts the notion of 5hmC deamination to 5hmU, and more so favours the other possibility of 5mC deamination to thymine. The hope is that future research will work towards eliminating such discrepancies amongst multiple lines of work as we gain a better understanding of the plausibility of these pathways.

3.1.5. DNMT dehydroxymethylation

In addition to AID and APOBEC, the activity of DNMTs themselves has recently been proposed as a possible 5mC demethylation mechanism. In 2012, Chen *et al.* demonstrated that DNMT enzymes can remove the hydroxymethyl group of 5hmC *in vitro* [155]. Hence, 5hmC is directly converted to cytosine [156]. Although it is still unknown whether such a reaction takes place in cells [84], it has been established that reducing conditions favour the generally accepted methyltransferase activity of DNMT3A and 3B while oxidizing conditions are ideal for dehydroxymethylation activity [155]. Participation in both methylation and demethylation results in rapid cycling between the removal and replacement of methylation patterns – a phenomenon that has been reported in two papers to date [157, 158]. In spite of our analysis of a limited number of experiments, both papers refer to the interplay of TDG and BER in this transcriptional cycling. Particular repair proteins were, in fact, recruited to site-specific locations, likely assisting in the reconstruction of the site [140]. Physiological implications must also be taken into account. S-adenosylmethionine (SAM) is required, not only at low levels for the DNMT3A/B mediated reaction, but also at specific levels for other biochemical reactions

[140]. Scientists continue to ponder the other biological effects which would result from rapid SAM level fluctuations.

Quite clearly, numerous potential active demethylation pathways do exist and the validity of one over the other is constantly being reassessed. Further oxidation to 5fC or 5caC, direct removal of the methyl group, AID/APOBEC, TDG, and BER pathways have all been proposed and are now under scientific scrutiny. Numerous sources highlight the possibility of more than one of these pathways operating simultaneously with one or more of the others.

4. Case study I: vitamin C

4.1. Scurvy

Lethargy, extreme muscle and joint pain, gum disease, loosening of teeth, and emotional instability. Often mistaken for syphilis, leprosy, or dysentery, such were the symptoms that characterized "the plague of the sea" [159].Now a rare disease, scurvy took the lives of two-thirds of Vasco de Gama's men, eighty per cent of Magellan's mates, and terrorized many of those who took to the sea during the Age of Exploration. Little did the famed 15th century explorers know that they were losing members of their crew to a vitamin deficiency. Sailors who boarded ships destined for long journeys relied mainly on cured and salted meats as well as dried grains, and suffered greatly for their deprivation of perishable fruits and vegetables. It was not until its identification and isolation in the 1930s that the association between vitamin C (ascorbate) and its role in scurvy was made. In fact, ascorbic acid, from which the L-enantiomer, ascorbate, is derived, actually means "anti-scurvy" [160].

Unlike many animals, primates, humans, guinea pigs, and a few varieties of fish, cannot synthesize vitamin C *de novo* in the liver [161]. In humans, for instance, the final step of vitamin C biosynthesis cannot be performed: the conversion of L-gulono-gamma-lactone into ascorbic acid. The gene that encodes gulonolactone, the enzyme which catalyzes this reaction, is present in the human genome, but is inactive as a result of mutation accumulation that turned it into a pseudogene [162]. Vitamin C is known to be a critical component of health, while lack of it is truly a detriment to the body because of its dual function in a number of enzymatic reactions as well as its role as an antioxidant.

4.2. Collagen biosynthesis

Without a doubt, vitamin C presence is absolutely vital in the regular synthesis of collagen. Being the most abundant protein in mammals and composed mainly of connective tissue [163], the triple helical construction of collagen requires the successful completion of a number of biochemical events. One of these is the essential enzymatic hydroxylation of proline (Pro) residues into hydroxyproline (Hyp) by prolyl-4-hydroxylase (P4H) [164]. A member of a dioxygenase superfamily, P4H decarboxylates the co-substrate, α-ketoglutarate, and utilizes Fe^{2+}as a co-factor, yielding hydroxyproline and an oxidized Fe^{3+}[165]. For full catalytic activity, ascorbate is required as another co-factor in the reaction [166, 167]. In the absence of ascorbate, this reaction can perform at a maximal rate, but only to a certain extent [164]. A buildup of Fe^{3+}requires the activity of ascorbate as a potent reducing agent to regenerate the reduced form of iron: Fe^{2+}[168, 169]. In this way, the catalytic potential of P4H is maintained at an efficient level.

Ascorbate deficiency, the situation which arose when sailors went to sea for several months at a time, leads to the incomplete hydroxylation of proline residues in collagen, which results in its improper folding [170]. Non-functional collagen in blood vessels and bones has been attributed to the severe bone and blood vessel related symptoms that came to characterize scurvy. As a point of interest, the symptoms that extended beyond the changes in bones and blood vessels, have also been linked to vitamin C deficiency. Prolyl hydroxylases are only one of a number of enzymes whose mechanism of action relies on this vitamin. The synthesis of norepinephrine from dopamine, for instance, is catalyzed by dopamine beta hydroxylase, another enzyme which utilizes vitamin C as a co-factor [171]. Required for the generation of metabolic energy via mitochondrial breakdown of fatty acids, carnitine synthesis [172], also necessitates the utilization of ascorbate. Thus, the neurological dysfunctioning of the sailors and their symptoms of lassitude can both be attributed to a lack of this indispensable vitamin.

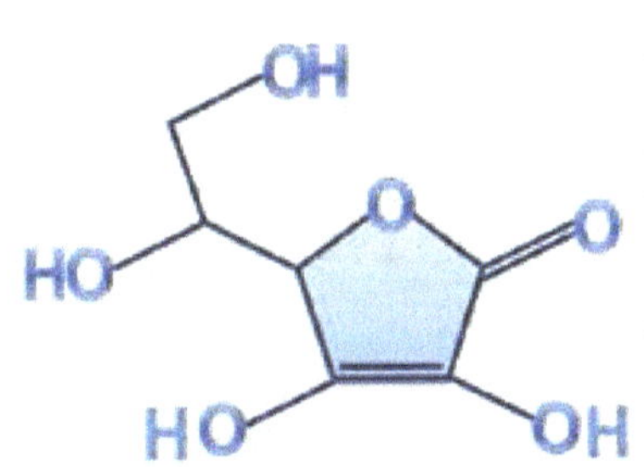

Figure 4. Structure of ascorbate. The vital nature of vitamin C (ascorbate) is exemplified by its dual function in the human body, acting as both a cofactor as well as an antioxidant. Collagen biosynthesis necessitates the hydroxylation of proline residues by prolyl-4-hydroxylase – one of a number of biochemical reactions that require the presence of vitamin C. Belonging to the same family as P4H, TET proteins were proposed as possible enzymes whose catalytic action might also have been augmented by the presence of vitamin C. Recent studies have found that ascorbate is responsible for widespread, yet specific demethylation, by way of inducing the generation of 5hmC by TET enzymes

Thus far, we have explored an interesting historical event that revealed the enormous impact of vitamin C on human health. The indisputably important role of vitamin C is further highlighted by its role in collagen biosynthesis. What's more intriguing is the fact that prolyl hydroxylases belong to the same family as the TET enzymes and share numerous structural features. The possibility of vitamin C interacting with the TET proteins and potentially contributing to the epigenetic landscape of modifications has become an area of scientific interest.

A recent report from Minor *et al.* conclusively stated that ascorbate induces the generation of 5hmC by TET enzymes, likely acting as a co-factor in the reaction [173]. Utilizing mouse embryonic fibroblasts (MEFs), the addition of ascorbate in a time-and dose-dependent manner was unmistakably seen to correlate with increased 5hmC levels. A novel role for vitamin C in epigenetic modifications has been brought to the forefront. In cells with knocked down TET expression, ascorbate still enhanced the generation of 5hmC by at least 3 fold above basal levels [173]. Rather than protein synthesis, it was shown that the mere accumulation of ascorbate inside the cells was all that was necessary in order to observe increased 5hmC levels. The researchers noted that a detailed mechanism for ascorbate's interaction with the TET enzymes has yet to be elucidated, but the similarity between TET and P4H catalytic action, points towards ascorbate performing a comparable role in TETs as it does for P4H [173].

Due to its enhancement of cell proliferation, vitamin C is a commonly used medium supplement in ES cell culture. A *Stem Cells* report from Chung *et al.* showed that vitamin C, at the concentration used in commercial media (50 μg/mL), promotes widespread DNA demethylation of human ES cells, yet, with remarkable specificity for the location of demethylation [174]. This study showed that the ascorbate-mediated hypomethylation of CpG island shores was highly correlated with gene expression at these sites. A precise set of 1,847 genes experienced altered gene expression as a result of ascorbate addition. From this, researchers speculated that DNA topology may have been changed such that histone demethylase and acetylase activity subsequently altered the accessibility of DNA to other factors [174].

Clearly, numerous connections are being made between vitamin C and the epigenetic landscape. Not only does the vitamin act as a co-factor in enzymatic reactions, but its biochemistry allows it to participate in an even wider array of interactions (Figure 4). As its demethylation potential is remarkably specific in locale, it was first speculated that this vitamin must be interacting with other enzymes to execute its action. Indeed, this interaction has been confirmed in the way that TET enzymes are thought to modulate the actual demethylation with ascorbate acting as a co-factor. Although the exact antioxidant behavior of vitamin C is not thoroughly illuminated here, the potential role of the general class of antioxidants is revealed in the context of the pathogenesis of atherosclerosis. Hence, vitamin C is intricately linked with another underlying theme of this chapter: cardiovascular disease.

4.3. Epigenetic mechanisms and the vascular endothelium

Endothelial cells, those that line the lumen of all blood vessels in mammals, mark the interface between blood flow and the entrance of substances into tissues and organs. The endothelium, itself, is composed of a thin layer of endothelial cells and an even thinner layer of basal lamina beneath the cells. Vascular smooth muscle cells neighbour the endothelial cells, but, as will be discussed later, exhibit remarkably distinct gene expression. Vasorelaxation was argued, by Furchgott and Zawadzki, to rely on an intact endothelial lining, from which an endothelium-derived relaxing factor (EDRF) would be released [175]. Soon after, the EDRF was recognized to be nitric oxide (NO) [176, 177]. Nitric oxide is now considered to be an incredibly vital component for maintaining vasculature tone due to its antiatherogenic and antithrombotic properties [177]. Nitric oxide generation is highly implicated in vasodilation, as well as its inhibition of platelet aggregation, leukocyte adhesion, and vascular smooth muscle cell proliferation [178-180].

A number of biochemical pathways in aerobic cells produce oxygen-derived free radicals as by-products. Free radicals are molecules with a single unpaired electron, exhibiting great chemical instability and high reactivity. Donating or accepting an electron normally results in the generation of another free radical. Normal cellular respiration produces $O_2^{\cdot}$, the superoxide anion, while the hydroxyl radical $OH^{\cdot}$ is the by-product of the reaction intended to eliminate $O_2^{\cdot}$. Humans have evolved a number of strategies to combat the production of these reactive oxygen species (ROS). For this purpose, humans are able to utilize diet-derived or *de novo* antioxidants in an effort to convert the damaging species into less toxic substances. Despite this effort, when the levels of reactive oxygen species are appreciably greater than antioxidant levels, a condition known as oxidative stress results. Free radicals, which are further generated from oxidative stress, induce tissue damage and are responsible for detrimental modification of lipids and proteins in the vasculature.

The damaging impacts of oxidative stress are seen nowhere as vividly as they are in the endothelium. Endothelial function is impaired by the conditions and NO production is diminished. The effects are disastrous: reduced vasodilation, enhanced platelet activation, and increased vascular smooth muscle migration and proliferation [181]. In the way that each of these outcomes lead to dysfunctioning of the endothelium, all have severe consequences for the pathogenesis of atherosclerosis. A condition primarily of the intima and a pre-cursor for a number of severe organismal dysfunctions, atherosclerosis can affect arteries as large as the aorta or as small as the tertiary branches of coronary arteries [182].

4.4. Pathogenesis of atherosclerosis

The lipid deposition associated with atherosclerosis is derived from an excess of low-density lipoprotein (LDL), the so-called "bad cholesterol," in the plasma. Endothelial damage, such that would occur during oxidative stress conditions, allows for the leakage of LDL into the sub-endothelial space via LDL receptors in endothelial cells [183, 184]. There, the free radical and other oxidized agents attack incoming LDL molecules and generate oxidized LDL (ox-LDL) [184]. Endothelial cells and smooth muscle cells have the capacity to oxidize LDL utilizing free radicals, the presence of which initiated the oxidative stress conditions [185-187]. Expression of adhesive cell surface glycoproteins such as VCAM-1 and ICAM-1 is induced as a result of mildly oxidized LDL [188-190]. Moreover, a variety of molecules within the intravascular space are responsible for attracting and modifying monocytes. An environment such as this, is now rich in modified lipoproteins, chemoattractants, and growth factors, all facilitating the differentiation of incoming monocytes into macrophages. These macrophages are quite powerful in that they are capable of a more relentless oxidation of LDL, acting as phagocytes and promoting smooth muscle cell migration and proliferation [188-191]. These lipid filled macrophages accumulate rapidly and begin to form the foam cells that characterize an atherosclerotic lesion on its way to becoming a clinically significant and potentially severe condition. Because LDL leakage is un-regulated, greater accumulation will lead to the bursting of the cell and an explosion of free radicals and ox-LDL – an event which upholds the cycling of cytoxicity, worsening the damage to the endothelium.

Clearly, the oxidation of LDL exhibits an enormously harmful effect on the endothelium and drastically alters the dynamics of its cellular function. Hence, endothelial injury and dysfunction have been proposed as the initiating events of atherosclerosis. In the presence of cardiovascular risk factors including hyperlipidemia, hypercholesterolemia, smoking, diabetes, and hypertension, the likelihood of cardiovascular disease is highly augmented.

For quite some time, increased antioxidant intake has been investigated for its potential biochemical role in reducing the levels of ROS. Antioxidants are known to protect cells from the effects of free radical damage either by disturbing their mode of production or by attenuating their proliferation once they have formed. They accomplish the former by converting free radical reactants into stable species and the latter takes place via neutralizing the effects of free radical molecules. More precisely, these antioxidants often act by donating an unpaired electron to the unstable free radical, themselves now in the position of becoming a pro-oxidative species. Yet, the structure of antioxidants is usually such that their unpaired electron can be stabilized by adapting one of several possible resonance structures [192-194]. Hence, antioxidants appear to be a very viable preventative measure towards the onset of atherosclerosis and potentially subsequent cardiovascular disease. Long-term studies must be conducted to judge the dose-and time-dependency of the plethora of potential antioxidants. Many of these substances play several integral roles in the body and any beneficial outcomes may not be a direct result of a substance's anti-atherosclerotic properties, *per se*. Furthermore, atherosclerosis pathogenesis is outstandingly complicated and it is now known that the condition's progression is linked to a number of redox-sensitive events that extend beyond the oxidation of LDL [195]. A great deal more investigation will have to be undertaken in an attempt to determine which components of the oxidative stress state are critical for atherosclerosis and the precise mechanism by which antioxidants function.

4.5. Epigenetic regulation of eNOS

Until this point, nitric oxide production and inhibition have been discussed in the context of atherosclerotic plaque formation and their potential role in cardiovascular disease. Moreover, from an epigenetic perspective, the endothelium and its biochemical properties also present an incredibly fascinating model. In mammals, three isoforms of nitric oxide synthase (NOS), encoded by genes on distinct chromosomes: neuronal NOS (nNOS), inducible NOS (iNOS), and endothelial NOS (eNOS), are responsible for the production of nitric oxide [196-198]. The latter of these, eNOS, is known to be the dominant producer of NO and has been found to be constitutively expressed in the endothelium [199]. The eNOS gene, itself, contains 26 exons over the length of 21 kb of genomic DNA, maps to chromosome 7q35-36, and is present as a single copy in the haploid genome [196-198, 200]. Additionally, the gene's promoter has no proximal CpG island and a TATA box is also absent [201]. eNOS deficiency, in animals, has been linked to pulmonary hypertension, atypical vascular remodeling, and flawed angiogenesis [181, 202]. eNOS deficiency in humans has been observed in pulmonary hypertensive individuals and in the coating of advanced plaques [203]. Much attention has been given to discovering and documenting the regulation of eNOS *in vitro* as well as *in vivo*.

Transcriptional, posttranscriptional, and posttranslational pathways have been linked to the intriguing regulation of eNOS [199]. In addition to von Willebrand factor (vWF), vascular-endothelial cadherin (VE-cadherin), intercellular adhesion molecule-2 (ICAM-2), and the vascular endothelial growth factor receptors (VEGFR1 and VEGFR2), eNOS is one of many proteins whose expression is largely endothelial-cell specific [181]. This remarkable nuance has allowed for gene regulation study, from a predominantly epigenetic perspective.

The classic *cis/trans* mentality would be the simplest way to account for the endothelial-cell specificity that is observed in eNOS and the other abovementioned proteins. By this way of thinking, the *cis*-acting elements would bind the 5` regulatory regions of target genes in near proximity. *Trans*-acting factors would be recruited, but they themselves, would have to be cell-restricted in expression. This arrangement would describe gene expression regulated by a master transcription factor. Several well documented instances of master regulation, in mammalian biology, include NeuroD in neurons [204], smooth muscle cell myocardin [205], peroxisome proliferator-actived receptor-γ in adipocytes [206], with the most profound example being MyoD in skeletal muscle cells [207]. In spite of all of these examples, a master regulator in endothelial cells has yet to be discovered [181]. There are some transcription factors, such as Hey2, Vezf1, HoxA9 [181], and KLF2 [208] which are preferentially expressed in the vascular endothelium, but can also be found in other locales. Much research is dedicated to establishing the prominence of each of these in the vascular endothelium, especially KLF2 (kruppel-like factor 2). *Cis*-DNA binding elements in the 5`-regulatory regions have been found in a number of the endothelial-cell restricted genes, and the current train of thought tends towards the cooperative activity of a unique combination of transcription factors present in endothelial cells and not in any other cell type [181].

4.6. Role of DNA methylation & eNOS expression

A differentially methylated region (DMR) that had been detected in the proximal promoter of eNOS in expressing cell types has been observed to be unmethylated or lightly methylated whereas that same DMR in nonexpressing cell types was heavily methylated [209]. Combination of chromatin immunoprecipitation (ChIP) and quantitative real-time PCR revealed the preferential attraction of transcription factors Sp1, Sp3, and Ets1 to the eNOS proximal promoter of endothelial cells, even though they were also present in the tested nonexpressing cell type: vascular smooth muscle cells (VSMC) [209]. Not only did RNA polymerase II preferentially bind to the proximal promoter of eNOS in endothelial cells, but the transcriptionally repressive methyl-CpG-binding domain protein, MeCP2, was attracted to the promoter of VSMCs [210]. Upon treatment with the DNMT inhibitor, 5-azacytidine, those heavily methylated CpG sites were found to be unmethylated, while expression of the eNOS mRNA was seen to increase [209]. Hence, human eNOS is the first identified constitutively expressed vascular endothelium gene whose specificity in expression, is at least partially dictated by DNA methylation [209].

4.7. A histone code for the endothelium

Despite the prominence of DNA methylation pathways in these intricate biochemical sequences, other chromatin based mechanisms, especially histone posttranslational modifications, have been studied in the context of eNOS. Transcriptionally activating marks such as the acetylation of H3 and H4 as well as the di-and tri-methylation of H3K4 have been experimentally detected in nucleosomes of the eNOS proximal promoter in expressing, but not nonexpressing human cell types [211]. As would be predicted, histone deacetylases (HDAC1 but not HDAC 2 or 3) were found at the promoter region of nonendothelial cell types [211]. We used ChIP analysis which recognized, at the eNOS promoter in endothelial cells, the discernible enrichment of acetylated H3K9 and H4K12. The above observations support the existence of a histone code unique to the endothelium, whose precise posttranslational modifications are, to a degree, responsible for gene expression regulation in the endothelium [209, 211].

In summary, current studies are attempting to decipher the relative importance of both DNA methylation and histone posttranslational modifications in gene expression regulation in the vascular endothelium. The ways in which these patterns are initially laid down in development are likely complex and understanding them is still well into the future. It has been speculated that disturbances of these epigenetic pathways may have implications for human health and disease. As we have seen, decreased eNOS expression, and hence, reduced NO production, can have profound consequences for conditions such as atherosclerosis.

4.8. LncRNA and the cardiovascular system

With the traditional four base static genetic code failing to account for the missing heritability of complex genetic disease phenotypes, the dynamic epigenetic code is becoming widely accepted as an important determinant of cardiovascular pathologies [212]. Epigenetics provides a heritable link between our environment and diseases classically linked to genetics. It should come as no surprise, then, that if lncRNAs can act as epigenetic regulators they might have a crucial role to play in the development and homeostasis of the cardiovascular system (Figure 5).

Advances in genome sequencing have allowed for new genetic screening techniques that are more accurate than ever. Within the last decade, genome wide association studies (GWAS) have paved the way for understanding genetic variation in common complex diseases. While traditional family based and linkage analysis studies are effective in identifying rare disease causing mutations, they fail to uncover genetic variation amongst common diseases such as cardiovascular disease [213]. Advances in genomic sequencing have lead to the establishment of databases like the Human Genome Project and the Human Haplotype Map Project that have allowed GWAS to become a useful and accurate tool for correlating single nucleotide polymorphisms (SNPs) to disease phenotype when implemented correctly. Using microarray technologies, up to a million SNPs can be assessed.

Interest in cardiovascular epidemiology has led to a number of GWA studies examining coronary artery disease (CAD) [214]. These studies found an unexpected risk association at the 9p21 locus, a locus with few protein coding genes. This locus showed the strongest genetic correlation to CAD, with ~20-25% of the Caucasian population homozygous for the risk haplotype corresponding to a 30-40% increase in CAD development [215]. Interestingly, however, the sequence of a recently described lncRNA, ANRIL (antisense non-coding RNA in the INK4 locus), was found to overlap with this genomic region [216]. These discoveries put the spotlight on ANRIL as a new potential regulator of cardiovascular integrity. As such, many recent studies have shed light on the functions of ANRIL. ANRIL is expressed in endothelial cells, vascular smooth muscle cells, and leukocytes, all of which are involved in the pathogenesis of atherosclerosis [217]. One of the key findings from studies with ANRIL was its function as an epigenetic regulator of the *INK4a/ARF/INK4b* locus. This locus encodes three proteins, p15, p14ARF, and p16, all with important implications as cell cycle regulators, which together slow cell proliferation. Initiation and maintenance of *INK4a/ARF/INK4b* gene repression is mediated by PRC2 and PRC1, respectively. As demonstrated by *Xist* and HOTAIR, PRC complexes seem to have a common relation to lncRNAs. ANRIL is no exception, and interacts with the SUZ12 subunit of PRC2 and the chromobox 7 (CBX7) subunit of PRC1, recruiting them in *cis* to the INK4a/ARF/INK4b locus. Indeed, knockdowns of ANRIL show a decrease in CBX7 and a subsequent increase in *INK4a/ARF/INK4b* gene expression. Although the exact mechanism of ANRIL's association to cardiovascular diseases has yet to be elucidated, the preliminary correlation has been made and further work may yet confirm ANRIL as the important regulatory molecule it is hypothesized to be.

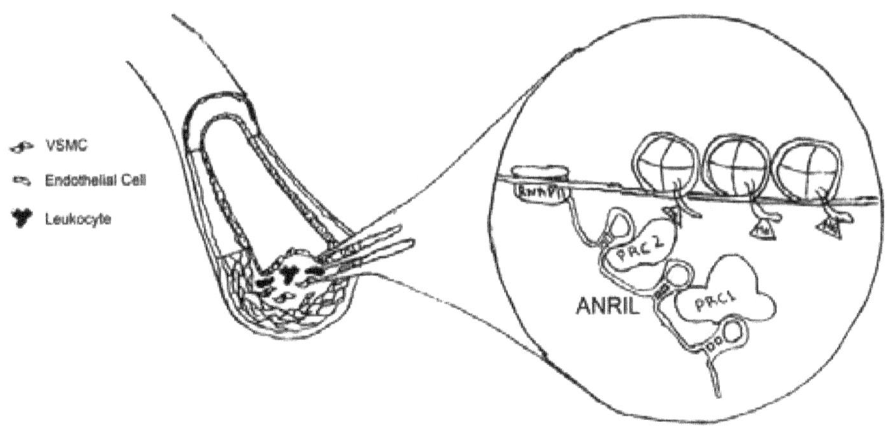

Figure 5. ANRIL is expressed in tissues associated with atherosclerosis. Expression of ANRIL in leukocytes, VSMCs, and endothelial cells acts in *cis* to repress the neighboring INK4a/ARF/INK4b locus harboring important cell cycle regulators. Silencing occurs via the recruitment of PRC1 and PRC2 complexes and subsequent increase in the repressive H3K27me3 histone modification.

More recently, new studies have identified a number of lncRNAs associated with the cardiovascular system. Specifically, two lncRNA have emerged as potential regulators of murine cardiogenesis. One group of researchers has identified a novel lncRNA, deemed Braveheart

(Bvht), which plays a role in cardiac development [218]. Bvht is an ~590 nucleotide mouse-specific transcript that has been shown to be an essential regulator of cardiac commitment in embryonic stem cells. Knockdown of Bvht in mouse ES cells, which were allowed to differentiate into cardiomyocytes, showed a substantial decrease in the percent of contractile cells compared to the control. Although the mechanism is unclear, evidence suggests that Bvht functions upstream of the MesP1 pathway, a known regulator of cardiac mesoderm development [219]. Notably, Bvht, in agreement with an emerging theme among lncRNAs, was also shown to interact with PRC complexes [218]. Bvht interacts with the SUZ12 component of the PRC2 complex. This provides some insight into its function as a possible epigenetic regulator of cardiac gene expression, although it is not known whether this interaction acts to keep PRC2 from repressing genes needed for cardiogenesis, or if it functions to recruit the repressive complex to genes that inhibit this process.

Shortly after the discovery of Bvht, another group reported an lncRNA in mice, named Fendrr, which was similarly involved in the development of the heart [220]. Fendrr is expressed in the lateral mesoderm of the developing embryo, where it is required for differentiation into lateral mesoderm derivatives, most notably the cardiac mesoderm and ventral body wall. Accordingly, Fendrr null mutant embryos are embryonic lethal and display distinct phenotypic changes in the heart, such as cardiac hypoplasia and impaired function. Once again, epigenetic regulation by an lncRNA is the likely culprit for these outcomes. Fendrr null mutants show an increase in the activating H3K4me3 mark, laid down by the TrxG/MLL complex, at the promoters of the cardiac development regulators GATA6 and Nkx2-5. Co-immunoprecipitation assays also show an interaction between Fendrr and TrxG/MLL. Additionally, co-immunoprecipitation assays also show an interaction of Fendrr with TrxG/MLL and PRC2. Fendrr interacts with the PRC2 complex in both *cis* and *trans* to regulate transcription factors in the lateral and cardiac mesoderm. Fendrr is able to bind to a region near the neighbouring Foxf1 gene, where it is believed to anchor and guide PRC2 to the promoter region and increase H3K27me3.

The lncRNAs mentioned are likely only scratching the surface of important regulators of cardiovascular function. In fact, one recent study using high-throughput sequencing techniques to study VSMC in rats has identified 24 novel lncRNA differentially expressed in response to AngII [221]. Similarly, another study has shown, using high throughput RNA-seq techniques, that 135 non-coding genes show differential expression in failing murine hearts [222]. Together, these studies illustrate the complexity of the cardiovascular transcriptome. With thousands of putative lncRNAs, more studies will no doubt uncover similar associations to the cardiovascular system. Further insight into the function of these lncRNAs is crucial to realizing their contribution to epigenetics, and is a probable direction of many future studies.

4.9. Epigenetic inheritance

A vital component of the definition of epigenetics and one which has briefly been mentioned in this chapter is that of the heritability of epigenetic patterns. These patterns carry great significance for the determination and preservation of defined and consistent gene expression programs that underlie cell fate decisions during and beyond early development. Despite flexibility of these patterns in totipotent and pluripotent stages, this plasticity wanes as development continues. The inheritance of such patterns is, therefore, of the utmost importance. The following section will explore the transmission of such information during the replication stages that take place in mitosis and meiosis, specifically analyzing DNA methylation and histone modification patterns within the context of these two processes.

DNA methylation is a significant epigenetic process that nicely fulfills the criterion for heritability. It has been proposed that DNA methylation may in fact act as a source of epigenetic memory, via the mitotic pathway. Previously, we offered a widely accepted and elegant sequence of events to describe the generational inheritance of DNA methylation patterns. *De novo* methyltransferases initially place methylation marks on DNA and, following replication, the maintenance DNMT marks the nascent strand with the same patterns exhibited by the original parent strand. Quite simply, DNA methylation absence demarcates active promoter regions, namely CpG islands, such that the promoters in which they are found remain potentially transcriptionally active throughout development and maturity. Conversely, segments of the genome that lack promoter activity become methylated and carry the flags of repression throughout the life of the organism. Our understanding of methylation pattern inheritance through mitosis is becoming relatively well elucidated, while more studies must be dedicated to comprehending the ways in which these patterns are initially laid down.

The semi-conservative model of inheritance that applies to both DNA replication and the transmission of DNA methylation patterns, had been speculated [223], and is now seldom conceived to be the main mode of transmission of histone modifications. Although compelling, this model relies on inherent symmetry within mono-nucleosomes as well as the semi-conservative separation of H3-H4 tetramers [224] (which, together with H2A and H2B dimers, make up the nucleosome core). Although two copies of each of the core histones are present within the nucleosome, it is unknown, yet highly doubted, that histone modifications exist in a symmetric manner [224]. Given the observation that the vast majority of H3-H4 tetramers actually segregate in a conservative manner [225-228], the more likely candidates to act as templates for new patterns would actually be adjacent, pre-existing nucleosomes on the same strand [224]. A possible mechanism for this may be envisioned whereby a neighbouring nucleosome that will be used as a template, is marked by a chromatin binding protein or reader protein [229] which would recruit a writer protein. Such a system may act in repetitive sequences where a number of nucleosomes all require the same replication. A self-cycling process has been proposed for up keeping repressive H3K27me3 marks, whereby polycomb repressive complex 2 (PRC2) binds to its own methylation site [230].

Based on these observations, the literal notion of copying a code during the S phase of the cell cycle does not seem to be applicable to the intricate system of histone modifications. In the next section, we mention that DNA methylation patterns likely influence the propagation of histone modifications. It may be speculated that the semi-conservative model applies well to DNA methylation pattern transmission, and the flags installed on the newly synthesized strand then act as markers for prompting the appropriate histone modifications.

Histone variant inheritance outside of S phase has suggested that histone modification inheritance can be replication-independent, unlike the events described above that would predominate at the replication fork. Histone variants are altered versions of one of the four core histone proteins. For example, H3.3 has been shown to be associated with transcriptionally active segments and is found abundantly in active histone marks [231-233]. H3.3 nucleosomes are known to be more dynamic and susceptible to displacement during transcription [234]. Consequently, the density of H3.3 nucleosomes is reduced during transcription. The replication-independent re-incorporation of H3.3 appears to be mediated by chaperone proteins, such as HIRA (Hir-related protein A) following the completion of transcription [235, 236]. Hence, this particular epigenetic modification can be maintained, despite dilution by replication.

4.10. Histone code dispute

Occasionally, the "histone code" is discussed as an entity whose existence is well established, while, at other times, it proves to be a highly debated topic. In the following, we will briefly touch upon these disputable characteristics and why a consensus has yet to be reached in this matter. Numerous tables have been compiled in an attempt to categorize the diverse range of possible histone modifications and the assortment of amino acid residues that are subject to these alterations. In contrast to the genetic code, the universality and predictability of the potential histone code seem to be much less clear-cut. In stark contrast to the genetic code, the consistency of histone patterns seems to vary dramatically from lower to higher eukaryotes [237]. Evidence has accumulated which argues against the notion of a simple binary relationship between modification and effect.

Turner thoroughly reviewed the concept of a histone code, in light of the extensive possibilities that result from combinations of modification and amino acid, from the perspective of semiotics: the study of signs and their use or meaning [237]. The genetic code is highlighted as the quintessential semiotic code in the way that following the central dogma of molecular biology (DNA→RNA→protein) requires the utilization of symbols, their meaning, and a code to make known their meaning. Even though the symbols of an epigenetic code would likely be combinations of histone modifications with DNA methylation marks, the number of these is far from being known. Such arrangements would increase in quantity with increasing number of cell types and would have to be pinpointed at different moments in differentiation. At this point, we can only speculate as to the number of different outcomes based on the indefinite capacity for combination. Thus, it can be seen that, in order to accurately describe the transmission of histone modifications as a "code," a much more comprehensive synthesis of the variable arrangements must be attained.

4.11. Relationships between epigenetic pathways

Several attempts have been made at identifying the relationships between the discussed epigenetic pathways. DNA methylation and histone posttranslational modifications have been implicated in a wide variety of instances, many of which have been discussed in this chapter. Biochemical and genetic evidence have tended towards a bidirectional relationship between the two systems: histone methylation has been seen to guide DNA methylation and a DNA methylation template likely influences the reversible placement of histone modifications [238].

In the following, both of these options, in addition to the joint roles they play in repression, will be discussed.

We can now appreciate the dynamic nature of methylation patterns during early development. At approximately the implantation stage, a wave of *de novo* methylation inputs the methylation patterns that will be transferred to somatic cells in subsequent generations. At the same time, there is a mechanism, speculated to be the combinatorial binding of *cis*-acting elements and active demethylation, which serves to protect CpG islands from indiscriminate *de novo* methylation (40, 239-241). Interestingly, there is support for the notion that it is the presence of H3K4 mono-, di-, or tri-methylation that appears to protect CpG islands before the round of *de novo* DNA methylation begins (63, 242). Recent studies suggest that H3K4 methylation protects DNA from *de novo* methylation [243, 244]. RNA polymerase II is known to be bound primarily to CpG islands in the early embryo and is responsible for recruiting H3K4 methyltransferases (Table 1) (63, 243-246). Therefore, it is these regions that remain unmethylated as a result of early histone modifications.

Another significant event of early development occurs at the time of gastrulation when targeted repression and *de novo* methylation of pluripotency preserving genes such as *Oct3/4*, takes place [247]. A sequential process ensues: binding of repressor molecules with the *Oct3/4* promoter turns off transcription [248-250] and a complex containing the histone methyltransferase G9a as well as histone deacetylases are recruited. Deacetylation, one of the histone modifications associated with transcriptional repression, is the next step, resetting the lysine residues so that G9a is able to catalyze H3K9 methylation [251]. From here, the successive binding of heterochromatin protein 1 (HP1) facilitates the formation of heterochromatin [251]. Finally, G9a binding also recruits DNMT3A and 3B [252], meaning that the final stages of silencing are completed. Gastrulation is the time at which the embryo begins to separate into germ layers, losing the ability to maintain pluripotency. Accordingly, it is histone modifications, working in conjunction with DNA methylation pathways that direct the repression of the expression of pluripotency-associated genes.

In the above two examples, HP1 was discussed in the context of deacetylation, whereas H3K4 methylation was said to protect CpG islands from *de novo* DNA methylation in early development. There are other instances, however, where H3K4me acts as a binding site for HP1 [253, 254]. A major component of heterochromatin, HP1, is well known to contribute to the establishment and maintenance of transcriptionally silent heterochromatin [255].

In addition to these instances of histone modifications guiding DNA methylation patterns, there is evidence to suggest that, through cell division, DNA methylation is important for maintaining many histone modifications [251]. As discussed previously, DNA methylation patterns are faithfully transmitted to the next generation by means of the maintenance methyltransferase DNMT1 and prior UHRF1and PCNA DNA binding. However, despite the importance of chromatin structure and composition in initiating transcriptional patterns, these same structures are liable to disruption as the replication fork and associated complexes make their way along the DNA during replication [251]. It has been inferred that DNA methylation patterns may act as an important indicator for the reconstruction of epigenetic patterns. That is, the more or less accurate transmission is likely necessary for the reproduction of chromatin conformation after replication has occurred.

Several studies have found that regions rich in unmethylated DNA are reformed in a rather open conformation, while those regions with more methylated DNA tend to be restructured in a sealed configuration [256, 257]. Acetylated (activating) histones are the primary component of those unmethylated, open regions. Conversely, it has also been shown that the nucleosomes of the compact, closed chromatin contain histones which are primarily non-acetylated [258, 259]. Also worth noting is the fact that methyl-CpG binding domain proteins such as MeCP2 and MBD2 also demonstrate the ability to attract histone deacetylases to methylated DNA regions [260, 261]. There is evidence that, in plants, DNA methylation may inhibit H3K4 methylation, a mark of activation, while perhaps also directing H3K9 dimethylation, a repressive indicator (259, 262, 263). Thus, even though the mechanism of action may still be relatively unknown for a number of these hypotheses, evidence does suggest the potential of a DNA methylation template guiding the placement of histone modifications.

Earlier in this chapter, upon describing the structure of nucleosomes, we mentioned the fact that ATP-dependent chromatin remodeling complexes often execute an action of nucleosome sliding. We revisit this topic here, in light of our exploration of the relationships amongst epigenetic pathways. The regulation of gene expression has also been found to be affected by these chromatin remodelers, namely the SNF2 family. Containing helical domains but executing no helicase activity, these proteins disturb the histone/DNA contacts and are believed to function in both transcriptional activation and repression, depending on the context [238]. Briefly, we will highlight a few key avenues of research. Jeddeloh *et al.* were the first to link DNA methylation with these SNF2 helicases [264]. In *A. thaliana,* mutation in a protein called DDM1 (decreased in DNA methylation) resulted in 70% diminishment in global DNA methylation levels [264]. The mammalian lymphoid specific helicase (Lsh) has been found to be the most closely related SNF2 member and has been linked to cell proliferation [238, 265]. Murine knockout experiments have demonstrated normal development until birth, but death occurs soon after because of renal lesions, as well as defects in lymphoid development and proliferation [238, 266].

Based on the above examples, there certainly seems to be some sort of connectivity between the epigenetic pathways. Crosstalk is clearly happening between histone posttranslational modifications and DNA methylation patterns, despite the fact that they are often studied independently. Future research would certainly focus on deciphering both the direct and indirect ways in which these processes act in tandem with one another.

5. Case study II: Dutch winter famine

It is a rare and tragic instance when a serious famine strikes an urban and industrialized setting, but exactly this happened in the winter of 1944-45 in West Netherlands. Excellent documentation of the event and the people most affected by it has allowed for the study of nutritional deprivation, in the form of famine, on human reproduction. Under German occupation, the

Western Netherlands suffered an unusually harsh winter, the effects of which were exacerbated by fuel shortages. Homes were not heated, grass and tulip bulbs were consumed, and every scrap of furniture was burned in a desperate effort to stay alive [267]. Food rationing has become an inevitably direct consequence of wartime events, and the Dutch Winter Famine was no exception to this phenomenon. A 1,800 calorie limit had been upheld for four years before mid-1944 when it was reduced to 1,600. A stark decline placed the limit at 400 calories in April of 1945 [267]. Although children as well as expectant and nursing mothers did receive slightly greater quantities, essentially every person suffered from severe hunger [268].

Case studies dedicated to investigating the impact of malnourished mothers on their offspring came about as a result of the initial Dutch Famine Birth Cohort Study. There are 2414 singletons born between November of 1943 and February of 1947 in Amsterdam for whom detailed birth records were collected and who, at the ages of 50 to 58, were surveyed as to their physical and mental health [268]. In general, low birth weight has been correlated with a number of conditions later in life: hypertension, insulin resistance, and obesity [268-271]. A decline in birth weight of up to 300g was seen among those exposed to maternal malnutrition in the third trimester [272]. The results of the Cohort study clearly demonstrated that exposure to famine at any point of gestation was associated with glucose intolerance [273]. Interestingly, the first trimester proved to be the most decisive stage of gestation at which maternal malnutrition impacts offspring health. Increased rates of coronary artery disease, atherogenic lipid accumulation, disturbed blood coagulation, type II diabetes, and cardiovascular disease were exhibited by those exposed to famine in early gestation. This Cohort Study clearly demonstrated that, not only is maternal famine exposure during gestation associated with chronic disease in offspring later life, but that effects varied based on the timing in gestation of famine exposure.

How can the solitary existence of the static DNA code account for such remarkable differences witnessed over the course of a single generation? Changes outside of the genome are needed to explain this trans-generational variation. To address this issue in more detail, Heijmans *et al.* focused on insulin-like growth factor 2 (IGF2), a maternally imprinted gene and a crucial factor in human growth and development, especially during gestation [274].To investigate whether maternal famine exposure was associated with differences in methylation of IGF2, 60 periconceptionally exposed people were compared with their same-sex sibling. Overall, exposure was found to be associated with an average reduction of 5.2% methylation in the DMR of IGF2. All CpG sites, except for one, were seen to be less methylated in those who had been exposed [274]. Statistically significant data showed periconceptional exposure, but not later exposure, was associated with this decrease. It is hypothesized that the deficiency of methyl donors such as the amino acid methionine, from reduced caloric intake, may account for the hypomethylation of IGF2 [274]. This study was the first to record persistent epigenetic changes in response to transient environmental conditions.

6. Concluding remarks

In this chapter, we have aimed to excite readers about the emerging field of epigenetics and the potential role it will play in future research initiatives. Without underscoring the importance of the genetic code, we have attempted to describe epigenetics in such a way that its significance is comparatively equivalent to that of genetics. The birth of the current molecular biological paradigm occurred relatively recently in the history of science, especially the history of scientific revolutions. Whether or not epigenetics is paving the way for a new paradigm in biology, is a debate that is best left to the philosophers of science. Yet, the relevancy of epigenetics cannot be understated as we embark on future investigations into human health and disease.

Known histone posttranslational modifications were explored first, and the repressive, activating, or joint consequences of a majority of alterations were delineated. Due to its duration of study, great emphasis was placed on DNA methylation, its consequences, mediators, and mechanisms of action. Then, we introduced the re-discovery of the promising 6th base pair: 5hmC. Although its role remains highly elusive, a great deal of research has been devoted to understanding the demethylation pathways in which this base is likely involved. Many of these options and their respective caveats were explored in the text. The observations that have been made about TET enzyme, DNA methylation, and DNA hydroxymethylation levels in zygotic development and PGC formation were also elucidated in this chapter and concisely summarized in Figure 3. Long non coding RNAs were discussed in their broad context as well as the role they play in the cardiovascular system.

Connections across the entire scope of the chapter were highlighted in our exploration of vitamin C. Its fascinating role in the human body cannot be understated. In scurvy, this vitamin's deficiency results in devastating physiological and psychological outcomes. Acting as both a co-factor for enzymatic reactions and as an antioxidant, the biochemical activity of ascorbate is also relevant in the context of cell culture and demethylation. Discovering the connections between P4H and TET enzyme structure has allowed the multi-faceted role of vitamin C in the epigenome, to also be elucidated. The pathogenesis of atherosclerosis was mechanized in such a way that the potential role of increased antioxidant intake was highlighted. Epigenetic regulation in the endothelium proves to be dynamic and highly changeable in the case of cardiovascular disease. eNOS gene regulation was thoroughly investigated as a representative case of highly endothelial-cell specific expression. Epigenetic inheritance at the replication fork was addressed in a DNA methylation and histone modification context. Crosstalk between these two pathways was discussed in the context of both DNA methylation patterns impacting those of histone modifications and vice versa. Finally, the Dutch Winter Famine was our second case study, this time further evaluating the role of transgenerational epigenetic inheritance in the context of severe maternal nutritional deprivation during pregnancy.

List of non-standard Abbreviations and Acronyms

5caC	5-carboxylcytosine
5hmC	5-hydroxymethylcytosine
5fC	5-formylcytosine
5mC	5-methylcytosine
ATP	adenosine triphosphate
AID	activation-induced cytidine deaminase
APOBEC	apolipoprotein B mRNA editing enzymes, catalytic polypeptide
BER	base excision repair
ChIP	chromatin immunoprecipitation
CD domain	Cys-rich and double stranded-helix DSBH region
CpG	cytosine - phosphate - guanine
CGIs	CpG islands
DPPA3	developmental pluripotency-associated 3 protein
DNMTs	DNA methyltransferases
DMR	differentially methylated region
ES cell	embryonic stem cell
EC	endothelial cell
eNOS	endothelial nitric oxide synthase
EDRF	endothelium-derived relaxing factor
ES cell	embryonic stem cell
GWAS	genome-wide association studies
HATs	histone acetyltransferases
HDACs	histone deacetylases
HDMTs	histone demethylases
HOXC	homeobox X
IGF2	insulin-like growth factor
ICAM-2	intercellular cell adhesion molecule-2
IAPs	intracisternal A particles
lnc-RNA	long non-coding RNA
MBDs	methyl CpG binding domain proteins
miRNA	micro RNA
MEFs	mouse embryonic fibroblasts
NO	nitric oxide
PRC2	polycomb repressive complex 2
PGCs	primordial germ cells

PCNA	proliferating cell nuclear antigen
P4H	prolyl 4-hydroxylase
ROS	reactive oxygen species
SAM	S-adenosylmethionine
SMUG1	selective monofunctional uracil-DNA glycosylase 1
SNP	single nucleotide polymorphism
SUMO	small ubiquitin-like modifier
TET enzymes	ten-eleven translocation enzymes
TDG	thymine DNA glycosylase
TSS	transcription start site
Ub	ubiquitin
UHRF1	ubiquitin-like with PHD and ring finger domains 1
VE-cadherin	vascular endothelial cadherin
VEGFR	vascular endothelial growth factor receptor
VSMC	vascular smooth muscle cell
vWF	von Willebrand factor

Acknowledgements

We gratefully thank members of the Marsden lab for the critical review of this manuscript. P.A. Marsden holds the Keenan Chair in Medical Research and is a recipient of a Career Investigator Award from the Heart and Stroke Foundation of Canada and is supported by a grant from the Canadian Institutes of Health Research (CIHR MOP 79475) and a grant from the National Institutes of Health (NIH/HHLBI P01 HL076540-06A1).

Author details

Alexandra A. Majerski[1], Anthony C. Quinton[1] and Philip A. Marsden[1,2*]

*Address all correspondence to: p.marsden@utoronto.ca

1 The Keenan Research Centre and Li Ka Shing Knowledge Institute, St. Michael's Hospital, Toronto, Canada

2 Department of Laboratory Medicine and Pathobiology, University of Toronto, Toronto, Canada

The authors have no conflicts of interest to disclose.

References

[1] Bernstein BE, Meissner A, Lander ES. The mammalian epigenome. Cell. 2007 Feb 23;128(4):669-81.

[2] Nightingale KP, O'Neill LP, Turner BM. Histone modifications: signalling receptors and potential elements of a heritable epigenetic code. Curr Opin Genet Dev. 2006 Apr;16(2):125-36.

[3] Kornberg RD. Chromatin structure: a repeating unit of histones and DNA. Science. 1974 May 24;184(4139):868-71.

[4] Alberts B, Johnson A, Lewis J, Raff M, Roberts K, Walter P. Molecular Biology of the Cell. 5th ed. Masson S, Jeffcock E, Anderson M, Granum S, Goatly B, editors. New York, NY; Abingdon, UK: Garland Science, Taylor & Francis Group, LLC.; 2008.

[5] Li G, Widom J. Nucleosomes facilitate their own invasion. Nat Struct Mol Biol. 2004 Aug;11(8):763-9.

[6] Allfrey VG, Faulkner R, Mirsky AE. Acetylation and Methylation of Histones and Their Possible Role in the Regulation of Rna Synthesis. Proc Natl Acad Sci U S A. 1964 May;51:786-94.

[7] Vaquero A, Loyola A, Reinberg D. The constantly changing face of chromatin. Sci Aging Knowledge Environ. 2003 Apr 9;2003(14):RE4.

[8] Shogren-Knaak M, Ishii H, Sun JM, Pazin MJ, Davie JR, Peterson CL. Histone H4-K16 acetylation controls chromatin structure and protein interactions. Science. 2006 Feb 10;311(5762):844-7.

[9] Vettese-Dadey M, Grant PA, Hebbes TR, Crane-Robinson C, Allis CD, Workman JL. Acetylation of histone H4 plays a primary role in enhancing transcription factor binding to nucleosomal DNA in vitro. EMBO J. 1996 May 15;15(10):2508-18.

[10] Dhalluin C, Carlson JE, Zeng L, He C, Aggarwal AK, Zhou MM. Structure and ligand of a histone acetyltransferase bromodomain. Nature. 1999 Jun 3;399(6735): 491-6.

[11] Owen DJ, Ornaghi P, Yang JC, Lowe N, Evans PR, Ballario P, et al. The structural basis for the recognition of acetylated histone H4 by the bromodomain of histone acetyltransferase gcn5p. EMBO J. 2000 Nov 15;19(22):6141-9.

[12] Jenuwein T, Allis CD. Translating the histone code. Science. 2001 Aug 10;293(5532): 1074-80.

[13] Lee DY, Teyssier C, Strahl BD, Stallcup MR. Role of protein methylation in regulation of transcription. Endocr Rev. 2005 Apr;26(2):147-70.

[14] Zhang Y, Reinberg D. Transcription regulation by histone methylation: interplay between different covalent modifications of the core histone tails. Genes Dev. 2001 Sep 15;15(18):2343-60.

[15] Martin C, Zhang Y. The diverse functions of histone lysine methylation. Nat Rev Mol Cell Biol. 2005 Nov;6(11):838-49.

[16] Langley E, Pearson M, Faretta M, Bauer UM, Frye RA, Minucci S, et al. Human SIR2 deacetylates p53 and antagonizes PML/p53-induced cellular senescence. EMBO J. 2002 May 15;21(10):2383-96.

[17] Wang H, Huang ZQ, Xia L, Feng Q, Erdjument-Bromage H, Strahl BD, et al. Methylation of histone H4 at arginine 3 facilitating transcriptional activation by nuclear hormone receptor. Science. 2001 Aug 3;293(5531):853-7.

[18] Fabbrizio E, El Messaoudi S, Polanowska J, Paul C, Cook JR, Lee JH, et al. Negative regulation of transcription by the type II arginine methyltransferase PRMT5. EMBO Rep. 2002 Jul;3(7):641-5.

[19] Pal S, Yun R, Datta A, Lacomis L, Erdjument-Bromage H, Kumar J, et al. mSin3A/histone deacetylase 2-and PRMT5-containing Brg1 complex is involved in transcriptional repression of the Myc target gene cad. Mol Cell Biol. 2003 Nov;23(21):7475-87.

[20] Kouzarides T, Berger SL. In: Allis CD, Jenuwein T, Reinberg D, Caparros M-L, editors. Epigenetics. Cold Spring Harbor, NY: Cold Spring Harbor Laboratory Press; 2007. p. 191-206.

[21] Wang H, Wang L, Erdjument-Bromage H, Vidal M, Tempst P, Jones RS, et al. Role of histone H2A ubiquitination in Polycomb silencing. Nature. 2004 Oct 14;431(7010):873-8.

[22] Ehrlich M, Gama-Sosa MA, Huang LH, Midgett RM, Kuo KC, McCune RA, et al. Amount and distribution of 5-methylcytosine in human DNA from different types of tissues of cells. Nucleic Acids Res. 1982 Apr 24;10(8):2709-21.

[23] Bird AP. CpG-rich islands and the function of DNA methylation. Nature. 1986 May 15-21;321(6067):209-13.

[24] Razin A, Riggs AD. DNA methylation and gene function. Science. 1980 Nov 7;210(4470):604-10.

[25] Wolf SF, Jolly DJ, Lunnen KD, Friedmann T, Migeon BR. Methylation of the hypoxanthine phosphoribosyltransferase locus on the human X chromosome: implications for X-chromosome inactivation. Proc Natl Acad Sci U S A. 1984 May;81(9):2806-10.

[26] Li E, Bird A. In: Allis CD, Jenuwein T, Reinberg D, Caparros M-L, editors. Epigenetics. Cold Spring Harbor, NY: Cold Spring Harbor Laboratory Press; 2007. p. 341-53.

[27] Watt F, Molloy PL. Cytosine methylation prevents binding to DNA of a HeLa cell transcription factor required for optimal expression of the adenovirus major late promoter. Genes Dev. 1988 Sep;2(9):1136-43.

[28] Hendrich B, Bird A. Identification and characterization of a family of mammalian methyl-CpG binding proteins. Mol Cell Biol. 1998 Nov;18(11):6538-47.

[29] Boyes J, Bird A. DNA methylation inhibits transcription indirectly via a methyl-CpG binding protein. Cell. 1991 Mar 22;64(6):1123-34.

[30] Hendrich B, Guy J, Ramsahoye B, Wilson VA, Bird A. Closely related proteins MBD2 and MBD3 play distinctive but interacting roles in mouse development. Genes Dev. 2001 Mar 15;15(6):710-23.

[31] Meehan RR, Lewis JD, McKay S, Kleiner EL, Bird AP. Identification of a mammalian protein that binds specifically to DNA containing methylated CpGs. Cell. 1989 Aug 11;58(3):499-507.

[32] Bird AP, Wolffe AP. Methylation-induced repression--belts, braces, and chromatin. Cell. 1999 Nov 24;99(5):451-4.

[33] Okano M, Xie S, Li E. Cloning and characterization of a family of novel mammalian DNA (cytosine-5) methyltransferases. Nat Genet. 1998 Jul;19(3):219-20.

[34] Sharif J, Muto M, Takebayashi S, Suetake I, Iwamatsu A, Endo TA, et al. The SRA protein Np95 mediates epigenetic inheritance by recruiting Dnmt1 to methylated DNA. Nature. 2007 Dec 6;450(7171):908-12.

[35] Bostick M, Kim JK, Esteve PO, Clark A, Pradhan S, Jacobsen SE. UHRF1 plays a role in maintaining DNA methylation in mammalian cells. Science. 2007 Sep 21;317(5845): 1760-4.

[36] Chuang LS, Ian HI, Koh TW, Ng HH, Xu G, Li BF. Human DNA-(cytosine-5) methyltransferase-PCNA complex as a target for p21WAF1. Science. 1997 Sep 26;277(5334): 1996-2000.

[37] Riggs AD. X inactivation, differentiation, and DNA methylation. Cytogenet Cell Genet. 1975;14(1):9-25.

[38] Holliday R, Pugh JE. DNA modification mechanisms and gene activity during development. Science. 1975 Jan 24;187(4173):226-32.

[39] Li E, Bestor TH, Jaenisch R. Targeted mutation of the DNA methyltransferase gene results in embryonic lethality. Cell. 1992 Jun 12;69(6):915-26.

[40] Okano M, Bell DW, Haber DA, Li E. DNA methyltransferases Dnmt3a and Dnmt3b are essential for de novo methylation and mammalian development. Cell. 1999 Oct 29;99(3):247-57.

[41] Qiu C, Sawada K, Zhang X, Cheng X. The PWWP domain of mammalian DNA methyltransferase Dnmt3b defines a new family of DNA-binding folds. Nat Struct Biol. 2002 Mar;9(3):217-24.

[42] Lukasik SM, Cierpicki T, Borloz M, Grembecka J, Everett A, Bushweller JH. High resolution structure of the HDGF PWWP domain: a potential DNA binding domain. Protein Sci. 2006 Feb;15(2):314-23.

[43] Bird AP. DNA methylation and the frequency of CpG in animal DNA. Nucleic Acids Res. 1980 Apr 11;8(7):1499-504.

[44] Coulondre C, Miller JH, Farabaugh PJ, Gilbert W. Molecular basis of base substitution hotspots in Escherichia coli. Nature. 1978 Aug 24;274(5673):775-80.

[45] Gardiner-Garden M, Frommer M. CpG islands in vertebrate genomes. J Mol Biol. 1987 Jul 20;196(2):261-82.

[46] Takai D, Jones PA. Comprehensive analysis of CpG islands in human chromosomes 21 and 22. Proc Natl Acad Sci U S A. 2002 Mar 19;99(6):3740-5.

[47] Larsen F, Gundersen G, Lopez R, Prydz H. CpG islands as gene markers in the human genome. Genomics. 1992 Aug;13(4):1095-107.

[48] Zhu J, He F, Hu S, Yu J. On the nature of human housekeeping genes. Trends Genet. 2008 Oct;24(10):481-4.

[49] Saxonov S, Berg P, Brutlag DL. A genome-wide analysis of CpG dinucleotides in the human genome distinguishes two distinct classes of promoters. Proc Natl Acad Sci U S A. 2006 Jan 31;103(5):1412-7.

[50] Ramirez-Carrozzi VR, Braas D, Bhatt DM, Cheng CS, Hong C, Doty KR, et al. A unifying model for the selective regulation of inducible transcription by CpG islands and nucleosome remodeling. Cell. 2009 Jul 10;138(1):114-28.

[51] Tazi J, Bird A. Alternative chromatin structure at CpG islands. Cell. 1990 Mar 23;60(6):909-20.

[52] Schones DE, Cui K, Cuddapah S, Roh TY, Barski A, Wang Z, et al. Dynamic regulation of nucleosome positioning in the human genome. Cell. 2008 Mar 7;132(5):887-98.

[53] Choi JK. Contrasting chromatin organization of CpG islands and exons in the human genome. Genome Biol.11(7):R70.

[54] Carninci P, Sandelin A, Lenhard B, Katayama S, Shimokawa K, Ponjavic J, et al. Genome-wide analysis of mammalian promoter architecture and evolution. Nat Genet. 2006 Jun;38(6):626-35.

[55] Juven-Gershon T, Hsu JY, Theisen JW, Kadonaga JT. The RNA polymerase II core promoter-the gateway to transcription. Curr Opin Cell Biol. 2008 Jun;20(3):253-9.

[56] Blackledge NP, Zhou JC, Tolstorukov MY, Farcas AM, Park PJ, Klose RJ. CpG islands recruit a histone H3 lysine 36 demethylase. Mol Cell. Apr 23;38(2):179-90.

[57] Strahl BD, Grant PA, Briggs SD, Sun ZW, Bone JR, Caldwell JA, et al. Set2 is a nucleosomal histone H3-selective methyltransferase that mediates transcriptional repression. Mol Cell Biol. 2002 Mar;22(5):1298-306.

[58] Youdell ML, Kizer KO, Kisseleva-Romanova E, Fuchs SM, Duro E, Strahl BD, et al. Roles for Ctk1 and Spt6 in regulating the different methylation states of histone H3 lysine 36. Mol Cell Biol. 2008 Aug;28(16):4915-26.

[59] Li B, Jackson J, Simon MD, Fleharty B, Gogol M, Seidel C, et al. Histone H3 lysine 36 dimethylation (H3K36me2) is sufficient to recruit the Rpd3s histone deacetylase complex and to repress spurious transcription. J Biol Chem. 2009 Mar 20;284(12):7970-6.

[60] Wang Z, Zang C, Rosenfeld JA, Schones DE, Barski A, Cuddapah S, et al. Combinatorial patterns of histone acetylations and methylations in the human genome. Nat Genet. 2008 Jul;40(7):897-903.

[61] Lee JH, Skalnik DG. CpG-binding protein (CXXC finger protein 1) is a component of the mammalian Set1 histone H3-Lys4 methyltransferase complex, the analogue of the yeast Set1/COMPASS complex. J Biol Chem. 2005 Dec 16;280(50):41725-31.

[62] Thomson JP, Skene PJ, Selfridge J, Clouaire T, Guy J, Webb S, et al. CpG islands influence chromatin structure via the CpG-binding protein Cfp1. Nature. Apr 15;464(7291):1082-6.

[63] Guenther MG, Levine SS, Boyer LA, Jaenisch R, Young RA. A chromatin landmark and transcription initiation at most promoters in human cells. Cell. 2007 Jul 13;130(1): 77-88.

[64] Mikkelsen TS, Ku M, Jaffe DB, Issac B, Lieberman E, Giannoukos G, et al. Genome-wide maps of chromatin state in pluripotent and lineage-committed cells. Nature. 2007 Aug 2;448(7153):553-60.

[65] Tahiliani M, Koh KP, Shen Y, Pastor WA, Bandukwala H, Brudno Y, et al. Conversion of 5-methylcytosine to 5-hydroxymethylcytosine in mammalian DNA by MLL partner TET1. Science. 2009 May 15;324(5929):930-5.

[66] Penn NW, Suwalski R, O'Riley C, Bojanowski K, Yura R. The presence of 5-hydroxymethylcytosine in animal deoxyribonucleic acid. Biochem J. 1972 Feb;126(4):781-90.

[67] Kriaucionis S, Heintz N. The nuclear DNA base 5-hydroxymethylcytosine is present in Purkinje neurons and the brain. Science. 2009 May 15;324(5929):929-30.

[68] Munzel M, Globisch D, Bruckl T, Wagner M, Welzmiller V, Michalakis S, et al. Quantification of the sixth DNA base hydroxymethylcytosine in the brain. Angew Chem Int Ed Engl. Jul 19;49(31):5375-7.

[69] Szwagierczak A, Bultmann S, Schmidt CS, Spada F, Leonhardt H. Sensitive enzymatic quantification of 5-hydroxymethylcytosine in genomic DNA. Nucleic Acids Res. Oct;38(19):e181.

[70] Ito S, Shen L, Dai Q, Wu SC, Collins LB, Swenberg JA, et al. Tet proteins can convert 5-methylcytosine to 5-formylcytosine and 5-carboxylcytosine. Science. Sep 2;333(6047):1300-3.

[71] Globisch D, Munzel M, Muller M, Michalakis S, Wagner M, Koch S, et al. Tissue distribution of 5-hydroxymethylcytosine and search for active demethylation intermediates. PLoS One.5(12):e15367.

[72] Ficz G, Branco MR, Seisenberger S, Santos F, Krueger F, Hore TA, et al. Dynamic regulation of 5-hydroxymethylcytosine in mouse ES cells and during differentiation. Nature. May 19;473(7347):398-402.

[73] Szulwach KE, Li X, Li Y, Song CX, Han JW, Kim S, et al. Integrating 5-hydroxymethylcytosine into the epigenomic landscape of human embryonic stem cells. PLoS Genet. Jun;7(6):e1002154.

[74] Branco MR, Ficz G, Reik W. Uncovering the role of 5-hydroxymethylcytosine in the epigenome. Nat Rev Genet. Jan;13(1):7-13.

[75] Ng HH, Zhang Y, Hendrich B, Johnson CA, Turner BM, Erdjument-Bromage H, et al. MBD2 is a transcriptional repressor belonging to the MeCP1 histone deacetylase complex. Nat Genet. 1999 Sep;23(1):58-61.

[76] Ng HH, Jeppesen P, Bird A. Active repression of methylated genes by the chromosomal protein MBD1. Mol Cell Biol. 2000 Feb;20(4):1394-406.

[77] Kass SU, Landsberger N, Wolffe AP. DNA methylation directs a time-dependent repression of transcription initiation. Curr Biol. 1997 Mar 1;7(3):157-65.

[78] Fujita N, Watanabe S, Ichimura T, Ohkuma Y, Chiba T, Saya H, et al. MCAF mediates MBD1-dependent transcriptional repression. Mol Cell Biol. 2003 Apr;23(8): 2834-43.

[79] Sarraf SA, Stancheva I. Methyl-CpG binding protein MBD1 couples histone H3 methylation at lysine 9 by SETDB1 to DNA replication and chromatin assembly. Mol Cell. 2004 Aug 27;15(4):595-605.

[80] Valinluck V, Tsai HH, Rogstad DK, Burdzy A, Bird A, Sowers LC. Oxidative damage to methyl-CpG sequences inhibits the binding of the methyl-CpG binding domain (MBD) of methyl-CpG binding protein 2 (MeCP2). Nucleic Acids Res. 2004;32(14): 4100-8.

[81] Jin SG, Kadam S, Pfeifer GP. Examination of the specificity of DNA methylation profiling techniques towards 5-methylcytosine and 5-hydroxymethylcytosine. Nucleic Acids Res. Jun;38(11):e125.

[82] Hashimoto H, Liu Y, Upadhyay AK, Chang Y, Howerton SB, Vertino PM, et al. Recognition and potential mechanisms for replication and erasure of cytosine hydroxymethylation. Nucleic Acids Res. Jun;40(11):4841-9.

[83] Choy JS, Wei S, Lee JY, Tan S, Chu S, Lee TH. DNA methylation increases nucleosome compaction and rigidity. J Am Chem Soc. Feb 17;132(6):1782-3.

[84] Pastor WA, Aravind L, Rao A. TETonic shift: biological roles of TET proteins in DNA demethylation and transcription. Nat Rev Mol Cell Biol. Jun;14(6):341-56.

[85] He YF, Li BZ, Li Z, Liu P, Wang Y, Tang Q, et al. Tet-mediated formation of 5-carboxylcytosine and its excision by TDG in mammalian DNA. Science. Sep 2;333(6047): 1303-7.

[86] Pfaffeneder T, Hackner B, Truss M, Munzel M, Muller M, Deiml CA, et al. The discovery of 5-formylcytosine in embryonic stem cell DNA. Angew Chem Int Ed Engl. Jul 25;50(31):7008-12.

[87] Iyer LM, Tahiliani M, Rao A, Aravind L. Prediction of novel families of enzymes involved in oxidative and other complex modifications of bases in nucleic acids. Cell Cycle. 2009 Jun 1;8(11):1698-710.

[88] Ito S, D'Alessio AC, Taranova OV, Hong K, Sowers LC, Zhang Y. Role of Tet proteins in 5mC to 5hmC conversion, ES-cell self-renewal and inner cell mass specification. Nature. Aug 26;466(7310):1129-33.

[89] Ko M, An J, Bandukwala HS, Chavez L, Aijo T, Pastor WA, et al. Modulation of TET2 expression and 5-methylcytosine oxidation by the CXXC domain protein IDAX. Nature. May 2;497(7447):122-6.

[90] Loenarz C, Schofield CJ. Physiological and biochemical aspects of hydroxylations and demethylations catalyzed by human 2-oxoglutarate oxygenases. Trends Biochem Sci. Jan;36(1):7-18.

[91] Upadhyay AK, Horton JR, Zhang X, Cheng X. Coordinated methyl-lysine erasure: structural and functional linkage of a Jumonji demethylase domain and a reader domain. Curr Opin Struct Biol. Dec;21(6):750-60.

[92] Tan L, Shi YG. Tet family proteins and 5-hydroxymethylcytosine in development and disease. Development. Jun;139(11):1895-902.

[93] Zhang H, Zhang X, Clark E, Mulcahey M, Huang S, Shi YG. TET1 is a DNA-binding protein that modulates DNA methylation and gene transcription via hydroxylation of 5-methylcytosine. Cell Res. Dec;20(12):1390-3.

[94] Xu Y, Wu F, Tan L, Kong L, Xiong L, Deng J, et al. Genome-wide regulation of 5hmC, 5mC, and gene expression by Tet1 hydroxylase in mouse embryonic stem cells. Mol Cell. May 20;42(4):451-64.

[95] Bestor TH. Activation of mammalian DNA methyltransferase by cleavage of a Zn binding regulatory domain. EMBO J. 1992 Jul;11(7):2611-7.

[96] Khachane AN, Harrison PM. Mining mammalian transcript data for functional long non-coding RNAs. PLoS One.5(4):e10316.

[97] Webster AL, Yan MS, Marsden PA. Epigenetics and cardiovascular disease. Can J Cardiol. Jan;29(1):46-57.

[98] Saxena A, Carninci P. Long non-coding RNA modifies chromatin: epigenetic silencing by long non-coding RNAs. Bioessays. Nov;33(11):830-9.

[99] Brown CJ, Ballabio A, Rupert JL, Lafreniere RG, Grompe M, Tonlorenzi R, et al. A gene from the region of the human X inactivation centre is expressed exclusively from the inactive X chromosome. Nature. 1991 Jan 3;349(6304):38-44.

[100] Wutz A. Gene silencing in X-chromosome inactivation: advances in understanding facultative heterochromatin formation. Nat Rev Genet. Aug;12(8):542-53.

[101] Lee JT. Epigenetic regulation by long noncoding RNAs. Science. Dec 14;338(6113): 1435-9.

[102] Zhao J, Sun BK, Erwin JA, Song JJ, Lee JT. Polycomb proteins targeted by a short repeat RNA to the mouse X chromosome. Science. 2008 Oct 31;322(5902):750-6.

[103] Sado T, Wang Z, Sasaki H, Li E. Regulation of imprinted X-chromosome inactivation in mice by Tsix. Development. 2001 Apr;128(8):1275-86.

[104] Sun BK, Deaton AM, Lee JT. A transient heterochromatic state in Xist preempts X inactivation choice without RNA stabilization. Mol Cell. 2006 Mar 3;21(5):617-28.

[105] Rinn JL, Kertesz M, Wang JK, Squazzo SL, Xu X, Brugmann SA, et al. Functional demarcation of active and silent chromatin domains in human HOX loci by noncoding RNAs. Cell. 2007 Jun 29;129(7):1311-23.

[106] Grier DG, Thompson A, Kwasniewska A, McGonigle GJ, Halliday HL, Lappin TR. The pathophysiology of HOX genes and their role in cancer. J Pathol. 2005 Jan;205(2): 154-71.

[107] Woo CJ, Kingston RE. HOTAIR lifts noncoding RNAs to new levels. Cell. 2007 Jun 29;129(7):1257-9.

[108] Lane N, Dean W, Erhardt S, Hajkova P, Surani A, Walter J, et al. Resistance of IAPs to methylation reprogramming may provide a mechanism for epigenetic inheritance in the mouse. Genesis. 2003 Feb;35(2):88-93.

[109] Morgan HD, Santos F, Green K, Dean W, Reik W. Epigenetic reprogramming in mammals. Hum Mol Genet. 2005 Apr 15;14 Spec No 1:R47-58.

[110] McLay DW, Clarke HJ. Remodelling the paternal chromatin at fertilization in mammals. Reproduction. 2003 May;125(5):625-33.

[111] van der Heijden GW, Dieker JW, Derijck AA, Muller S, Berden JH, Braat DD, et al. Asymmetry in histone H3 variants and lysine methylation between paternal and maternal chromatin of the early mouse zygote. Mech Dev. 2005 Sep;122(9):1008-22.

[112] Mayer W, Niveleau A, Walter J, Fundele R, Haaf T. Demethylation of the zygotic paternal genome. Nature. 2000 Feb 3;403(6769):501-2.

[113] Oswald J, Engemann S, Lane N, Mayer W, Olek A, Fundele R, et al. Active demethylation of the paternal genome in the mouse zygote. Curr Biol. 2000 Apr 20;10(8): 475-8.

[114] Santos F, Peters AH, Otte AP, Reik W, Dean W. Dynamic chromatin modifications characterise the first cell cycle in mouse embryos. Dev Biol. 2005 Apr 1;280(1):225-36.

[115] Dean W, Santos F, Stojkovic M, Zakhartchenko V, Walter J, Wolf E, et al. Conservation of methylation reprogramming in mammalian development: aberrant reprogramming in cloned embryos. Proc Natl Acad Sci U S A. 2001 Nov 20;98(24):13734-8.

[116] Santos F, Hendrich B, Reik W, Dean W. Dynamic reprogramming of DNA methylation in the early mouse embryo. Dev Biol. 2002 Jan 1;241(1):172-82.

[117] Wossidlo M, Nakamura T, Lepikhov K, Marques CJ, Zakhartchenko V, Boiani M, et al. 5-Hydroxymethylcytosine in the mammalian zygote is linked with epigenetic reprogramming. Nat Commun.2:241.

[118] Iqbal K, Jin SG, Pfeifer GP, Szabo PE. Reprogramming of the paternal genome upon fertilization involves genome-wide oxidation of 5-methylcytosine. Proc Natl Acad Sci U S A. Mar 1;108(9):3642-7.

[119] Gu TP, Guo F, Yang H, Wu HP, Xu GF, Liu W, et al. The role of Tet3 DNA dioxygenase in epigenetic reprogramming by oocytes. Nature. Sep 29;477(7366):606-10.

[120] Borgel J, Guibert S, Li Y, Chiba H, Schubeler D, Sasaki H, et al. Targets and dynamics of promoter DNA methylation during early mouse development. Nat Genet. Dec; 42(12):1093-100.

[121] Olek A, Walter J. The pre-implantation ontogeny of the H19 methylation imprint. Nat Genet. 1997 Nov;17(3):275-6.

[122] Nakamura T, Liu YJ, Nakashima H, Umehara H, Inoue K, Matoba S, et al. PGC7 binds histone H3K9me2 to protect against conversion of 5mC to 5hmC in early embryos. Nature. Jun 21;486(7403):415-9.

[123] Reik W. Stability and flexibility of epigenetic gene regulation in mammalian development. Nature. 2007 May 24;447(7143):425-32.

[124] Hackett JA, Sengupta R, Zylicz JJ, Murakami K, Lee C, Down TA, et al. Germline DNA demethylation dynamics and imprint erasure through 5-hydroxymethylcytosine. Science. Jan 25;339(6118):448-52.

[125] Carlson LL, Page AW, Bestor TH. Properties and localization of DNA methyltransferase in preimplantation mouse embryos: implications for genomic imprinting. Genes Dev. 1992 Dec;6(12B):2536-41.

[126] Hata K, Okano M, Lei H, Li E. Dnmt3L cooperates with the Dnmt3 family of de novo DNA methyltransferases to establish maternal imprints in mice. Development. 2002 Apr;129(8):1983-93.

[127] Kaneda M, Sado T, Hata K, Okano M, Tsujimoto N, Li E, et al. Role of de novo DNA methyltransferases in initiation of genomic imprinting and X-chromosome inactivation. Cold Spring Harb Symp Quant Biol. 2004;69:125-9.

[128] Pastor WA, Pape UJ, Huang Y, Henderson HR, Lister R, Ko M, et al. Genome-wide mapping of 5-hydroxymethylcytosine in embryonic stem cells. Nature. May 19;473(7347):394-7.

[129] Wu H, Zhang Y. Tet1 and 5-hydroxymethylation: a genome-wide view in mouse embryonic stem cells. Cell Cycle. Aug 1;10(15):2428-36.

[130] Dawlaty MM, Ganz K, Powell BE, Hu YC, Markoulaki S, Cheng AW, et al. Tet1 is dispensable for maintaining pluripotency and its loss is compatible with embryonic and postnatal development. Cell Stem Cell. Aug 5;9(2):166-75.

[131] Ko M, Bandukwala HS, An J, Lamperti ED, Thompson EC, Hastie R, et al. Ten-Eleven-Translocation 2 (TET2) negatively regulates homeostasis and differentiation of hematopoietic stem cells in mice. Proc Natl Acad Sci U S A. Aug 30;108(35):14566-71.

[132] Li Z, Cai X, Cai CL, Wang J, Zhang W, Petersen BE, et al. Deletion of Tet2 in mice leads to dysregulated hematopoietic stem cells and subsequent development of myeloid malignancies. Blood. Oct 27;118(17):4509-18.

[133] Moran-Crusio K, Reavie L, Shih A, Abdel-Wahab O, Ndiaye-Lobry D, Lobry C, et al. Tet2 loss leads to increased hematopoietic stem cell self-renewal and myeloid transformation. Cancer Cell. Jul 12;20(1):11-24.

[134] Quivoron C, Couronne L, Della Valle V, Lopez CK, Plo I, Wagner-Ballon O, et al. TET2 inactivation results in pleiotropic hematopoietic abnormalities in mouse and is a recurrent event during human lymphomagenesis. Cancer Cell. Jul 12;20(1):25-38.

[135] Hajkova P, Erhardt S, Lane N, Haaf T, El-Maarri O, Reik W, et al. Epigenetic reprogramming in mouse primordial germ cells. Mech Dev. 2002 Sep;117(1-2):15-23.

[136] Hackett JA, Zylicz JJ, Surani MA. Parallel mechanisms of epigenetic reprogramming in the germline. Trends Genet. Apr;28(4):164-74.

[137] Hajkova P, Jeffries SJ, Lee C, Miller N, Jackson SP, Surani MA. Genome-wide reprogramming in the mouse germ line entails the base excision repair pathway. Science. Jul 2;329(5987):78-82.

[138] Vincent JJ, Huang Y, Chen PY, Feng S, Calvopina JH, Nee K, et al. Stage-specific roles for tet1 and tet2 in DNA demethylation in primordial germ cells. Cell Stem Cell. Apr 4;12(4):470-8.

[139] Reik W, Dean W, Walter J. Epigenetic reprogramming in mammalian development. Science. 2001 Aug 10;293(5532):1089-93.

[140] Wu SC, Zhang Y. Active DNA demethylation: many roads lead to Rome. Nat Rev Mol Cell Biol. Sep;11(9):607-20.

[141] Maiti A, Drohat AC. Thymine DNA glycosylase can rapidly excise 5-formylcytosine and 5-carboxylcytosine: potential implications for active demethylation of CpG sites. J Biol Chem. Oct 14;286(41):35334-8.

[142] Zhang L, Lu X, Lu J, Liang H, Dai Q, Xu GL, et al. Thymine DNA glycosylase specifically recognizes 5-carboxylcytosine-modified DNA. Nat Chem Biol. Apr;8(4):328-30.

[143] Morgan MT, Bennett MT, Drohat AC. Excision of 5-halogenated uracils by human thymine DNA glycosylase. Robust activity for DNA contexts other than CpG. J Biol Chem. 2007 Sep 21;282(38):27578-86.

[144] Sibghat U, Gallinari P, Xu YZ, Goodman MF, Bloom LB, Jiricny J, et al. Base analog and neighboring base effects on substrate specificity of recombinant human G:T mismatch-specific thymine DNA-glycosylase. Biochemistry. 1996 Oct 1;35(39):12926-32.

[145] Waters TR, Swann PF. Kinetics of the action of thymine DNA glycosylase. J Biol Chem. 1998 Aug 7;273(32):20007-14.

[146] Abu M, Waters TR. The main role of human thymine-DNA glycosylase is removal of thymine produced by deamination of 5-methylcytosine and not removal of ethenocytosine. J Biol Chem. 2003 Mar 7;278(10):8739-44.

[147] Maiti A, Morgan MT, Pozharski E, Drohat AC. Crystal structure of human thymine DNA glycosylase bound to DNA elucidates sequence-specific mismatch recognition. Proc Natl Acad Sci U S A. 2008 Jul 1;105(26):8890-5.

[148] Schiesser S, Hackner B, Pfaffeneder T, Muller M, Hagemeier C, Truss M, et al. Mechanism and stem-cell activity of 5-carboxycytosine decarboxylation determined by isotope tracing. Angew Chem Int Ed Engl. Jun 25;51(26):6516-20.

[149] Morgan HD, Dean W, Coker HA, Reik W, Petersen-Mahrt SK. Activation-induced cytidine deaminase deaminates 5-methylcytosine in DNA and is expressed in pluripotent tissues: implications for epigenetic reprogramming. J Biol Chem. 2004 Dec 10;279(50):52353-60.

[150] Zhu JK. Active DNA demethylation mediated by DNA glycosylases. Annu Rev Genet. 2009;43:143-66.

[151] Chen ZX, Riggs AD. DNA methylation and demethylation in mammals. J Biol Chem. May 27;286(21):18347-53.

[152] Nabel CS, Jia H, Ye Y, Shen L, Goldschmidt HL, Stivers JT, et al. AID/APOBEC deaminases disfavor modified cytosines implicated in DNA demethylation. Nat Chem Biol. Sep;8(9):751-8.

[153] Guo JU, Su Y, Zhong C, Ming GL, Song H. Hydroxylation of 5-methylcytosine by TET1 promotes active DNA demethylation in the adult brain. Cell. Apr 29;145(3): 423-34.

[154] Cortellino S, Xu J, Sannai M, Moore R, Caretti E, Cigliano A, et al. Thymine DNA glycosylase is essential for active DNA demethylation by linked deamination-base excision repair. Cell. Jul 8;146(1):67-79.

[155] Chen CC, Wang KY, Shen CK. The mammalian de novo DNA methyltransferases DNMT3A and DNMT3B are also DNA 5-hydroxymethylcytosine dehydroxymethylases. J Biol Chem. Sep 28;287(40):33116-21.

[156] Liutkeviciute Z, Lukinavicius G, Masevicius V, Daujotyte D, Klimasauskas S. Cytosine-5-methyltransferases add aldehydes to DNA. Nat Chem Biol. 2009 Jun;5(6): 400-2.

[157] Metivier R, Gallais R, Tiffoche C, Le Peron C, Jurkowska RZ, Carmouche RP, et al. Cyclical DNA methylation of a transcriptionally active promoter. Nature. 2008 Mar 6;452(7183):45-50.

[158] Kangaspeska S, Stride B, Metivier R, Polycarpou-Schwarz M, Ibberson D, Carmouche RP, et al. Transient cyclical methylation of promoter DNA. Nature. 2008 Mar 6;452(7183):112-5.

[159] Lamb J. Captain Cook and the Scourge of Scurvy. [BBC historical piece] 2011 [updated February 17 2011August 15 2013]; Available from: http://www.bbc.co.uk/history/british/empire_seapower/captaincook_scurvy_01.shtml#top.

[160] Davies MB, Austin J, Partridge DA. Vitamin C: Its Chemistry and Biochemistry. Cambridge: The Royal Society of Chemistry; 1991.

[161] Grollman AP, Lehninger AL. Enzymic synthesis of L-ascorbic acid in different animal species. Arch Biochem Biophys. 1957 Jul;69:458-67.

[162] Nishikimi M, Yagi K. Molecular basis for the deficiency in humans of gulonolactone oxidase, a key enzyme for ascorbic acid biosynthesis. Am J Clin Nutr. 1991 Dec;54(6 Suppl):1203S-8S.

[163] Shoulders MD, Raines RT. Collagen structure and stability. Annu Rev Biochem. 2009;78:929-58.

[164] Gorres KL, Raines RT. Prolyl 4-hydroxylase. Crit Rev Biochem Mol Biol. Apr;45(2): 106-24.

[165] Westbye MP, Feyzi E, Aas PA, Vagbo CB, Talstad VA, Kavli B, et al. Human AlkB homolog 1 is a mitochondrial protein that demethylates 3-methylcytosine in DNA and RNA. J Biol Chem. 2008 Sep 5;283(36):25046-56.

[166] Myllyla R, Kuutti-Savolainen ER, Kivirikko KI. The role of ascorbate in the prolyl hydroxylase reaction. Biochem Biophys Res Commun. 1978 Jul 28;83(2):441-8.

[167] Nietfeld JJ, Kemp A. The function of ascorbate with respect to prolyl 4-hydroxylase activity. Biochim Biophys Acta. 1981 Jan 15;657(1):159-67.

[168] de Jong L, Albracht SP, Kemp A. Prolyl 4-hydroxylase activity in relation to the oxidation state of enzyme-bound iron. The role of ascorbate in peptidyl proline hydroxylation. Biochim Biophys Acta. 1982 Jun 4;704(2):326-32.

[169] De Jong L, Kemp A. Stoicheiometry and kinetics of the prolyl 4-hydroxylase partial reaction. Biochim Biophys Acta. 1984 May 31;787(1):105-11.

[170] Peterkofsky B. Ascorbate requirement for hydroxylation and secretion of procollagen: relationship to inhibition of collagen synthesis in scurvy. Am J Clin Nutr. 1991 Dec;54(6 Suppl):1135S-40S.

[171] Padh H. Vitamin C: newer insights into its biochemical functions. Nutr Rev. 1991 Mar;49(3):65-70.

[172] Rebouche CJ. Ascorbic acid and carnitine biosynthesis. Am J Clin Nutr. 1991 Dec;54(6 Suppl):1147S-52S.

[173] Minor EA, Court BL, Young JI, Wang G. Ascorbate induces ten-eleven translocation (Tet) methylcytosine dioxygenase-mediated generation of 5-hydroxymethylcytosine. J Biol Chem. May 10;288(19):13669-74.

[174] Chung TL, Brena RM, Kolle G, Grimmond SM, Berman BP, Laird PW, et al. Vitamin C promotes widespread yet specific DNA demethylation of the epigenome in human embryonic stem cells. Stem Cells. Oct;28(10):1848-55.

[175] Furchgott RF, Zawadzki JV. The obligatory role of endothelial cells in the relaxation of arterial smooth muscle by acetylcholine. Nature. 1980 Nov 27;288(5789):373-6.

[176] Ignarro LJ, Buga GM, Wood KS, Byrns RE, Chaudhuri G. Endothelium-derived relaxing factor produced and released from artery and vein is nitric oxide. Proc Natl Acad Sci U S A. 1987 Dec;84(24):9265-9.

[177] Palmer RM, Ferrige AG, Moncada S. Nitric oxide release accounts for the biological activity of endothelium-derived relaxing factor. Nature. 1987 Jun 11-17;327(6122): 524-6.

[178] Lefer AM. Nitric oxide: nature's naturally occurring leukocyte inhibitor. Circulation. 1997 Feb 4;95(3):553-4.

[179] Gauthier TW, Scalia R, Murohara T, Guo JP, Lefer AM. Nitric oxide protects against leukocyte-endothelium interactions in the early stages of hypercholesterolemia. Arterioscler Thromb Vasc Biol. 1995 Oct;15(10):1652-9.

[180] de Graaf JC, Banga JD, Moncada S, Palmer RM, de Groot PG, Sixma JJ. Nitric oxide functions as an inhibitor of platelet adhesion under flow conditions. Circulation. 1992 Jun;85(6):2284-90.

[181] Fish JE, Marsden PA. Endothelial nitric oxide synthase: insight into cell-specific gene regulation in the vascular endothelium. Cell Mol Life Sci. 2006 Jan;63(2):144-62.

[182] Gallo R, Fuster V. In: Tardif J-C, Bourassa MG, editors. Antioxidants and Cardiovascular Disease. Dordrecht, The Netherlands: Kluwer Academic Publishers; 2000. p. 19-46.

[183] Stary HC. The sequence of cell and matrix changes in atherosclerotic lesions of coronary arteries in the first forty years of life. Eur Heart J. 1990 Aug;11 Suppl E:3-19.

[184] Stary HC, Chandler AB, Glagov S, Guyton JR, Insull W, Jr., Rosenfeld ME, et al. A definition of initial, fatty streak, and intermediate lesions of atherosclerosis. A report from the Committee on Vascular Lesions of the Council on Arteriosclerosis, American Heart Association. Circulation. 1994 May;89(5):2462-78.

[185] Cathcart MK, Morel DW, Chisolm GM, 3rd. Monocytes and neutrophils oxidize low density lipoprotein making it cytotoxic. J Leukoc Biol. 1985 Aug;38(2):341-50.

[186] Parthasarathy S, Printz DJ, Boyd D, Joy L, Steinberg D. Macrophage oxidation of low density lipoprotein generates a modified form recognized by the scavenger receptor. Arteriosclerosis. 1986 Sep-Oct;6(5):505-10.

[187] Morel DW, DiCorleto PE, Chisolm GM. Endothelial and smooth muscle cells alter low density lipoprotein in vitro by free radical oxidation. Arteriosclerosis. 1984 Jul-Aug;4(4):357-64.

[188] Navab M, Hama SY, Nguyen TB, Fogelman AM. Monocyte adhesion and transmigration in atherosclerosis. Coron Artery Dis. 1994 Mar;5(3):198-204.

[189] Ross R. The pathogenesis of atherosclerosis--an update. N Engl J Med. 1986 Feb 20;314(8):488-500.

[190] Ross R. The pathogenesis of atherosclerosis: a perspective for the 1990s. Nature. 1993 Apr 29;362(6423):801-9.

[191] Guyton JR, Klemp KF. Development of the lipid-rich core in human atherosclerosis. Arterioscler Thromb Vasc Biol. 1996 Jan;16(1):4-11.

[192] Mason RP, Walter MF, Trumbore MW, Olmstead EG, Jr., Mason PE. Membrane antioxidant effects of the charged dihydropyridine calcium antagonist amlodipine. J Mol Cell Cardiol. 1999 Jan;31(1):275-81.

[193] Mason RP, Rhodes DG, Herbette LG. Reevaluating equilibrium and kinetic binding parameters for lipophilic drugs based on a structural model for drug interaction with biological membranes. J Med Chem. 1991 Mar;34(3):869-77.

[194] Mason RP, Campbell SF, Wang SD, Herbette LG. Comparison of location and binding for the positively charged 1,4-dihydropyridine calcium channel antagonist amlodipine with uncharged drugs of this class in cardiac membranes. Mol Pharmacol. 1989 Oct;36(4):634-40.

[195] John F. Keaney J. In: Tardif J-C, Bourassa MG, editors. Antioxidants and Cardiovascular Disease. Dordrecht, The Netherlands: Kluwer Academic Publishers; 2000. p. 101-16.

[196] Marsden PA, Heng HH, Scherer SW, Stewart RJ, Hall AV, Shi XM, et al. Structure and chromosomal localization of the human constitutive endothelial nitric oxide synthase gene. J Biol Chem. 1993 Aug 15;268(23):17478-88.

[197] Nadaud S, Bonnardeaux A, Lathrop M, Soubrier F. Gene structure, polymorphism and mapping of the human endothelial nitric oxide synthase gene. Biochem Biophys Res Commun. 1994 Feb 15;198(3):1027-33.

[198] Robinson LJ, Weremowicz S, Morton CC, Michel T. Isolation and chromosomal localization of the human endothelial nitric oxide synthase (NOS3) gene. Genomics. 1994 Jan 15;19(2):350-7.

[199] Tai SC, Robb GB, Marsden PA. Endothelial nitric oxide synthase: a new paradigm for gene regulation in the injured blood vessel. Arterioscler Thromb Vasc Biol. 2004 Mar; 24(3):405-12.

[200] Marsden PA, Schappert KT, Chen HS, Flowers M, Sundell CL, Wilcox JN, et al. Molecular cloning and characterization of human endothelial nitric oxide synthase. FEBS Lett. 1992 Aug 3;307(3):287-93.

[201] Matouk CC, Marsden PA. Epigenetic regulation of vascular endothelial gene expression. Circ Res. 2008 Apr 25;102(8):873-87.

[202] Liu VW, Huang PL. Cardiovascular roles of nitric oxide: a review of insights from nitric oxide synthase gene disrupted mice. Cardiovasc Res. 2008 Jan;77(1):19-29.

[203] Wilcox JN, Subramanian RR, Sundell CL, Tracey WR, Pollock JS, Harrison DG, et al. Expression of multiple isoforms of nitric oxide synthase in normal and atherosclerotic vessels. Arterioscler Thromb Vasc Biol. 1997 Nov;17(11):2479-88.

[204] Bertrand N, Castro DS, Guillemot F. Proneural genes and the specification of neural cell types. Nat Rev Neurosci. 2002 Jul;3(7):517-30.

[205] Wang Z, Wang DZ, Pipes GC, Olson EN. Myocardin is a master regulator of smooth muscle gene expression. Proc Natl Acad Sci U S A. 2003 Jun 10;100(12):7129-34.

[206] Lehrke M, Lazar MA. The many faces of PPARgamma. Cell. 2005 Dec 16;123(6):993-9.

[207] Tapscott SJ. The circuitry of a master switch: Myod and the regulation of skeletal muscle gene transcription. Development. 2005 Jun;132(12):2685-95.

[208] Atkins GB, Jain MK. Role of Kruppel-like transcription factors in endothelial biology. Circ Res. 2007 Jun 22;100(12):1686-95.

[209] Chan Y, Fish JE, D'Abreo C, Lin S, Robb GB, Teichert AM, et al. The cell-specific expression of endothelial nitric-oxide synthase: a role for DNA methylation. J Biol Chem. 2004 Aug 13;279(33):35087-100.

[210] Teichert AM, Karantzoulis-Fegaras F, Wang Y, Mawji IA, Bei X, Gnanapandithen K, et al. Characterization of the murine endothelial nitric oxide synthase promoter. Biochim Biophys Acta. 1998 Dec 22;1443(3):352-7.

[211] Fish JE, Matouk CC, Rachlis A, Lin S, Tai SC, D'Abreo C, et al. The expression of endothelial nitric-oxide synthase is controlled by a cell-specific histone code. J Biol Chem. 2005 Jul 1;280(26):24824-38.

[212] Matouk CC, Turgeon PJ, Marsden PA. Epigenetics and stroke risk-beyond the static DNA code. Advances in Genomics and Genetics. 2012;2012:2:67-84.

[213] Bush WS, Moore JH. Chapter 11: Genome-wide association studies. PLoS Comput Biol.8(12):e1002822.

[214] Samani NJ, Erdmann J, Hall AS, Hengstenberg C, Mangino M, Mayer B, et al. Genomewide association analysis of coronary artery disease. N Engl J Med. 2007 Aug 2;357(5):443-53.

[215] McPherson R, Pertsemlidis A, Kavaslar N, Stewart A, Roberts R, Cox DR, et al. A common allele on chromosome 9 associated with coronary heart disease. Science. 2007 Jun 8;316(5830):1488-91.

[216] Bown MJ, Braund PS, Thompson J, London NJ, Samani NJ, Sayers RD. Association between the coronary artery disease risk locus on chromosome 9p21.3 and abdominal aortic aneurysm. Circ Cardiovasc Genet. 2008 Oct;1(1):39-42.

[217] Broadbent HM, Peden JF, Lorkowski S, Goel A, Ongen H, Green F, et al. Susceptibility to coronary artery disease and diabetes is encoded by distinct, tightly linked SNPs in the ANRIL locus on chromosome 9p. Hum Mol Genet. 2008 Mar 15;17(6):806-14.

[218] Klattenhoff CA, Scheuermann JC, Surface LE, Bradley RK, Fields PA, Steinhauser ML, et al. Braveheart, a long noncoding RNA required for cardiovascular lineage commitment. Cell. Jan 31;152(3):570-83.

[219] Lindsley RC, Gill JG, Murphy TL, Langer EM, Cai M, Mashayekhi M, et al. Mesp1 coordinately regulates cardiovascular fate restriction and epithelial-mesenchymal transition in differentiating ESCs. Cell Stem Cell. 2008 Jul 3;3(1):55-68.

[220] Grote P, Wittler L, Hendrix D, Koch F, Wahrisch S, Beisaw A, et al. The tissue-specific lncRNA Fendrr is an essential regulator of heart and body wall development in the mouse. Dev Cell. Jan 28;24(2):206-14.

[221] Leung A, Trac C, Jin W, Lanting L, Akbany A, Saetrom P, et al. Novel Long Non-Coding RNAs Are Regulated by Angiotensin II in Vascular Smooth Muscle Cells. Circ Res. May 22.

[222] Lee JH, Gao C, Peng G, Greer C, Ren S, Wang Y, et al. Analysis of transcriptome complexity through RNA sequencing in normal and failing murine hearts. Circ Res. Dec 9;109(12):1332-41.

[223] Annunziato AT. Split decision: what happens to nucleosomes during DNA replication? J Biol Chem. 2005 Apr 1;280(13):12065-8.

[224] Zhu B, Reinberg D. Epigenetic inheritance: uncontested? Cell Res. Mar;21(3):435-41.

[225] Leffak IM, Grainger R, Weintraub H. Conservative assembly and segregation of nucleosomal histones. Cell. 1977 Nov;12(3):837-45.

[226] Jackson V. In vivo studies on the dynamics of histone-DNA interaction: evidence for nucleosome dissolution during replication and transcription and a low level of dissolution independent of both. Biochemistry. 1990 Jan 23;29(3):719-31.

[227] Yamasu K, Senshu T. Conservative segregation of tetrameric units of H3 and H4 histones during nucleosome replication. J Biochem. 1990 Jan;107(1):15-20.

[228] Xu M, Long C, Chen X, Huang C, Chen S, Zhu B. Partitioning of histone H3-H4 tetramers during DNA replication-dependent chromatin assembly. Science. Apr 2;328(5974):94-8.

[229] Taverna SD, Li H, Ruthenburg AJ, Allis CD, Patel DJ. How chromatin-binding modules interpret histone modifications: lessons from professional pocket pickers. Nat Struct Mol Biol. 2007 Nov;14(11):1025-40.

[230] Hansen KH, Bracken AP, Pasini D, Dietrich N, Gehani SS, Monrad A, et al. A model for transmission of the H3K27me3 epigenetic mark. Nat Cell Biol. 2008 Nov;10(11):1291-300.

[231] Loyola A, Bonaldi T, Roche D, Imhof A, Almouzni G. PTMs on H3 variants before chromatin assembly potentiate their final epigenetic state. Mol Cell. 2006 Oct 20;24(2):309-16.

[232] McKittrick E, Gafken PR, Ahmad K, Henikoff S. Histone H3.3 is enriched in covalent modifications associated with active chromatin. Proc Natl Acad Sci U S A. 2004 Feb 10;101(6):1525-30.

[233] Ahmad K, Henikoff S. The histone variant H3.3 marks active chromatin by replication-independent nucleosome assembly. Mol Cell. 2002 Jun;9(6):1191-200.

[234] Probst AV, Dunleavy E, Almouzni G. Epigenetic inheritance during the cell cycle. Nat Rev Mol Cell Biol. 2009 Mar;10(3):192-206.

[235] Tagami H, Ray-Gallet D, Almouzni G, Nakatani Y. Histone H3.1 and H3.3 complexes mediate nucleosome assembly pathways dependent or independent of DNA synthesis. Cell. 2004 Jan 9;116(1):51-61.

[236] Ray-Gallet D, Quivy JP, Scamps C, Martini EM, Lipinski M, Almouzni G. HIRA is critical for a nucleosome assembly pathway independent of DNA synthesis. Mol Cell. 2002 May;9(5):1091-100.

[237] Turner BM. Defining an epigenetic code. Nat Cell Biol. 2007 Jan;9(1):2-6.

[238] Geiman TM, Robertson KD. Chromatin remodeling, histone modifications, and DNA methylation-how does it all fit together? J Cell Biochem. 2002;87(2):117-25.

[239] Brandeis M, Frank D, Keshet I, Siegfried Z, Mendelsohn M, Nemes A, et al. Sp1 elements protect a CpG island from de novo methylation. Nature. 1994 Sep 29;371(6496):435-8.

[240] Siegfried Z, Eden S, Mendelsohn M, Feng X, Tsuberi BZ, Cedar H. DNA methylation represses transcription in vivo. Nat Genet. 1999 Jun;22(2):203-6.

[241] Macleod D, Charlton J, Mullins J, Bird AP. Sp1 sites in the mouse aprt gene promoter are required to prevent methylation of the CpG island. Genes Dev. 1994 Oct 1;8(19): 2282-92.

[242] Ooi SK, Qiu C, Bernstein E, Li K, Jia D, Yang Z, et al. DNMT3L connects unmethylated lysine 4 of histone H3 to de novo methylation of DNA. Nature. 2007 Aug 9;448(7154):714-7.

[243] Meissner A, Mikkelsen TS, Gu H, Wernig M, Hanna J, Sivachenko A, et al. Genome-scale DNA methylation maps of pluripotent and differentiated cells. Nature. 2008 Aug 7;454(7205):766-70.

[244] Weber M, Hellmann I, Stadler MB, Ramos L, Paabo S, Rebhan M, et al. Distribution, silencing potential and evolutionary impact of promoter DNA methylation in the human genome. Nat Genet. 2007 Apr;39(4):457-66.

[245] Mohn F, Weber M, Rebhan M, Roloff TC, Richter J, Stadler MB, et al. Lineage-specific polycomb targets and de novo DNA methylation define restriction and potential of neuronal progenitors. Mol Cell. 2008 Jun 20;30(6):755-66.

[246] Okitsu CY, Hsieh CL. DNA methylation dictates histone H3K4 methylation. Mol Cell Biol. 2007 Apr;27(7):2746-57.

[247] Gidekel S, Bergman Y. A unique developmental pattern of Oct-3/4 DNA methylation is controlled by a cis-demodification element. J Biol Chem. 2002 Sep 13;277(37): 34521-30.

[248] Fuhrmann G, Chung AC, Jackson KJ, Hummelke G, Baniahmad A, Sutter J, et al. Mouse germline restriction of Oct4 expression by germ cell nuclear factor. Dev Cell. 2001 Sep;1(3):377-87.

[249] Ben-Shushan E, Sharir H, Pikarsky E, Bergman Y. A dynamic balance between ARP-1/COUP-TFII, EAR-3/COUP-TFI, and retinoic acid receptor:retinoid X receptor heterodimers regulates Oct-3/4 expression in embryonal carcinoma cells. Mol Cell Biol. 1995 Feb;15(2):1034-48.

[250] Sylvester I, Scholer HR. Regulation of the Oct-4 gene by nuclear receptors. Nucleic Acids Res. 1994 Mar 25;22(6):901-11.

[251] Cedar H, Bergman Y. Linking DNA methylation and histone modification: patterns and paradigms. Nat Rev Genet. 2009 May;10(5):295-304.

[252] Feldman N, Gerson A, Fang J, Li E, Zhang Y, Shinkai Y, et al. G9a-mediated irreversible epigenetic inactivation of Oct-3/4 during early embryogenesis. Nat Cell Biol. 2006 Feb;8(2):188-94.

[253] Bannister AJ, Zegerman P, Partridge JF, Miska EA, Thomas JO, Allshire RC, et al. Selective recognition of methylated lysine 9 on histone H3 by the HP1 chromo domain. Nature. 2001 Mar 1;410(6824):120-4.

[254] Lachner M, O'Carroll D, Rea S, Mechtler K, Jenuwein T. Methylation of histone H3 lysine 9 creates a binding site for HP1 proteins. Nature. 2001 Mar 1;410(6824):116-20.

[255] Bachman KE, Rountree MR, Baylin SB. Dnmt3a and Dnmt3b are transcriptional repressors that exhibit unique localization properties to heterochromatin. J Biol Chem. 2001 Aug 24;276(34):32282-7.

[256] Suzuki MM, Bird A. DNA methylation landscapes: provocative insights from epigenomics. Nat Rev Genet. 2008 Jun;9(6):465-76.

[257] Weber M, Schubeler D. Genomic patterns of DNA methylation: targets and function of an epigenetic mark. Curr Opin Cell Biol. 2007 Jun;19(3):273-80.

[258] Eden S, Hashimshony T, Keshet I, Cedar H, Thorne AW. DNA methylation models histone acetylation. Nature. 1998 Aug 27;394(6696):842.

[259] Hashimshony T, Zhang J, Keshet I, Bustin M, Cedar H. The role of DNA methylation in setting up chromatin structure during development. Nat Genet. 2003 Jun;34(2): 187-92.

[260] Nan X, Ng HH, Johnson CA, Laherty CD, Turner BM, Eisenman RN, et al. Transcriptional repression by the methyl-CpG-binding protein MeCP2 involves a histone deacetylase complex. Nature. 1998 May 28;393(6683):386-9.

[261] Jones PL, Veenstra GJ, Wade PA, Vermaak D, Kass SU, Landsberger N, et al. Methylated DNA and MeCP2 recruit histone deacetylase to repress transcription. Nat Genet. 1998 Jun;19(2):187-91.

[262] Lande-Diner L, Zhang J, Ben-Porath I, Amariglio N, Keshet I, Hecht M, et al. Role of DNA methylation in stable gene repression. J Biol Chem. 2007 Apr 20;282(16): 12194-200.

[263] Zilberman D, Coleman-Derr D, Ballinger T, Henikoff S. Histone H2A.Z and DNA methylation are mutually antagonistic chromatin marks. Nature. 2008 Nov 6;456(7218):125-9.

[264] Jeddeloh JA, Stokes TL, Richards EJ. Maintenance of genomic methylation requires a SWI2/SNF2-like protein. Nat Genet. 1999 May;22(1):94-7.

[265] Raabe EH, Abdurrahman L, Behbehani G, Arceci RJ. An SNF2 factor involved in mammalian development and cellular proliferation. Dev Dyn. 2001 May;221(1): 92-105.

[266] Geiman TM, Muegge K. Lsh, an SNF2/helicase family member, is required for proliferation of mature T lymphocytes. Proc Natl Acad Sci U S A. 2000 Apr 25;97(9):4772-7.

[267] Hart N. Famine, maternal nutrition and infant mortality: a re-examination of the Dutch hunger winter. Popul Stud (Camb). 1993 Mar;47(1):27-46.

[268] Roseboom T, de Rooij S, Painter R. The Dutch famine and its long-term consequences for adult health. Early Hum Dev. 2006 Aug;82(8):485-91.

[269] Newsome CA, Shiell AW, Fall CH, Phillips DI, Shier R, Law CM. Is birth weight related to later glucose and insulin metabolism?--A systematic review. Diabet Med. 2003 May;20(5):339-48.

[270] Curhan GC, Chertow GM, Willett WC, Spiegelman D, Colditz GA, Manson JE, et al. Birth weight and adult hypertension and obesity in women. Circulation. 1996 Sep 15;94(6):1310-5.

[271] de Rooij SR, Painter RC, Roseboom TJ, Phillips DI, Osmond C, Barker DJ, et al. Glucose tolerance at age 58 and the decline of glucose tolerance in comparison with age 50 in people prenatally exposed to the Dutch famine. Diabetologia. 2006 Apr;49(4): 637-43.

[272] Lumey LH, Stein AD, Kahn HS, van der Pal-de Bruin KM, Blauw GJ, Zybert PA, et al. Cohort profile: the Dutch Hunger Winter families study. Int J Epidemiol. 2007 Dec;36(6):1196-204.

[273] Ravelli AC, van der Meulen JH, Michels RP, Osmond C, Barker DJ, Hales CN, et al. Glucose tolerance in adults after prenatal exposure to famine. Lancet. 1998 Jan 17;351(9097):173-7.

[274] Heijmans BT, Tobi EW, Stein AD, Putter H, Blauw GJ, Susser ES, et al. Persistent epigenetic differences associated with prenatal exposure to famine in humans. Proc Natl Acad Sci U S A. 2008 Nov 4;105(44):17046-9.

4

Methylomes

Minghua Wu

1. Introduction

Epigenetic modifications stably influence gene expression without changing the underlying DNA sequence [1]. The epigenomic era has revealed a well-connected network of molecular processes. These processes comprise abnormal methylomes, transcriptosomes, genome-wide histone post-transcriptional modifications patterns, histone variants, and noncoding RNAs [2]. The genome-wide DNA methylation status of cells exists in a methylated, hydroxymethylated or unmethylated state, collectively referred to as the DNA methylome [3]. Methylation of the DNA (DNAme) occurs in position 5 in cytosine residues. In mammals, the vast majority (98%) of DNA methylation occurs in CpG (cytosine-phosphate-guanine) dinucleotides in somatic cells [4]. In embryomic stem (ES) cells, however, about one-quarter of all DNA methylation occurs in non-CpG context [4]. The haploid human genome contains approximately 29 million CpGs, DNA methylation involves the transfer of a methyl group to cytosine in a CpG dinucleotide through DNA methyltransferases that creates or maintains methylation patterns [3]. Hydroxymethylation of cytosines has also been reported, though its biological functions are unknown. Several methods have been developed which enable capture of genome-wide profiling of DNA methylation. The complete DNA methylomes for several organisms are now available, helping clarify the evolutionary story of this epigenetic mark and its distribution in key genomic elements. The variation of DNA methylome plays an important role in regulating normal development and differentiation. DNA methylation patterns can be inherited and influenced by the environment, diet and aging, and disrupted in diseases [5]. From a functional perspective, the DNA methylome variation is a stable change in a transcriptional regulatory element, which changes the expression of a gene without any change in DNA sequence or in the intracellular environment. However, a change in environmental conditions could perturb the stability profile of the methylome at a locus, changing the probability of variant states arising, even making a variant state more stable than the previous reference state [6].

2. Methylomes and evolution

DNA methylation is a typical characteristic of most eukaryotes and some of its features are conserved in many species. The methylation states that present in the germline are heritable and participate in evolution. Boffelli D and Martin DI [6] combined phylogenomic and somatic methylation data to infer germline methylation states. Methylated CGs undergo mutation to TG much more frequently than unmethylated CGs, but only CG decay that occurs in the germline results in heritable sequence changes that can become fixed within a species. The predominant trend within the genome is to lose methylated cytosines and this destrucrion of a CpG dinucleotide by a SNP has been shown to lead to significant cis-methylation effects [7]. The loss and gain of CpGs over time is proposed to be a significant evolutionary device, the polymorphic nature of CpG-SNP dinucleotide sequences will help define human population epigenomics [8].

Currently, by the base-resolution sequencing, the complete methylomes for 25 organisms are available (10 animals, 8 plants, 2 insect and 5 fungi). These eukaryotic methylomes have provided initial insights into the evolutionary history of DNA methylation (Figure 1). Since the density of possible methylation sites, and the distribution of 5-methyl-cytosines (5meC) is not uniform in the genome contexts, the role of DNA methylation in promoters, gene bodies, regulatory features, and transposable and repetitive elements can be remarkably different. Such as, the evolutionary history of DNA methylation in gene bodies and transposons is independent. Zemach et al. quantified DNA methylation in 17 eukaryotic genomes and found that gene body methylation is an ancient property of eukaryotic genomes, and is conserved between plants and animals, whereas selective methylation of transposons is not [9]. The transposon methylation is only conserved in fungi [10], and appears to be related to the degree of sexual outcrossing [11]. In general, the DNA methylation landscape can be either continuous along the genome, or constituted by a series of heavily methylated DNA domains interspersed with domains that are methylation free, and the methylation pattern is quite conserved [5].

3. Human methylomes

Because of its association with human development and disease, DNA methylation has stayed in the research focus for almost half a century. The development of methods for whole-genome methylation profiling has now enabled acquisition of the complete human methylomes, especially powerful are methylome profiling techniques with single-base resolution sequencing. Genome-wide, tissue-specific or cell type-specific DNA methylation profiling has begun to shift the focus of DNA methylation research from mostly promoters and immediate upstream enhancers to including intragenic regions and distal intergenetic regions [12]. These revealed that methylation of gene bodies is more frequent than in promoters in the vertebrate genomes [13]. Shen et al [14] characterized the methylome in purified peripheral blood monocytes (PBMs) by using methylated DNA immunoprecipitation combined with high-throughput sequencing, and found that promoters were commonly (58%) found to be

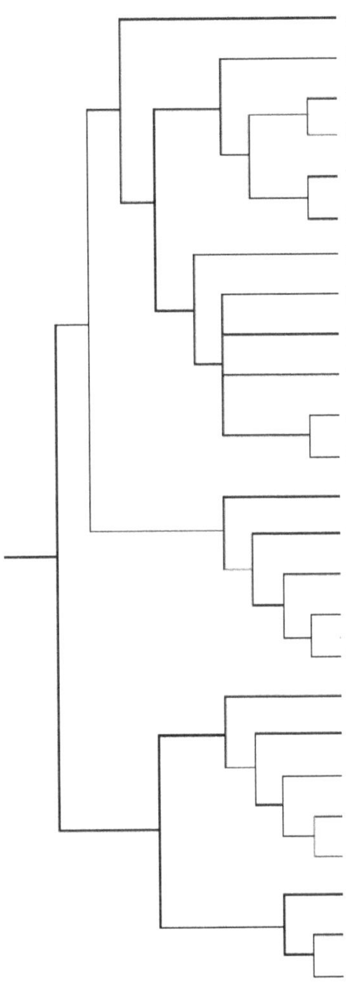

	Genome Size/Mb	mCG%	mCHG%	mCHH%
Nematostella vectensis	356.6	9.40	.16	.15
Ciona intestinalis	116.7	21.60	.28	.15
Mus musculus	2798.8	74.20	.30	.29
Homo sapiens	3234.8	67-72	.09-2.80	.04-.90
Tetraodon nigroviridis	342.4	65.20	.25	.34
Danio rerio	1412.5	80.30	1.22	.91
Schistocerca gregaria(brain)	11.1	92.0		
Drosophila melanogaster	139.5	.12	.11	.11
Bombyx mori	481.8	.71	.08	.09
Tribolium castaneum	210.3	.11	.12	.12
Apis mellifera	250.3	.51	.11	.16
Nasonia vitripennis	297.7	64.9		
Phycomyces blakesleeanus	51.1	4.90		
Uncinocarpus reesii	22.4	.67		
Postia placenta	90.9	12.1		
Laccaria bicolor	64.9	20.3		
Coprinopsis cinerea	36.2	12.2		
Physcomitrella patens	478.0	29.5	29.7	23.2
Selaginella moellendorffii	212.5	12.5	9.0	23.2
Oryza sativa	382.6	50.00	27.40	5.20
Arabidopsis thaliana	119.6	22.30	5.92	1.51
Populus trichocarpa	485.7	41.9	20.9	3.25
Chlorella sp. NC64A	46.4	80.5	2.2	0.25
Volvox carteri	137.7	2.6	.08	.08
Chlamydomonas reinhardtii	120.4	5.4	2.59	2.49

Figure 1. Methylation levels in 25 eukaryotic organisms. The organisms are organized according to their evolutionary distance. Tree topology is determined from the NCBI Taxonomy (http://www.ncbi.nlm.nih.gov/guide/taxonomy/) and displayed using TreeView X (http://darwin.zoology.gla.ac.uk/~rpage/treeviewx/index.html). The genome size is indicated together with the percentage of methylated sites within three sequence contexts: CpG, CHG and CHH (H being A, C or T).

unmethylated; whereas protein coding regions were largely (84%) methylated. Zilbauer et al [15] provide detailed functional genome-wide methylome maps of five primary peripheral blood leukocyte subsets including T-cells, B-cells, monocytes/ macrophages and neutrophils obtained from healthy individuals and identified important cell-type specific hypomethylated regions (HMRs) that strongly correlate with gene transcription levels. SNPs associated with immune-mediated disease in genome-wide association studies (GWAS) preferentially localised to these cell-specific regulatory HMRs, offering insight into the pathogenesis role of DNA hypomethylation in regulating immune mediated disease. Recent insights into tissue-specific intra-and intergenic methylation and into cancer methylomes suggest that both cancer-associated DNA hypomethylation and hypermethylation are found throughout the genome [16]. The hypermethylation includes promoters of tumor suppressor genes whose expression becomes repressed, thereby facilitating cancer formation. Cancer-associated DNA hypomethylation from intergenic enhancers, promoter regions, silencers, and chromatin boundary elements may alter transcription rates. Whereas, the intragenic DNA hypomethylation might modulate alternative promoter usage, production of intragenic noncoding RNA transcripts, cotranscriptional splicing, and transcription initiation or elongation [16].The new discoveries that genomic 5-hydroxymethylcytosine is an intermediate in DNA demethylation and exhibits cancer-associated losses.

4. Methylomes in cell differentiation and reprogramming

During embryonic development, cells become gradually restricted in their developmental potential and start elaborating lineage-specific transcriptional networks to ultimately acquire a unique differentiated state [17].That is, cell differentiation is a process characterized by the progressive loss of developmental potential and gain in functional specialization. During this process, DNA methylation plays an important role in epigenetic programming by silencing developmental genes and activating tissue-specific genes, thus establishing a cellular memory that defines both cell lineage and cell type.

4.1. DNA methylation remodeling in the embryo development

Over the course of mammalian development, the genome undergo nearly complete remodeling of DNA methylation patterns. Primordial germ cells begin with very low DNA methylation levels, then with gametogenesis parental imprinting tags are established, with substantially methylated but differing methylomes in the sperm and egg. In the preimplantation early embryo there is a wave of genome-wide demethylation that occurs, which is rapid in the paternal genome, except for centromeric, repetitive and paternally imprinted genes, with a comparative slow process occurring in the maternal genome [18].This is then followed by heavy de novo methylation, DNA methylation patterns are then progressively re-established, marking gradual commitment towards lineage-specific differentiation [19].

4.2. DNA methylomes in embryonic stem cells

Embryonic stem cells (ESCs) are a special population of pluripotent cells derived from the inner cell mass (ICM) of a blastocyst during mammalian development. ESCs retain the ability to indefinitely self-renew and differentiate into all cell types found in the adult body. The importance of DNA methylation in ESC stemness maintenance and differentiation is indicated by diverse studies demonstrating the following: (1) DNA methylation is essential for pluripotency but not self-renewal in ESCs. Embryonic stem cells deficient in Dnmt1 and/or Dnmt3a/3b or lacking CpG-binding proteins show a loss of pluripotency and severe impairment of differentiation potential, but still maintain self-renew [20-23]. (2) CpG methylation contributes to differentiation of ESCs. In a search for differentially methylated (DM) regions (DMRs) by reduced-representation bisulfite sequencing(RRBS), Meissner et al [24] found that approximately 8% of CpGs that were unmethylated in ESCs became methylated in ESC-derived neural progenitor cells and approximately 2% of CpGs methylated in ESCs were unmethylated in the neural progenitor derivatives; Genomic analysis provides supporting evidence for the CpG methylation of gene promoters to selectively silence differentiation genes in ESCs, and global DNA demethylation is mostly linked with the upregulation of tissue-specific genes [25]. (3) ESCs are enriched in non-CpG methylation. A recent major study using Methyl-Seq technology reports significant non-CpG methylation in human ESCs, estimating nearly 25% of total cytosine methylation to be non-CpG sites, with CHG and CHH as the major motifs (where H=A, C, or T). Genomic regions enriched in non-CpG methylation are associated with genes involved in RNA processing, RNA splicing and RNA metabolic processes. Interestingly, enrichment of non-CpG methylation in gene bodies correlates with significantly more intronic RNA.

4.3. DNA methylation remodeling in multipotent stem cells

Multipotent stem cells provide a unique intermediate between pluripotent ESCs and unipotent differentiated cells. Multipotent stem cells also show significant reprogramming variability, including somatic memory and aberrant reprogramming of DNA methylation [26].

4.3.1. Mesenchymal stem cells

Mesenchymal stem cells (MSCs) are multipotent stem cells of mesodermal origin that can be isolated from various sources and induced into different cell types [27]. Adipose tissue-derived stem cells (ADSCs) are isolated from liposuction material, which provide an abundant source of MSCs. Studies show that select adipogenic and nonadipogenic promoters in MSCs, ADSCs and hESCs are hypomethylated and hypermethylated, respectively, suggesting DNA methylation controls adipogenic differentiation by activating adipogenic-related genes and silencing nonspecific lineage genes[27]. In addition, epigenomic changes in DNA methylation and chromatin structure have been hypothesized to be critical in the determination of lineage-specific differentiation and tumorigenesis of MSCs [27]. Leu et al [27] applied a targeted DNA methylation method to methylate a polycomb group protein-governed gene, Trip10, in MSCs, which accelerated the cell fate determination of MSCs. However, targeted methylation of HIC1 and RassF1A, both tumor suppressor genes, transformed MSCs into tumor stem cell-like cells.

4.3.2. Hematopoietic stem cells

Hematopoietic stem cells (HSCs) are a special population of multipotent stem cells that are derived from the bone marrow and give rise to a subset of mature blood cells that directs all the immune responses. Accumulating evidence suggests that DNA methylation play critical roles in the maintenance of both self-renewing hematopoietic stem cells and leukemic stem cells [29]. Changes in the DNA methylation profile have a critical role in the division of these stem cells into the myeloid and lymphoid lineages and in the establishment of a specific phenotype and functionality in each terminally differentiated cell type [30]. HSCs deficient in both Dnmt3a and 3b show a loss of proliferative ability but retain differentiation potential, suggesting de novo methylation is important for self-renewal in HSCs [28]. The aberrant DNA methylation has been associated with several immune deficiencies and autoimmune disorders [30].

4.3.3. Multipotent neural progenitor cells

The central nervous system (CNS) is composed of three major cell types-neurons, astrocytes, and oligodendrocytes-which differentiate from common multipotent neural stem cells (NSCs). Comparisons between ESCs, NSCs and terminally differentiated neurons demonstrate that the majority of de novo methylated genes are already present in NSCs, suggesting that the bulk of DNA methylation changes during differentiation is associated with a loss of pluripotency and a commitment to a multipotent state, rather than terminal differentiation [28]. Interestingly, when NSCs further differentiate into astroglial lineage, selective promoter demethylation occurs in glial marker genes, including GFAP and S100B [31, 32]. Loss of methylation using 5-azacytidine (5-azaC) also triggers premature glial differentiation [31]. Consistently, Dnmt1-deficient NSCs precociously differentiate into astroglial cells, which have been linked to increase JAK-STAT signaling and demethylation of the STAT1 and GFAP promoters [32].

4.4. DNA methylations in cell reprogramming

Epigenetic marks can be reset and usually result in the gain of developmental potential, called epigenetic reprogramming. Researches indicated that mammalian somatic cells can be directly reprogrammed into induced pluripotent stem cells (iPSCs) by introducing defined sets of transcription factors Oct4, Sox2, Klf4 and c-Myc [33-35]. The ultimate aim of research on cell reprogramming is to create iPSC that is identical to embryonic stem cells (ESC) and differentiates into tissue specific cell types with intact function, which will pave the way for great advances in regenerative medicine in the future.

4.4.1. 5-hydroxymethylcytosine-mediated epigenetic modifications during reprogramming to pluripotency

Although 5-hydroxymethylcytosine (5hmC) was discovered several decades ago, it became a major focus of epigenomic research only after it was recently identified in murine brain and stem cell DNA. 5hmC is an oxidative product of 5-methylcytosine (5mC) which catalyzed by the ten eleven translocation (TET) family of enzymes [36]. TET1-mediated 5hmC modification could contribute to the epigenetic variation of iPSCs reprogramming and iPSC-hESC differences [37]. Wang et al [37] found that 5hmC levels is increased significantly during reprogramming to human iPSCs mainly owing to TET1 activation, and this hydroxymethylation change is critical for optimal epigentic reprogramming, but does not compromise primed pluripotency.

4.4.2. Non-CpG cytosine methylation in cells reprogramming

Although methylation mainly occurs on the cytosines in the CpG dinucleotide context, non-CG methylation (mCH:DNA methylation targeting CpA, CpT, and CpC dinucleotides) is prevalent in brain, oocytes and pluripotent stem cell [38-40]. Compared to non-growing oocytes (NGOs), germinal vesicle oocytes (GVOs) were over four times more methylated at non-CG sites, indicating that non-CG methylation accumulates during oocyte growth. Widespread methylome reconfiguration occurs during fetal to young adult development, coincident with synaptogenesis. During this period, highly conserved non-CG methylation (mCH) accumulates in neurons, but not glia, to become the dominant form of methylation in the human neuronal genome[38]. Shirane et al [39] found that nearly two-thirds of all methylcytosines occur in a non-CG context in GVOs. The distribution of non-CG methylation closely resembled that of CG methylation throughout the genome and showed clear enrichment in gene bodies. Ziller et al [40] reported a comprehensive analysis of non-CpG methylation in 76 genome-scale DNA methylation maps across pluripotent and differentiated human cell types, and confirm non-CpG methylation to be predominantly present in pluripotent cell types and observe a decrease upon differentiation and near complete absence in various somatic cell types. Non-CpG cytosine methylation has been identified at a high level in stem cells and reprogrammed progenitor cells, indicating that loss of this form of methylation may be critical in the path from pluripotency to differentiation. The total level of global methylation and the degree of non-CpG methylation is inversely proportional to the level of differentiation.

5. Methylomes in cancer

Carcinogenesis is a complex multifactorial process of the transformation of normal cells into malignant cells, and is characterized by many biologically significant and interdependent alterations triggered by the mutational and/or non-mutational (i.e., epigenetic) events. One of these events, specific to all types of cancer, is alterations in DNA methylation. Aberrant DNA methylation is frequently observed and considered to be a hallmark of cancers.

5.1. DNA methylome alterations induced by carcinogens

According to the mechanism of cancer causation, all carcinogenic agents may be divided into genotoxic (carcinogenic agents that interact with DNA) and non-genotoxic (carcinogenic agents causing tumor by mechanisms other than directly damaging DNA) carcinogens (Figure 2). Exposure to genotoxic carcinogens induces genotoxic and non-genotoxic effects in the DNA methylome, whereas exposure to non-genotoxic carcinogens causes non-genotoxic effects only. Genotoxic effects on the DNA methylome are consist of increased carcinogen–DNA-adduct formation at methylated CpG sites and subsequent elevated mutation rates; however, genotoxic effects may cause also non-genotoxic events in the DNA methylome by compromising ability of the DNA methylation machinery to methylate DNA accurately. Nongenotoxic effects of both genotoxic and non-genotoxic carcinogens consist of global loss of DNA methylation, gene-specific hypermethylation, and gene-specific hypomethylation. Non-genotoxic global DNA hypomethylation leads to genotoxic events such as elevated mutation rates and genome instability. Gene specific DNA hypermethylation of critical tumor suppressor genes causes transcriptional repression and the loss of gene function. In contrast, gene specific DNA hypomethylation induces activation of oncogenes and tumor-promoting genes. Silencing of DNA repair genes, e.g., MGMT, BRCA1 and MLH1, or activation of xenobiotic metabolizing genes, e.g., CYP1A1, may elevate mutation rates indirectly.

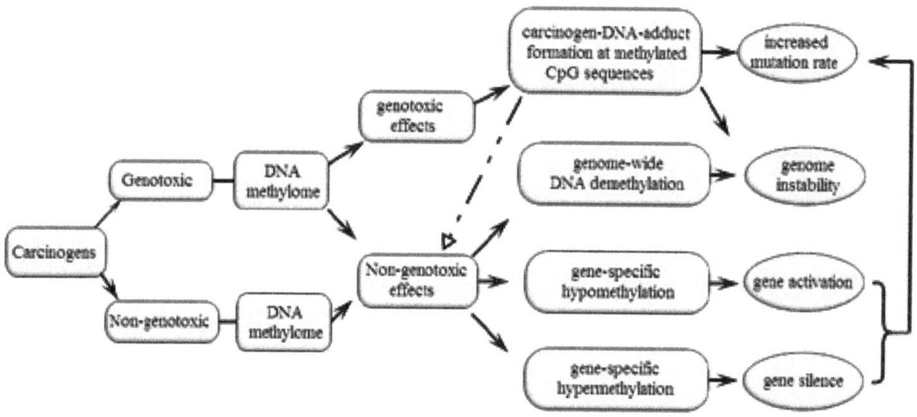

Figure 2. Alterations of the DNA methylome induced by carcinogens

5.1.1. Global DNA hypomethylation in cancer

DNA hypomethylation arises mainly from the loss of methylation at normally heavily methylated areas of genome. The loss of global DNA methylation is one of the most common DNA methylome alterations in human cancers, which is closely related to carcinogenesis. First, genomic demethylation causes a significant elevation in mutation rates] and aberrant activation of"normally"silenced tumor promoting genes [41-43]. Second, hypomethylation of DNA results in the loss of genomic imprinting (LOI), which is currently considered as one of the earliest and most frequent alterations in human tumors [44-46]. Third, demethylation of repetitive sequences, such as long interspersed nucleotide elements (LINE)-1, short interspersed nucleotide elements (SINE), and retroviral intracisternal. Alu elements may cause chromosomal abnormalities and genomic instability via the induction of permissive transcriptional activity of repetitive elements [47-48]. Finally, the recent research indicated that the loss of 5hmC has been found in a broad spectrum of solid tumors, including lung, breast, brain, gastric, and colorectal cancers [49-50].

5.1.2. Cancer-linked gene-specific DNA hypermethylation or hypomethylation

DNA hypermethylation is the most extensively studied epigenetic abnormality in cancer, and the hypermethylation of promoter CpG islands causes permanent and stable transcriptional silencing of a wide range of protein-coding genes and non-coding RNA genes. There is also growing evidence for the importance of non-CpG island-promoter methylation in cancer, including methylation of CpG island shores [51], non-CpG promoters [52], and coding regions [53], which results in gene silencing. A mechanistic link between DNA hypermethylation and carcinogenesis is epigenetic silencing of critical tumor-suppressor genes, such as cyclin-dependent kinase inhibitor 2A (CDKN2A; p16INK4A), secreted frizzled-related protein genes (SFRPs), adenomatous polyposis coli (APC), Ras association (RalGDS/AF-6) domain family member 1 (RASSF1A) [54], et al. It has been established unequivocally that role of epigenetically-driven gene silencing has been the main mechanism favoring tumor development and progression. This overshadowed the importance of gene-specific hypomethylation in cancer; however, accumulating evidence indicates that the hypomethylation of "normally" methylated CpG island-containing genes also plays a significant role in tumor development. Currently, several hypomethylated tumor-promoting genes, including S100 calcium binding protein A4 (S100A4), plasminogen activator, urokinase (UPA), heparanase (HPA), synuclein, gamma (SNCG), trefoil factor 3 (TFF3), and flap structure-specific endonuclease 1 (FEN1), have been identified in major human cancers [55].

Anyway, cancer-linked gene-specific DNA hypermethylation and hypomethylation are associated with the well-established hallmarks of cancer, including the acquisition of persistent proliferative signaling, resistance to cell death, evasion of growth suppression, replicative immortality, inflammation, deregulation of energy metabolism, induction of angiogenesis, and activation of invasion, complement and enhance each other in the disruption of cellular homeostasis favoring cancer development [56]. Next, as examples, the role of DNA methylation alterations in carcinogenesis was demonstrated in chronic lymphocytic leukemia and glioma.

5.2. Methylome in chronic lymphocytic leukemia

Chronic lymphocytic leukemia (CLL) is the most frequent leukemia of adults in western countries. Next-generation sequencing of whole genomes, exomes and DNA methylomes in CLL has provided the first comprehensive view of somatic mutations and methylation changes in this disease. Here, we mainly elaborate the change of DNA methylomes in CLL.

5.2.1. Hypomethylation contributes to the genomic instability and oncogene activation in CLL

Two decades ago, high-pressure liquid chromatography (HPLC) analysis revealed the genome DNA of CLL to be globally hypomethylated relative to healthy controls. The subsequent study found that aberrant hypomethylation of repetitive sequences, such as ALU, LINE and SATα leading to genomic instability may be a contributing factor in the increased propensity of TP53-deleted/mutated cases to acquire CLL genomic alterations [57]. Recently, next-generation sequencing of the DNA methylome has also noted gene body hypomethylation to be particularly widespread within enhancer regions in CLL patients [57-59]. After the CLL genome was discovered to be hypomethylated, hypomethylation of oncogene is found to correlate with increased protein expression in CLL. Such as, BCL2, a key anti-apoptotic gene, MDR1, the multiple drug resistance gene, and TCL1, an activator of NF-κB, were subsequently found to be hypomethylated and upregulated in CLL [57].

5.2.2. Cells origin and subtypes of CLL on basis of genome and methylome

Because of the differences in the immunoglobulin heavy variation (IGHV) mutational status and B-cell receptor reactivity, chronic lymphocytic leukemia was classified into two subtypes: chronic lymphocytic leukemia lacking significant somatic IGHV mutation (uCLL) and chronic lymphocytic leukemia with significant somatic IGHV mutation (mCLL), which was derived from naive B cells and memory B cells [60]. Most mutated genes cluster in a few molecular pathways that are also differentially represented in the two subtypes of CLL. Mutations in NOTCH1 signaling, mRNA splicing, processing and transport, and DNA damage response pathways are more common in uCLL, whereas mutations in the innate inflammatory pathway occur predominantly in mCLL.

B cells at different maturation stages require a different level of DNA methylation reprogramming to give rise to uCLL and mCLL. Microarray analysis of a large series of patients indicates that uCLLs acquire approximately seven times more DNA methylation changes than mCLL compared with their respective cells of origin. In particular, two-thirds of the DNA methylation changes that take place in the transformation of naive B cells into uCLL can also be detected in their physiological differentiation into memory B cells [58].

By genome-wide differential DNA methylation profile analysis in uCLL and mCLL, CLL was derived from three different B-cell subpopulations: uCLL resembles both native B cells (IgD $^{+}$and CD27^{-}) and CD5^{+} pregerminal center mature B cells (CD5^{+}, IgD^{+}, and CD27^{-}), whereas mCLL is more similar to non class-switched and class-switched memory B cells (IgM/ D^{+} or IgA/G^{+}, CD27^{+}). The third group of CLL was accompied with an intermediate DNA methylation pattern and enriched for mCLLs with a significantly lower level of somatic IGHV mutations [58]. This group might be derived from a third B-cell type, for example, an antigen-experienced, germinal center-independent B cell that has acquired low levels of somatic hypermutations [60].

5.3. Methylomes in glioma

Glioma is the most frequent and devastating primary brain tumor in adults. Aberrant DNA methylation contributes to glioma development and progression.We employed MeDIP-chip to investigate the whole-genome differential methylation patterns between glioma and normal brain samples. We identified 524 hypermethylated and 114 hypomethylated differential regions in the primary gliomas. Intriguingly, some of the human genome differential methylation regions (DMRs), 199 hypermethylation and 30 hypomethylated differential regions were mapped to genomic regions without any gene annotation (Fig 3A). Only 325 hypermethylation and 74 hypomethylation differential regions were mapped to annotated genes regions, including promoter, intragenic and downstream of genes (Fig3A). A great percentage of DMRs, 63.0% (216) of hypermethylated and 79.0% (60) of hypomethylated differential regions, was mapped to promoter regions of known genes (Fig 3B). 53 hypermethylated and 27 hypomethylated differential regions were mapped to the regions which were both promoter of known genes and CpG islands (Fig 3C). Thus, we identified many novel DMRs that reside in promoters, intragenic, downstream of known genes and unannotated genomic regions in primary gliomas. Since change of promoter methylation status may have close related with gene expression and involved in tumor development, we focused on the analysis of DMRs in glioma which were mapped to gene promoter regions. The 216 promoter hypermethylated genes and 60 promoter hypomethylated genes identified by MeDIP-chip were analyzed according to their chromosomal location and the physical distribution of these loci was further analyzed (Fig 3D). Except that there were intensive promoter hypermethylation genes in 1, 2, 3, 17 and X chromosomes, the promoter hypermethylated genes were found to be distributed evenly in other chromosomes. While promoter hypomethylated genes mainly distributed in 1, 11, 16, 19, 20 and 22 chromosomes, the number of genes in these chromosomes account for the majority of the total promoter hypomethylated genes [61].

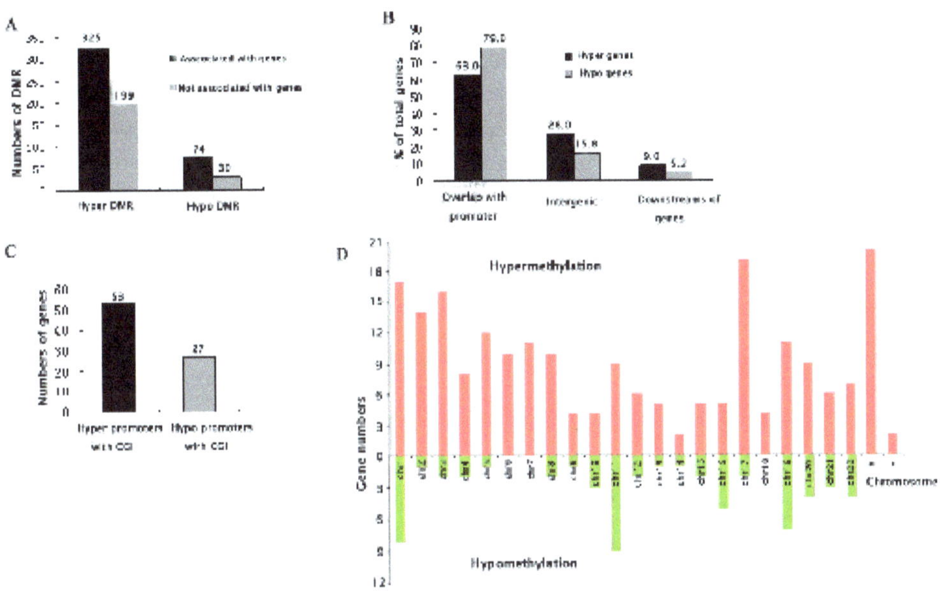

Figure 3. Genome-wide analysis of DMRs in primary glioma. (A) Number of differentially methylated regions that are associated with or without genes. (B) Distribution of diifferentially methylated regions associated with genes. Most of the identified DMRs associated with genes were mapped to gene promoters. (C) Number of DMRs which were both gene promoters and CpG islands. (D) Chromosomal distribution of 216 promoter hypermethylated genes and 60 promoter hypomethylated genes.

6. The connected networks of DNA methylation, histone modifications, transcript factor and miRNAs

Epigenetic mechanisms include: DNA methylation; histone tail modifications; chromatin remodeling; and noncoding RNA expression. DNA methylation is essential for a properly functioning genome through its roles in the maintenance of chromatin structure, chromosome stability and transcription. Histones are the protein moiety around which DNA is packaged within the chromatin, and they can suffer a variety of post-translational modifications of their

N-terminal tails, including acetylation, methylation, phosphorylation, sumoylation, ubiquitination and ADP ribosylation [62,63]. miRNAs are ~20–22 nucleotide non-coding RNA molecules that tend to negatively regulate genes by binding to the 3' untranslated region of the target mRNA via the RNA-induced silencing complex causing mRNA destabilization and/or translational inhibition [64,65]. Growing evidence supports a role for miRNAs as both targets and effectors in aberrant mechanisms of DNA methylation [66,67]. Meanwhile, miRNAs are also invovlved in the control of DNA methylation by targeting the DNA methylation machinery [68, 69]. In this section, we combined with our own work to demonstrate the connected networks of DNA methylation, histone modifications, transcript factor and miRNAs in glioma. On the basis DNA methylome of glioma, we identified fifteen new methylated genes including 9 hypermethylated genes(ANKDD1A, GAD1, SIX3, SST, PHOX2B, PCDHA8,PCDHA13, HIST1H3E and LRRC4) and 6 hypomethylated genes (F10, POTEH, CPEB1, LMO3, ELFN2 and PRDM16) were validated by the Sequenom MassARRAY platform and bisulfite sequencing (BSP) in glioma. Aberrant promoter methylation and changed histone modifications were associated with gene abnormal expression in glioma. miR-185 targets the DNA methyltransferases 1 and regulates global DNA methylation [61], however, miR-101 regulates histone methylation modication of hypomethylated gene CPEB1 by targeting EZH2 and EED, and DNMT3A, and affected their methylation level and expression in glioma [70].

6.1. The regulation networks between hypermethylated gene, miRNA, transcript factor and target gene in glioma

Leucine-rich repeat C4 (LRRC4) gene, a new hypermethylated gene identified by DNA methylome of glioma, are highly specific to brain tissue and it behaved as a tumor suppressor gene in the pathogenesis of gliomas. Methylation of the LRRC4 promoter has been considered as one of the important mechanisms inactivating LRRC4 in gliomas. Exogenous overexpression of LRRC4 could inhibit glioma cells growth and arrest glioma cells in the G0/G1 phase of the cell cycle. Induction of LRRC4 expression inhibited glioma cell proliferation and invasion by downregulating the ERK/MAPK and PI-3K/AKT signaling pathways [71-75].

6.1.1. LRRC4-AP-2-miR-182-LRRC4 loop played important role in the pathogenesis of glioma

It's known that miRNAs took part in proliferation and growth in glioma cells. miR-182 or miR-381 overexpression could promote glioma cell growth in vivo and in vitro. Therefore, they were considered to be potential therapeutic biomarker in glioma. miR-182 or miR-381 silencing could arrest glioma cells in the G0/G1 phase of the cell cycle and inhibit glioma cells growth by upregulating phosphorylated Rb and suppressing E2F3. LRRC4 was the co-target gene of miR-182 and miR-381. The expression of miR-182, miR-381 and BRD7 were inversely correlated with LRRC4 expression in gliomas. miR-182 and miR-381 silencing was found to inhibit the expression of BRD7, upregulate phosphorylated Rb, suppress E2F3, arrest glioma cells in the G0/G1 phase of the cell cycle, inhibit glioma cells growth and induce differentiation of glioma cells to astrocyte-like cell by upregulating LRRC4 and suppressing LRRC4-mediated binding of AP-2/SP1/E2F6/c-Myc to BRD7 in ERK/MAPK and PI-3K/AKT signal pathways [76].

Transcription of miR-182 was induced by transcription factor AP-2 predicted by online softwares and confimed by ChIP. According to our previous results, miR-182 was verified to inhibit the expression of LRRC4, and LRRC4 might inhibit the expression and transcription of AP-2 through negatively regulating the ERK/MAPK and PI-3K/AKT signaling pathways. It's indicated that the LRRC4-AP-2-miR-182-LRRC4 loop formed among LRRC4, miR-182 and AP-2 was involved in glioma development [77].

6.1.2. LRRC4-miR-185/SP1-DNMT1-LRRC4 loop played an important role in glioma

miR-185 could function as a tumor suppressor gene. It's certified that miR-185 could inhibit glioma cell growth, motility and invasion identified by MTT, scratch test and transwell test [78-80]. DNMT1 is one of the most important DNA methyltransferase which maintains methylation. Our research showed that overexpression of miR-185 could inhibit DNMT1 and reduce global methylation by HPLC-DAD, and decreased the expression of nine new hyper-methylated genes (LRRC4, ANKDD1A, GAD1, HIST1H3E, PCDHA8, PCDHA13, PHOX2B, SIX3 and SST) [61]. Hence, miR-185 was considered to inhibit glioma cells growth and migration by targeting DNMT1, reducing global methylation and recovering expression of such hypermethylation genes as LRRC4.

miR-185 also was predicted to participate in Rho GTPase activity based on GO analysis, while CDC42 and RhoA were the main elements regulating Rho GTPase. Then CDC42 and RhoA were identified to be the direct targets of miR-185[61]. Further, CDC42 and RhoA were inversely correlated with miR-185 expression in gliomas. miR-185 was clarified to mediate glioma cell growth and migration by inhibiting CDC42 and RhoA and VEGFA indirectly [61].

It's verified that overexpressing LRRC4 could increase the expression of miR-185, while miR-185 could regulate global methylation by inhibiting DNA methyltranferase DNMT1 and increasing the expression of such hypermethylation gene as LRRC4. There may be form LRRC4-miR-185-DNMT1-LRRC4 loop which LRRC4 are to be as core the loop, miR185 and DNMT1 that participating in glioma development. In addition,. DNMT1 was positively regulated by SP1, and it could increase the expression of LRRC4, while LRRC4 could also inhibit SP1 by negatively regulate ERK/MAPK and PI-3K/AKT signal pathway. So that the LRRC4-SP1-DNMT1-LRRC4 loop formed among LRRC4, SP1 and DNMT1 took part in the glioma formation.

In conclusion, development of glioma is the pathological processing with multiple genes and multi-stages. Genes, miRNAs and DNA methylation play an important role in glioma formation. They may support or antagonize each other and construct complicated network in glioma. In sum of above study, at the time of LRRC4 regulating miRNAs as a tumor suppressor, those miRNAs regulated by LRRC4 were found to regulate the binding of transcription factors to DNA in their targets mediated signaling pathways by directly targeting genes (such as LRRC4), or regulate methylation and expression of such hypermethylation genes as LRRC4 by directly targeting DNA methyltransferase and controlling global methylation. And multipases regulation loops which the core was LRRC4 were formed. They were LRRC4-AP-2-miR-182-LRRC4, LRRC4-miR-185-DNMT1-LRRC4 and LRRC4-SP1-DNMT1-LRRC4. These loops participated in glioma development with multiple positive feedback formation among them (Fig 4).

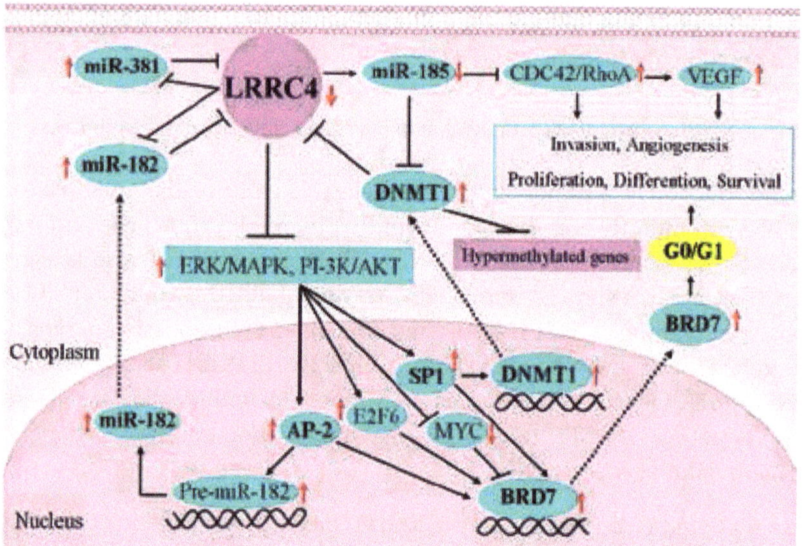

Figure 4. The regulation networks of hypermethylated genes, miRNA, DNMT, transcript factors and targets genes in glioma

6.2. miR-101 regulates the expression of hypomethylated/hpermethylated genes by different histone protein methylaiton modification

It's well-known that miRNAs play significant role by regulating gene expression in tumors. We assumed to analyze the upregulation mechanism of hypomethylation genes in the extent of gene regulation by miRNA. Subsequently, we predicted miRNAs which could regulate hypomethylation genes CPEB1. Interestedly, CPEB1was predicted to be a target of miR-101 by online software Targetscan6.0. It's confirmed that miR-101 could bind to the 3′UTR of CPEB1 and inhibit their expression [70].

6.2.1. miR-101 indirectly suppressed expression of CPEB1 and affected their methylation levels by targeting EZH2, EED and DNMT3A and regulating histone methylation in glioma cells

As miR-101 regulated the methylation status and expression of gene through histone modification, it may regulate the methylation status of CPEB1 in the same way. Hence, the effect of miR-101, EZH2 siRNA, EED siRNA and DNMT3A siRNA on histone methylation and expression of CPEB1 was detected. ChIP combining with qRT-PCR and BSP was used to verify that miR-101 decreased the H3K4me2 and H3K27me3 occupancy at CPEB1 core promoter and increased the H3K9me3 and H4K20me3 occupancy at CPEB1 core promoter by targeting

EZH2, EED and DNMT3A, then it recovered the methylation levels of CPEB1 gene promoter, and indirectly down-regulating the expression of these hypomethylation genes.

6.2.2. miR-101 recovered the expression of hypermethylation gene LRRC4 by down-regulating H3K27me3 occupancy and hypomethylation level of LRRC4 in glioma cells

LRRC4 has been a glioma suppressor gene and its hypermethylation and down-expression is common in glioma. In order to clarify the mechanism of LRRC4 regulation, miRNAs regulating LRRC4 were predicted. miR-101 was predicted to target LRRC4. Here, we indicated that miR-101 could not bind to 3′UTR of LRRC4, but it remain to upregulate the expression of LRRC4 in glioma cells. miR-101 decreased the occupancy of H3K27me3 at LRRC4 core promoter and induced hypomethylation of LRRC4 by targeting EZH2, EED and DNMT3A [81].

Token together, deregulation of gene methylation including hypermethylation and hypomethylation plays an important role in carcinogenesis of glioma. Hypermethylation or hypomethylation of genes and their deregulated expression could be applied to predict the early diagnosis and prognosis of glioma. miRNAs are small noncoding RNA, around 22-24 nucleotides in size. They could not only directly regulate expression hyper/hypo-methylation genes by binding to 3′-UTR of genes, but also regulate the methylation level and gene expression through histone and DNA methylation modification by targeting histone and DNA methyltransferases (Fig 5).

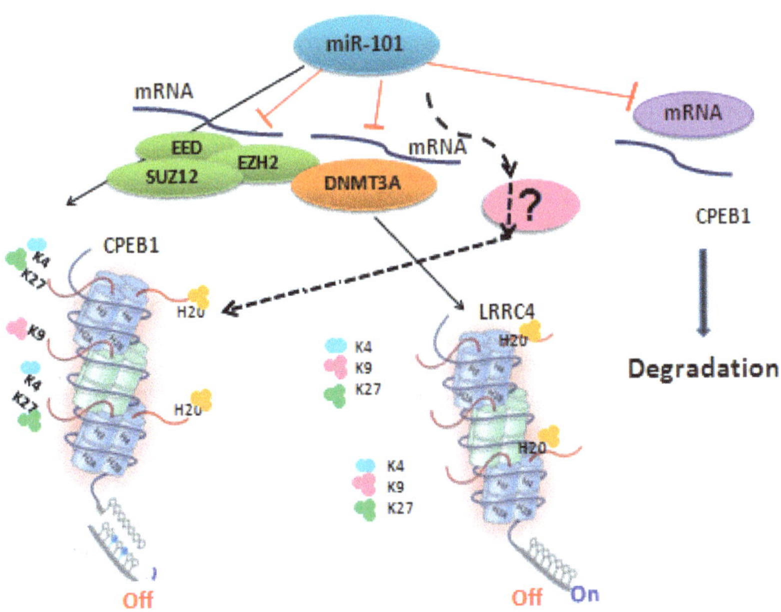

Figure 5. The regulation networks of miRNA, genes methylation and histone protein modification in glioma

7. Conclusion

The advances in next-generation sequencing technologies have allowed for mapping of DNA methylation and its derivatives: 5hmC and 5fC at base-pair resolution. These studies have provided key new insights into the function, dynamics and distribution of DNA methylation in vertebrate genomes. In the near future, studies of DM sites and focal DMRs will aid the discovery of transcription factors and transcription regulatory elements involved in controlling the expression of specific genes in vivo. More experiments in model systems will be done to directly test the functionality of DMRs or individual DM sites identified in epigenomic profiles. It is likely that intragenic and distant intergenic changes in DNA methylation will be studied much more than at present for their contribution to diseases involving epigenetic deregulation, especially cancer, immunological diseases and neurological diseases.

Acknowledgements

This work was supported by grants from National Natural Science Foundation of China (81272297; 81171932) and Hunan Province Natural Sciences Foundations (11JJ1013); Research Fund for the Doctoral Program of Higher Education of China (20110162110037). There are no financial or other relationships that might lead to a conflict of interest.

Author details

Minghua Wu[1,2,3*]

Address all correspondence to: wuminghua554@aliyun.com

1 Cancer Research Institute, Central South University, Changsha, Hunan, China

2 Disease genome Research Center, Central South University, Changsha, Hunan, China

3 Key Laboratory of Carcinogenesis and Cancer Invasion, Ministry of Education; Key Laboratory of Carcinogenesis, Ministry of Health; The Center for Skull Base Surgery and Neurooncology, Hunan Province, China

References

[1] Smirnova L, Sittka A, Luch A. On the role of low-dose effects and epigenetics in toxicology. EXS 2012; 101:499-550. doi: 10.1007/978-3-7643-8340-4_18.

[2] Guil S, Esteller M. DNA methylomes, histone codes and miRNAs: tying it all together. Int J Biochem Cell Biol. 2009; 1(41):87-95. doi: 10.1016/j.biocel.2008.09.005.

[3] Fouse SD, Nagarajan RO, Costello JF. Genome-scale DNA methylation analysis. Epigenomics 2010; 2(1):105-17. doi: 10.2217/epi.09.35.

[4] Blancafort P, Jin J, Frye S. Writing and rewriting the epigenetic code of cancer cells: from engineered proteins to small molecules. Mol Pharmacol 2013; 3(83):563-76. doi: 10.1124/mol.112.080697.

[5] Pelizzola M, Ecker J R. The DNA methylome. FEBS Lett 2011; 13(585):1994-2000. doi: 10.1016/j.febslet.2010.10.061.

[6] Boffelli D, Martin D I. Epigenetic inheritance: a contributor to species differentiation? DNA Cell Biol 2012; 31 Suppl 1):S11-6. doi: 10.1089/dna.2012.1643.

[7] Kerkel K, Spadola A, Yuan E, *et al.* Genomic surveys by methylation-sensitive SNP analysis identify sequence-dependent allele-specific DNA methylation. Nat Genet 2008; 7(40):904-8. doi: 10.1038/ng.174.

[8] Feinberg A P, Irizarry R A. Evolution in health and medicine sackler colloquium: stochastic epigenetic variation as a driving force of development, evolutionary adaptation, and disease. Proc Natl Acad Sci U S A 2010; 107(Suppl 1):1757-64. doi: 10.1073/pnas.0906183107.

[9] Zemach A, McDaniel I E, Silva P, *et al.* Genome-wide evolutionary analysis of eukaryotic DNA methylation. Science 2010; 5980(328):916-9. doi: 10.1126/science.1186366.

[10] Suzuki M M, Bird A. DNA methylation landscapes: provocative insights from epigenomics. Nat Rev Genet 2008; 6(9):465-76. doi: 10.1038/nrg2341.

[11] Jones P A, Liang G. Rethinking how DNA methylation patterns are maintained. Nat Rev Genet 2009; 11(10):805-11. doi: 10.1038/nrg2651.

[12] Ehrlich M, Lacey M. DNA hypomethylation and hemimethylation in cancer. Adv Exp Med Biol 2013; 754:31-56. doi: 10.1007/978-1-4419-9967-2_2.

[13] Bogdanovic O,Gomez-Skarmeta J L. Embryonic DNA methylation: insights from the genomics era. Brief Funct Genomics 2013; doi: 10.1093/bfgp/elt039.

[14] Shen H, Qiu C,Li J, *et al.* Characterization of the DNA methylome and its interindividual variation in human peripheral blood monocytes. Epigenomics 2013; 3(5): 255-69. doi: 10.2217/epi.13.18.

[15] Zilbauer M, Rayner T F, Clark C, *et al.* Genome-wide methylation analyses of primary human leukocyte subsets identifies functionally important cell-type specific hypomethylated regions. Blood 2013; doi: 10.1182/blood-2013-05-503201.

[16] Ehrlich M, Lacey M. DNA hypomethylation and hemimethylation in cancer. Adv Exp Med Biol 2013; 754: 31-56. doi: 10.1007/978-1-4419-9967-2_2.

[17] Cerda-Esteban N, Spagnoli F M. A glimpse into hox and tale regulation of cell differentiation and reprogramming. Dev Dyn 2013; doi: 10.1002/dvdy.24075.

[18] Shi W, Dirim F, Wolf E, *et al.* Methylation reprogramming and chromosomal aneuploidy in in vivo fertilized and cloned rabbit preimplantation embryos. Biol Reprod 2004; 1(71):340-7. doi: 10.1095/biolreprod.103.024554.

[19] Kwon G S, Viotti M, Hadjantonakis A K. The endoderm of the mouse embryo arises by dynamic widespread intercalation of embryonic and extraembryonic lineages. Dev Cell 2008; 4(15):509-20. doi: 10.1016/j.devcel.2008.07.017.

[20] Tucker K L, Beard C, Dausmann J, *et al.* Germ-line passage is required for establishment of methylation and expression patterns of imprinted but not of nonimprinted genes. Genes Dev 1996; 8(10):1008-20.

[21] Tsumura A, Hayakawa T, Kumaki Y, *et al.* Maintenance of self-renewal ability of mouse embryonic stem cells in the absence of DNA methyltransferases Dnmt1, Dnmt3a and Dnmt3b. Genes Cells 2006; 7(11):805-14. doi: 10.1111/j. 1365-2443.2006.00984.x.

[22] Jackson M, Krassowska A, Gilbert N, *et al.* Severe global DNA hypomethylation blocks differentiation and induces histone hyperacetylation in embryonic stem cells. Mol Cell Biol 2004; 20(24):8862-71. doi: 10.1128/MCB.24.20.8862-8871.2004.

[23] Carlone D L, Lee J H, Young S R, *et al.* Reduced genomic cytosine methylation and defective cellular differentiation in embryonic stem cells lacking CpG binding protein. Mol Cell Biol 2005; 12(25):4881-91. doi: 10.1128/MCB.25.12.4881-4891.2005.

[24] Meissner A, Mikkelsen TS, Gu H, et al.Genome-scale DNA methylation maps of pluripotent and differentiated cells. Nature 2008; 454(7205):766-70. doi: 10.1038/ nature07107.

[25] Laurent L, Wong E, Li G, *et al.* Dynamic changes in the human methylome during differentiation. Genome Res 2010; 3(20):320-31. doi: 10.1101/gr.101907.109.

[26] Lister R, Pelizzola M, Kida Y S, *et al.* Hotspots of aberrant epigenomic reprogramming in human induced pluripotent stem cells. Nature 2011; 7336(471):68-73. doi: 10.1038/nature09798.

[27] Lister R, Pelizzola M, Kida Y S, *et al.* Hotspots of aberrant epigenomic reprogramming in human induced pluripotent stem cells. Nature 2011; 7336(471):68-73. doi: 10.1038/nature09798.

[28] Huang K, Fan G. DNA methylation in cell differentiation and reprogramming: an emerging systematic view. Regen Med 2010; 4(5):531-44. doi: 10.2217/rme.10.35.

[29] Sashida G, Iwama A. Epigenetic regulation of hematopoiesis. Int J Hematol 2012; 4(96):405-12. doi: 10.1007/s12185-012-1183-x.

[30] Suarez-Alvarez B, Rodriguez R M, Fraga M F, *et al*. DNA methylation: a promising landscape for immune system-related diseases. Trends Genet 2012; 10(28):506-14. doi: 10.1016/j.tig.2012.06.005.

[31] Takizawa T, Nakashima K, Namihira M, *et al*. DNA methylation is a critical cell-intrinsic determinant of astrocyte differentiation in the fetal brain. Dev Cell 2001; 6(1): 749-58.

[32] Fan G, Martinowich K, Chin M H, *et al*. DNA methylation controls the timing of astrogliogenesis through regulation of JAK-STAT signaling. Development 2005; 15(132):3345-56. doi: 10.1242/dev.01912.

[33] Takahashi K, Yamanaka S. Induction of pluripotent stem cells from mouse embryonic and adult fibroblast cultures by defined factors. Cell 2006; 4(126):663-76. doi: 10.1016/j.cell.2006.07.024.

[34] Takahashi K, Tanabe K, Ohnuki M, *et al*. Induction of pluripotent stem cells from adult human fibroblasts by defined factors. Cell 2007; 5(131):861-72. doi: 10.1016/j.cell.2007.11.019.

[35] Yu J, Vodyanik M A, Smuga-Otto K, *et al*. Induced pluripotent stem cell lines derived from human somatic cells. Science 2007; 5858(318):1917-20. doi: 10.1126/science.1151526.

[36] Kinney S R, Pradhan S. Ten eleven translocation enzymes and 5-hydroxymethylation in mammalian development and cancer. Adv Exp Med Biol 2013; 754):57-79. doi: 10.1007/978-1-4419-9967-2_3.

[37] Wang T, Wu H, Li Y, *et al*. Subtelomeric hotspots of aberrant 5-hydroxymethylcytosine-mediated epigenetic modifications during reprogramming to pluripotency. Nat Cell Biol 2013; 6(15):700-11. doi: 10.1038/ncb2748.

[38] Lister R, Mukamel E A, Nery J R, *et al*. Global epigenomic reconfiguration during mammalian brain development. Science 2013; 6146(341):1237905. doi: 10.1126/science.1237905.

[39] Shirane K, Toh H, Kobayashi H, *et al*. Mouse oocyte methylomes at base resolution reveal genome-wide accumulation of non-CpG methylation and role of DNA methyltransferases. PLoS Genet 2013; 4(9):e1003439. doi: 10.1371/journal.pgen.1003439.

[40] Ziller M J, Muller F, Liao J, *et al*. Genomic distribution and inter-sample variation of non-CpG methylation across human cell types. PLoS Genet 2011; 12(7):e1002389. doi: 10.1371/journal.pgen.1002389.

[41] Chen R Z, Pettersson U, Beard C, *et al*. DNA hypomethylation leads to elevated mutation rates. Nature 1998; 6697(395):89-93. doi: 10.1038/25779.

[42] Rodriguez J, Frigola J,Vendrell E, *et al*. Chromosomal instability correlates with genome-wide DNA demethylation in human primary colorectal cancers. Cancer Res 2006; 17(66):8462-9468. doi: 10.1158/0008-5472.CAN-06-0293.

[43] Ehrlich M. DNA methylation in cancer: too much, but also too little. Oncogene 2002; 35(21):5400-13. doi: 10.1038/sj.onc.1205651.

[44] Feinberg A P, Cui H, Ohlsson R. DNA methylation and genomic imprinting: insights from cancer into epigenetic mechanisms. Semin Cancer Biol 2002; 5(12):389-98.

[45] Uribe-Lewis S, Woodfine K, Stojic L, *et al*. Molecular mechanisms of genomic imprinting and clinical implications for cancer. Expert Rev Mol Med 2011; 1:e2. doi: 10.1017/S1462399410001717.

[46] Jelinic P, Shaw P. Loss of imprinting and cancer. J Pathol 2007; 3(211):261-8. doi: 10.1002/path.2116.

[47] Eden A, Gaudet F, Waghmare A, *et al*. Chromosomal instability and tumors promoted by DNA hypomethylation. Science 2003; 5618(300):455. doi: 10.1126/science.1083557.

[48] Wong N C, Wong L H, Quach J M, *et al*. Permissive transcriptional activity at the centromere through pockets of DNA hypomethylation. PLoS Genet 2006; 2(2):e17. doi: 10.1371/journal.pgen.0020017.

[49] Yang H, Liu Y, Bai F, *et al*. Tumor development is associated with decrease of TET gene expression and 5-methylcytosine hydroxylation. Oncogene 2013; 5(32):663-9. doi: 10.1038/onc.2012.67.

[50] Kraus T F, Globisch D, Wagner M, *et al*. Low values of 5-hydroxymethylcytosine (5hmc), the "sixth base," are associated with anaplasia in human brain tumors. Int J Cancer 2012; 7(131):1577-90. doi: 10.1002/ijc.27429.

[51] Irizarry R A, Ladd-Acosta C,Wen B, *et al*. The human colon cancer methylome shows similar hypo-and hypermethylation at conserved tissue-specific CpG island shores. Nat Genet 2009; 2(41):178-86. doi: 10.1038/ng.298.

[52] Han H, Cortez C C, Yang X, *et al*. DNA methylation directly silences genes with non-CpG island promoters and establishes a nucleosome occupied promoter. Hum Mol Genet 2011; 22(20):4299-310. doi: 10.1093/hmg/ddr356.

[53] Tomasi M L, Li T W, Li M, *et al*. Inhibition of human methionine adenosyltransferase 1A transcription by coding region methylation. J Cell Physiol 2012; 4(227):1583-91. doi: 10.1002/jcp.22875.

[54] Baylin S B, Jones P A. A decade of exploring the cancer epigenome biological and translational implications. Nat Rev Cancer 2011; 10(11):726-34. doi: 10.1038/nrc3130.

[55] Pogribny I P, Beland F A. DNA hypomethylation in the origin and pathogenesis of human diseases. Cell Mol Life Sci 2009; 14(66):2249-61. doi: 10.1007/s00018-009-0015-5.

[56] Hanahan D, Weinberg R A. Hallmarks of cancer: the next generation. Cell 2011; 5(144):646-74. doi: 10.1016/j.cell.2011.02.013.

[57] Cahill N, Rosenquist R. Uncovering the DNA methylome in chronic lymphocytic leukemia. Epigenetics 2013; 2(8):138-48. doi: 10.4161/epi.23439.

[58] Martin-Subero J I, Lopez-Otin C, Campo E. Genetic and epigenetic basis of chronic lymphocytic leukemia. Curr Opin Hematol 2013; 4(20):362-8. doi: 10.1097/MOH. 0b013e32836235dc.

[59] Rahmatpanah F B, Carstens S, Hooshmand S I, *et al*. Large-scale analysis of DNA methylation in chronic lymphocytic leukemia. Epigenomics 2009; 1(1):39-61. doi: 10.2217/epi.09.10.

[60] Chiorazzi N, Ferrarini M. Cellular origin(s) of chronic lymphocytic leukemia: cautionary notes and additional considerations and possibilities. Blood 2011; 6(117): 1781-91. doi: 10.1182/blood-2010-07-155663.

[61] Zhang Z, Tang H, Wang Z, *et al*. Mir-185 targets the DNA methyltransferases 1 and regulates global DNA methylation in human glioma. Mol Cancer 2011; 10):124. doi: 10.1186/1476-4598-10-124.

[62] Bhaumik S R, Smith E, Shilatifard A. Covalent modifications of histones during development and disease pathogenesis. Nat Struct Mol Biol 2007; 11(14):1008-16. doi: 10.1038/nsmb1337.

[63] Kouzarides T. Chromatin modifications and their function. Cell 2007; 4(128):693-705. doi: 10.1016/j.cell.2007.02.005.

[64] Bartel D P. MicroRNAs: genomics, biogenesis, mechanism, and function. Cell 2004; 6):281-97.

[65] He L, Hannon G J. Micrornas: small RNAs with a big role in gene regulation. Nat Rev Genet 2004; 7(5):522-31. doi: 10.1038/nrg1379.

[66] Saito Y, Liang G, Egger G, *et al*. Specific activation of microRNA-127 with downregulation of the proto-oncogene bcl6 by chromatin-modifying drugs in human cancer cells. Cancer Cell 2006; 6(9):435-43. doi: 10.1016/j.ccr.2006.04.020.

[67] Fabbri M, Garzon R, Cimmino A, *et al*. MicroRNA-29 family reverts aberrant methylation in lung cancer by targeting dna methyltransferases 3a and 3b. Proc Natl Acad Sci U S A 2007; 40(104):15805-10. doi: 10.1073/pnas.0707628104.

[68] Benetti R, Gonzalo S, Jaco I, *et al*. A mammalian microrna cluster controls dna methylation and telomere recombination via rbl2-dependent regulation of DNA methyltransferases. Nat Struct Mol Biol 2008; 9(15):998. doi: 10.1038/nsmb0908-998b.

[69] Wu L, Zhou H, Zhang Q, *et al*. DNA methylation mediated by a microRNA pathway. Mol Cell 2010; 3(38):465-75. doi: 10.1016/j.molcel.2010.03.008.

5

Current Understanding of Epigenomics and Epigenetics in Neurodevelopmental Disorders

Takeo Kubota, Kunio Miyake and Takae Hirasawa

1. Introduction

Epigenetics is a mechanism that regulates gene expression not depending on the underlying DNA sequence, but on the chemical modification of DNA and histone proteins. It is known that several neurodevelopmental disorders are caused by congenital abnormalities in epigenetic mechanisms, including Prader-Willi and Angelman syndromes, which are genomic imprinting disorders [1-3]. The advances in understanding of the epigenetic gene regulation mechanisms and identification of proteins that participate in them have led to the identification of other neurodevelopmental disorders, such as ICF and Rett syndromes, caused by mutations in the genes that encode such proteins [4-8]. The discovery of Rett syndrome, a representative autistic disorder caused by mutations in *MECP2* that encodes an epigenetic regulatory protein, introduced to us a new paradigm that neurodevelopmental disorders are not only caused by mutations in the neuronal genes [9, 10], but also caused by abnormal epigenetic regulation of the neuronal genes.

Several lines of evidence suggest that various environmental factors, such as nutrition (e.g. folic acid and royal jelly), environmental chemicals, external electric stimuli to neurons, and mental stress, can change epigenomic status, which supports the hypothesis that the epigenome is more susceptible to environmental factors than the genome [11].

DNA methylation was initially believed to change gradually during the lifetime through studies in cancer. However, it has recently been shown that DNA methylation can be altered during the first week of life after birth in mice, and that the altered epigenomic status in the brain is prolonged throughout the lifetime long with abnormal behavior [12]. It is also reported that epigenetic changes can be induced by malnutrition during the fetal period, which introduces the origin of adult diseases in the fetus in rats [13, 14]. Recent comparative studies between monozygotic twins suggest that epigenomic changes also occur in humans [15, 16].

Epigenetic is a reversible mechanism and thus, it has been accepted as a mechanism for genomic imprinting in which the maternal expression pattern can be erased and reset to be the paternal expression pattern when the imprinted gene is transmitted from the mother to the offspring [17-20]. It has recently been shown that some drugs for mental disorders have an effect on restoration of the epigenetic status and the expression pattern of the neuronal genes based on this epigenomic reversibility [21-25]. It has also been reported that administration of folic acid is effective in treating autistic children possibly by restoring DNA methylation status at the disease-related gene regions [26-28]. Therefore, it is intriguing to think that advanced "epigenomic drug" can be designed that only target to disease-specific gene regions using recent technology such as pyrrole-imidazole polyamide [29, 30].

Epigenetics now challenge the biological dogma that "acquired nature cannot be transmitted to the next generation", because recent studies have shown that mental stress-induced epigenomic changes cannot be completely erased at the stage of spermatogenesis and can be transmitted to the third generation in mice [20, 31]. However, it is possible that appropriate intervention such as drug, nutrition, and environmental condition can be restore the abnormal epigenomic status and halt its inheritance, if such transmission is true in humans.

In this chapter, we present the epigenetic mechanisms that cause congenital disorders, show examples of environmental factors that can alter the epigenetic status, and discuss recent topics in epigenetics, such as strategies for the treatment of neurodevelopmental disorders utilizing epigenetic reversibility and the possibility of its transgenerational inheritance.

2. Importance of proper gene regulation in the brain

The brain is a gene-dosage sensitive organ in which either under-expression or over-expression of the same genes encoding proteins related to brain function results in a range of neurological disorders. For example, Pelizaeus-Merzbacher disease, a severe congenital disease is caused by either a deletion, mutation, or duplication of the proteolipid protein 1 (*PLP1*) gene [32]. Further, lissencephaly, a rare brain formation disorder, is caused by either deletion or duplication of the platelet-activating factor acetylhydrolase 1B subunit alpha (*PAFAH1B1*) gene that encodes a neuronal migration factor [33, 34]. Charcot-Marie-Tooth disease, an adult-onset neuromuscular disease is caused by a mutation or duplication of the peripheral myelin protein 22 (*PMP22*) gene [35], and Parkinson's disease is caused by a mutation or multiplication of the α-synuclein (*SNCA*) gene [36]. These are all neurological disorders, and such examples have not been observed in other clinical fields. Thus, these findings suggest that the brain is extremely sensitive to perturbations in gene regulation, and further indicate that the brain is an organ that requires a proper control system for gene expression.

Epigenetic mechanisms are one of the ways by which gene expression is controlled in higher vertebrates. These mechanisms are essential for normal development during embryogenesis [37], and for differentiation of neural cells [38] and other cell types [39]. Understanding of epigenetic mechanisms, including DNA methylation, histone modification, and regulation by microRNAs, is important in elucidating the pathogenic pathways in neurodevelopmental disorders [40-42].

3. Epigenetic mechanisms that cause congenital neurodevelopmental disorders

Genomic imprinting is an epigenetic phenomenon that was initially discovered in humans and mammals, which determines parental-specific monoallelic expression of a relatively small number of genes during development. Imprinting must be logically imparted in the germ line, where inherited maternal and paternal imprints are erased and new imprinting established according to the individual's sex (Figure 1) [17]. For example, before the maternal allele-specific DNA methylation that contribute to monoallelic expression is established in a differential methylated region 2 (DMR2) of mouse *Igf2* gene, DMR2 is demethylated in both male and female primordial gene cells (PGCs) by 13.5 days post coitum (dpc), indicating that the erasure of imprinting in this region occurs earlier in PGC development [18]. Although DNA methylation is the best established epigenetic mark that is critical for the allele-specific expression of imprinted genes, many aspects of the regulation of DNA methylation are unknown, including how methylation complexes are targeted and the molecular mechanisms underlying DNA demethylation [19]. In this context, one mechanism related to genome-wide DNA demethylation to reset the epigenome for totipotency was recently revealed that erasure of CpG methylation (5mC) in PGCs occurs via conversion to 5-hydroxymethylcytosine (5hmC), driven by high levels of TET1 and TET2, and that global conversion to 5hmC is initiated asynchronously in PGCs at embryonic days (E) 9.5 to E10.5 for imprint erasure [20].

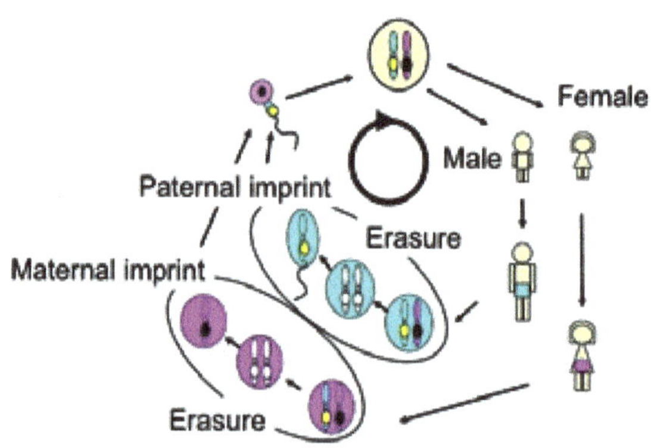

Figure 1. Erasure and establishment of genomic imprinting. Inherited maternal and paternal imprints are erased and new imprinting established according to the individual's sex during the process of spermatogenesis and oogenesis.

In an imprinted gene, one of the two parental alleles is active and the other is inactive due to an epigenetic mechanism such as DNA methylation. Therefore, a defect in the active allele of the imprinted gene results in the loss of expression. This has been found in the neurodevelopmental diseases, Prader-Willi syndrome and Angelman syndrome [2].

The X chromosome has a large number of genes, whereas the Y chromosome has relatively few. Thus, females (XX) have more genes than males (XY). To minimize this sex imbalance, one of the two X chromosomes in females is inactivated by an epigenetic mechanism [3]. Improper X chromosome inactivation (XCI) is thought to be an embryonic lethal condition, as suggested by the findings that a majority of aborted embryonic clones produced by somatic nuclear transfer showed failure of XCI [43, 44], although it is difficult to directly demonstrate failure of XCI in human aborted embryos. Even when failure of XCI occurs in women with one normal X chromosome and a small X chromosome due to a large terminal deletion, and thus the overdosage effect of X-linked genes is small, such affected women show severe congenital neurodevelopmental delays [3], indicating that proper epigenetic gene suppression is essential for normal development.

DNA methylation is a fundamental step in epigenetic gene control, and occurs by the DNA methyltransferase (DNMT)-mediated addition of a methyl group (CH_3) to CpG dinucleotides. A defect in one of the DNMTs (e.g., DNMT3B) can cause a syndrome characterized by immunodeficiency, centromere instability, facial anomalies (ICF), and mild mental retardation [4-6]. Methyl-CpG-binding domain proteins (MBDs) are also important molecules in the control of gene expression. Mutations in the methyl-CpG-binding protein 2 gene (*MECP2*), one of the genes that encodes for MBD protein, can cause Rett syndrome, which is characterized by seizures, ataxic gait, language dysfunction, and autistic behavior [7, 8]. Therefore, it is thought that MeCP2 dysfunction leads to aberrant expression of genes in the brain associated with neurological features of the disease. Recent studies have shown that MeCP2 controls a subset of neuronal genes [45-48] or a potentially large number of genes [49], suggesting that epigenetic dysregulation of multiple neuronal genes may cause neurological features of the disease.

4. Environmental factors that alter the epigenetic status associated with neurodevelopmental disorders

We have previously demonstrated that epigenetic instability at imprinting loci during the process of finding proper methylation sites for diagnosis of Prader-Willi / Angelman syndromes, the epigenetic disorders described above [50]. In our study, the imprinted DNA methylation status at the small nuclear ribonucleoprotein associated polypeptide N (*SNRPN*) promoter region (e.g., maternally methylated and paternally unmethylated) in chromosome 15q12 was stable among various tissues such as lymphocyte, amniotic fluid cells, cultured chorionic villus samples, various fetal tissues and Epstein-Barr virus lymphoblast cell lines established from lymphocytes. However, at the PW71 locus adjacent to the SNRPN locus, the imprinted methylation status was not consistent among these tissues. This indicates that epigenetic status at the loci associated with neurodevelopmental disorders are susceptible to environmental factors *in vitro*.

In neurodevelopmental disorders such as autism, both environmental factors (e.g., toxins, infections) and genetic factors (e.g., mutations in synaptic molecules) have historically been discussed [51]. However, a biological mechanism that links these two groups of factors has not been identified. Epigenetics may be the bridge between these factors, thereby contributing to disease development [11]. Besides the *intrinsic* (congenital) epigenetic defects (associated with disease as described above), several lines of evidence suggest that *extrinsic* (environmental) factors, such as malnutrition [13, 14], drugs [21-25], mental stress during the neonatal period [12], and neuronal stimulation [52], alter the epigenetic status and thereby affect brain function. Therefore, it is intriguing to speculate that acquired neurodevelopmental disorders, including autistic disorders, may be the result of epigenetic dysregulation caused by environmental factors (Figure 2).

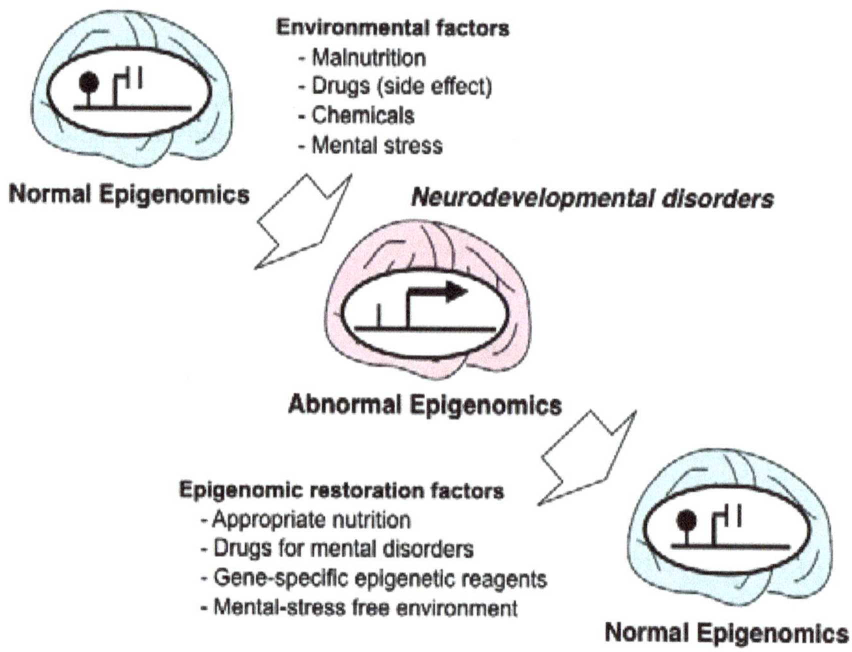

Figure 2. Current understanding of extrinsic mechanisms of neurodevelopmental disorders. Acquired neurodevelopmental disorders are caused by extrinsic mechanism via various environmental factors.

Short-term mental stress after birth may alter the epigenetic status in the brain and result in persistent abnormal behavior [12]. In rat pups from mothers exhibiting low levels of maternal care, DNA methylation at the promoter of the glucocorticoid receptor gene (*GR*), which is also known as the nuclear receptor subfamily 3 group C member 1 (*NR3C1*) gene, increased in the hippocampus, which suppressed expression of the gene within the first week of life. In contrast, promoter methylation decreased in the brains of the offspring with high maternal care during the same period [12]. This paradigm was suggested to provide a putative animal model for childhood neglect and maltreatment in humans. Postmortem analysis of the hippocampus of suicide victims with a history of childhood abuse revealed the presence of hypermethylation of the neuron-specific promoter of *NR3C1* in combination with a decrease in its expression [53].

This finding suggests that the adverse effects of early-life stress on DNA methylation may last throughout life [54], and also indicates that neurodevelopmental problems may arise from epigenetic dysregulation caused by environmental factors in early life.

Epigenetic mechanisms are also likely to be relevant to drug addiction. Gene expression in the dopaminergic and glutamatergic systems is mediated by epigenetic mechanisms, and cocaine and alcohol are known to alter the epigenetic state (e.g., cocaine induces either hyperacetylation or hypoacetylation of histone H3 or H4 in the nucleus accumbens of mice, and alcohol induces hyperacetylation of histones H3 and H4 in the frontal cortex and the nucleus accumbens of adolescent rats), which may be associated with permanent behavioral consequences [55, 56].

The findings above were mainly obtained in animal studies, and there is little evidence in humans. However, the fact that epigenomic differences are larger in older monozygotic twins than those in younger twins suggests that epigenetic status may be altered during aging by environmental factors in humans [15]. Likewise, in monozygotic twins with discordant severity of Rett syndrome, the epigenomic patterns and expression of neuronal genes have been shown to differ [16]. This indicates that environmental factors may affect the human epigenome and that epigenomic differences induced by environmental factors may contribute to mental phenotypes.

Another phenomenon that may be related to epigenomic changes is the decline in birth weights that has occurred during the past 20 years. This trend is thought to be a result of the popularity of dieting among young women and of the recommendation by obstetric physicians to minimize pregnancy weight gain in order to reduce the risk of gestational diabetes mellitus [57]. Based on current epidemiological studies of populations affected by famines in the Netherlands and China, the generation with lower birth weight is expected to have an increased risk of not only metabolic disorders (e.g., obesity, diabetes mellitus) [58], but also mental disorders [59]. This expectation is referred to as the Developmental Origin of Health and Diseases (DOHaD) [60]. Recent studies have demonstrated that malnutrition during the fetal period causes a hypomethylation imprint on the peroxisome proliferator-activated receptor alpha (*PPARa*) gene in the rat liver [61]. Similar DNA methylation changes have been identified in the peripheral tissues of people who suffered malnutrition during a period of famine in the Netherlands [62]. It has also been reported that assisted reproductive technologies (ART) (e.g., in vitro fertilization and intracytoplasmic sperm injection), which are now widely used due to increases in maternal age, lead to decreased DNA methylation status at multiple maternally methylated imprinted loci [63, 64]. Therefore, it is intriguing to think that current social factors, such as DOHaD and ART, may be involved in the recent increase of children with mild neurodevelopmental disorders in Japan and other countries [65-70] and that epigenetic alteration may underlie this social phenomenon.

5. Treatment of neurodevelopmental disorders by utilizing epigenetic reversibility

It has been reported that administration of folic acid to pregnant rats alters the DNA methylation status in the offspring [71]. Furthermore, folic acid supplementation in pregnant rats under malnutrition conditions prevents hypomethylation of a hepatic gene in the offspring [13]. In addition to folic acid, various environmental factors, such as royal jelly [72], drugs for mental disorders [21, 23, 25], environmental chemicals [73, 74], and external stimuli (electroconvulsive treatment for psychiatric diseases) [49], have also been reported to alter DNA methylation and histone modification status in the brain and other organs in mice or other species.

As mentioned above, mental stress in the first week of life causes epigenetic abnormalities in the brains of mice. Conversely, several mouse studies have demonstrated that appropriate educational conditions can ameliorate behavior abnormalities. Environmental enrichment (EE), consisting of larger-sized home cages with a variety of objects including running wheels, improved motor coordination and decreased anxiety-related behavior in heterozygous *Mecp2+/-*female mice, a model of Rett syndrome [75, 76]. EE also improved locomotor activity with reduced ventricular volume, and restored the expression of synaptic markers, such as synaptophysin and PSD95 in the hypothalamus and syntaxin 1a and synaptotagmin in the cortex of hemizygous *Mecp2-/y* male mice [77, 78].

It is generally thought to be difficult to cure patients with congenital mental disorders caused by mutations that encode neuronal molecules, since it is difficult to distribute gene products to the appropriate brain regions and at the appropriate time of brain development. However, it was recently demonstrated that the epigenetic disorder Rett syndrome may be an exception, partly because MeCP2 does not encode a product required for brain structure, but rather encodes a "lubricant" that works at a relatively later period of brain development. As a consequence, reintroduction of *MECP2* into *Mecp2* null mice not only before birth [79], but also after birth, is sufficient to rescue Rett-like neurological symptoms [80]. Furthermore, restoration of MeCP2 function in astrocytes substantially improves locomotion, anxiety levels, and respiratory abnormalities in hemizygous *Mecp2-/Y* male mice along with restoring dendritic morphology [81]. These results suggest that up-regulation of *MECP2*, possibly mediated by drug treatment, might help to improve brain function in Rett syndrome patients. Valproic acid, one of the most popular drugs for epileptic seizure and a known HDAC inhibitor, increases MeCP2 expression [82, 83], as well as fluoxetine, a drug for mental disorders, and cocaine [84]. Taken together, these results indicate that neurodevelopmental disorders caused by epigenetic abnormalities can be treatable.

6. The possibility of transgenerational epigenetic inheritance

According to current understanding in the field of biology, one's acquired character is not inherited by the next generation of offspring. Based on this notion of Darwinian inheritance, bad habits acquired during one's lifetime would not be transmitted to one's children. However, recent advances in epigenomics and epigenetics have revealed that such undesirable acquired traits might be transmitted into the next generation.

Epigenetic marks, either DNA methylation or histone modifications, allow the mitotic transmission of gene activity states from one cell to its daughter cells. A fundamental question in epigenetics is whether these marks can also be transmitted meiotically through the germline. In mammals, epigenetic marks should be cleared by demethylating factors such as the cytidine deaminases (e.g., AID, APOBEC1) and re-established in each generation, but this clearing is incomplete at some loci in the genome of several model organisms possibly due to deficiency of demethylating factors (e.g. AID) [85]. A recent study has demonstrated rare regulatory elements that escape systematic DNA demethylation in PGCs, providing a potential mechanistic basis for transgenerational epigenetic inheritance [20]. Therefore, based on this phenomenon, "transgenerational epigenetic inheritance", which refers to the germline transmission of an epigenetic mark [86, 87], may provide a direct biological proof for Lamarckism, hypothesis suggesting the heritability of acquired characteristics.

It is important to draw a distinction between transgenerational epigenetic inheritance and heritable germline epimutation. Transgenerational epigenetic inheritance is independent of the DNA sequence, whereas heritable germline epimutation is a direct consequence of a *cis*-acting epigenetic alteration, such as hypermethylation induced by an expansion of an unstable CGG repeat within exon 1 of the Fragile X Mental Retardation Syndrome 1 gene (*FMR1)*, hypermethylation induced by a deletion in an adjacent gene within the promoter of the globin gene, and hypermethylation induced by repetitive retrotransposons [87, 88]. Such specific-sequence driven-epimutation is observed in an affected mother and son in a family with fragile X syndrome, and it can be classified as a case of heritable germline epimutation [88]. This inheritance pattern is also observed in other species, such as *Caenorhabditis elegans*. Therefore, the heritability does not necessarily involve transgenerational epigenetic inheritance, as the methylated state could be cleared on passage through the germline and could be re-established according to a certain sequence during zygotic genome activation [88].

Transgenerational inheritance of epigenetic marks was first demonstrated in a specific mouse strain. The methylation status at the *Axin (Fu)* locus in mature sperm, which reflects the methylation state of the allele in the somatic tissue of the animal is linked to the shape of the animal's tail and does not undergo epigenetic reprogramming during gametogenesis [89]. Environmental factors, notably the fungicide vinclozilin, stress responses and nutritional challenges, have been associated with transgenerational epigenetic inheritance in animal models. However, it is often difficult to obtain direct evidence of transmission of epigenetic marks *per se* from transmission of the exposure itself [90, 91]. Therefore, transgenerational effects should be distinguished from parental and grandparental effects. In addition to contributing to their DNA, parents can influence their offspring in many ways: for example, by contributing bioactive molecules in the egg and sperm cytoplasm, and by providing nutrients and hormonal information during embyogenesis. For example, malnutrition during pregnancy does not only affect the pregnant mother and fetus but also the fetus's primordial germ cells, which can lead to phenotypic changes in the grandchildren (second generation).

In one study, a specific diet (supplementation of folic acid) induced methylation at the *Axin (Fu)* locus, which altered the hair color of the animals, and this alteration was inherited over 2 generations, but this status was lost by the third generation [92]. These findings indicate that while a specific diet leads to parental and grandparental effects, the acquired epigenetic information is not inherited transgenerationally, and that the *Axin (Fu)* locus is resistant to environmentally induced acquisition of new germ-line epigenetic information [92].

Transgenerational effects of environmental toxins – namely, the endocrine disruptors vinclozolin (an antiandrogenic compound) and methyoxychlor (estrogenic compound)-have been demonstrated in the fourth generation (F4) of rats resulting in decreased spermatogenic capacity and increased male infertility, and the effects on reproduction correlate with altered DNA methylation patterns in the germ line [93]. It has also been demonstrated that plastic-derived endocrine disrupters, including bisphenol A, increase the risk of pubertal abnormalities, testicular diseases and ovarian diseases in the F3 generation of rats, and that differential DNA methylated patterns were identified in the plastic-lineage F3 generation sperm in comparison with control-lineage F3 generation sperm [94]. Therefore, "true" transgenerational epigenetic inheritance up to third generation is suggested to exist in animals. This observation has also been confirmed in Drosophila, in which an aberrant epigenetic mark (defective chromatin state) acquired in one generation induced by environmental stress (e.g. heat shock) was inherited by the next generation [95].

It has also been demonstrated that an aberrant epigenetic mark acquired in one generation by mental stress (maternal separation in early life) can be inherited by the next generation (Figure 3, left) [31]. Chronic maternal separation alters behaviors as well as the profile of DNA methylation in the promoter of several candidate genes in both the germline of the separated mice and brains of the offspring with altered gene expression (e.g. decreases in the expression of corticotropin releasing factor receptor 2 (*Crfr2*) in the amygdala and the hypothalamus) [31]. In this study, abnormal behavior was observed in the third generation, and altered DNA methylation in the CpG islands of *Mecp2*, cannabinoid receptor-1 (*Cb1*), and *Crfr2* were observed in F1 sperm and F2 brain. It has also been reported that chronic maternal separation increases cytosine methylation of the estrogen receptor (Er)-alpha1b gene promoter, indicating that individual differences in maternal behavior are epigenetically transmitted from the mother to her female offspring [96]. Further, the third generation of male rats upon exposure to vinclozolin, a commonly-used fungicide, respond differently to chronic restraint (i.e., mental) stress during adolescence; they also show altered gene expression in the cortex and CA1 regions of the brain, although direct epigenetic alteration (e.g., DNA methylation) has not been confirmed [97]. These findings provide biological evidence suggesting that environmental factors, including traumatic experiences in early life, are risk factors for the development of behavioral and emotional disorders.

Environmental stress (e.g., maternal separation) in neonatal period induces epigenomic changes in the brain and sperm in mice. The changes are transmitted to the next generation along with abnormal behavior even when the offspring is reared by a normal mother. However, it is possible to ameliorate these epigenetic changes by providing appropriate environ-

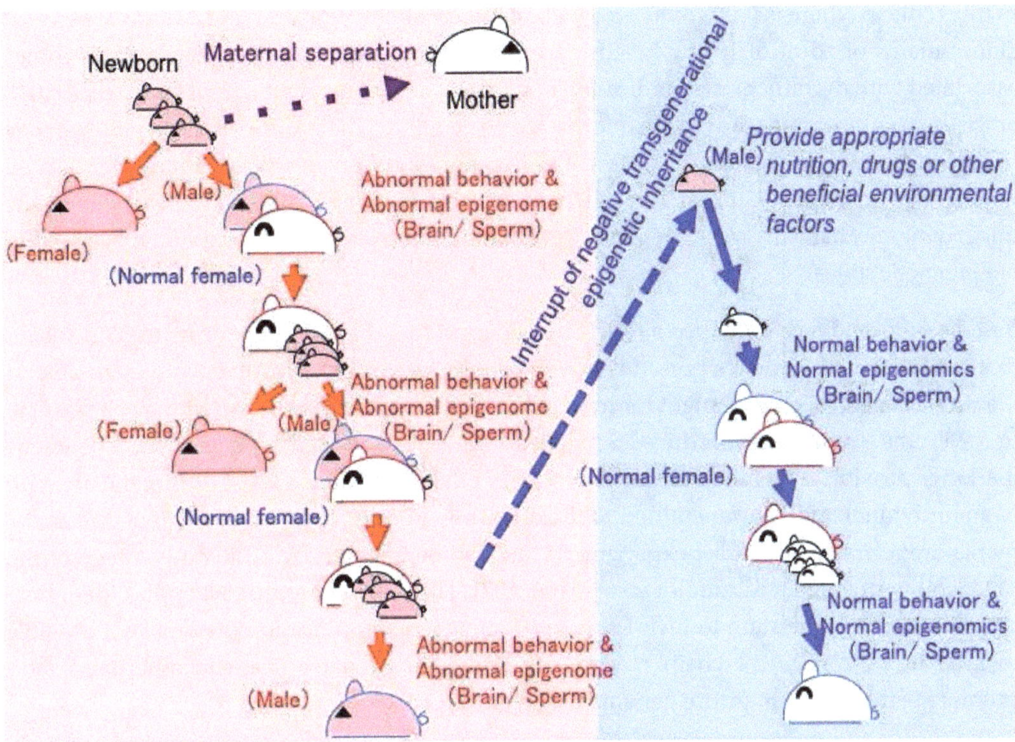

Figure 3. Transgenerational abnormal epigenomic inheritance along with abnormal phenotype.

mental factors (e.g., nutrition, neuropsychiatric drugs or brain-stimulating enriched environment).

Recent studies have suggested that epigenetic variations influenced by the environment occur spontaneously and that the specific epigenetic pattern created is inherited over several generations in plant populations. Understanding the emergence and heritability of epigenetic variants is critical for understanding how they might become subject to natural selection and thus affect genetic diversity [98]. In humans, clinical features can vary among family members who share the same disease-causing mutation-a phenomenon referred to as variable expressivity; however, the precise molecular mechanism is not known. Therefore, it is intriguing to speculate that the variable clinical expressivity is caused by the stochastic occurrence of epigenetic variation during development [99] or by the spontaneous epigenetic changes during the transmission to the next generation, as was observed in plants [98, 100].

It has been demonstrated that neuronal plasticity is determined by epigenetic plasticity, such as chromatin remodeling and dynamic DNA methylation changes during brain development [101, 102], and multiple lines of evidence that connect environmental factors to brain functions via epigenetic regulation have been accumulating [21-25]. However, little is known as to whether environment-induced epigenetic changes in the brain are transmitted to the next generation along with abnormal brain functions, including mental disorders [31, 103].

In this context, whereas it is widely known that maternal nutrition and metabolism are critical determinants of adult offspring health, recent reports describe adverse offspring outcomes associated with the father's diet, indicating nongenetic inheritance of paternal experience [104]. Since the results of this study were interpreted as "you are what your dad ate" [105], we may be able to interpret the results of studies of transgenerational epigenetic inheritance associated with a specific mental state [31, 103] as "you are how your dad behaved". Determining the underlying mechanisms may require a reevaluation of our understanding of the heritability of epigenetic states.

Based on the evidence described above, the readers of this chapter might draw the conclusion that the field of epigenetics portends adverse news for society. However, if we are able to identify a beneficial environment for human health in terms of epigenetics, it may be possible to sever the environment-induced epigenetic patterns across the generation. Epigenetic markings provide a "memory of past experiences"; these markings persist during the life span of an individual and are transmitted to the offspring. Recent reports indicate that epigenetic marks are a "memory of past experiences" that can be restored by taking advantage of the reversibility of epigenetic modifications [106, 107]. Therefore, drug discovery and identification of beneficial condition to revert abnormal epigenetic modification may make it possible to interrupt the negative chain reaction of transgenerational epigenetic inheritance and promote better health in future generations (Figure 3, right).

7. Conclusion

The failure of epigenetic gene regulation is known to cause various rare congenital disorders. However, this deregulation also cause common diseases that are induced by environmental factors, since the epigenetic status is affected and changed by various environmental factors. Furthermore, the altered epigenetic status in the genome can be transmitted to the succeeding generations. Therefore, precise understanding of gene-environment interactions in light of epigenomics and epigenetics is necessary, which will further our knowledge of neurodevelopmental disorders.

Acknowledgements

The research described in this chapter was partially supported by the Ministry of Education, Science, Sports and Culture (MEXT), Grants-in-Aid (KAKENHI) for Scientific Research (A) and (B) (#23390272; to TK), for Exploratory Research (#25670473; to TK), for Young Scientists (B) (#25860852; to KM), for Grant-in-Aid for Scientific Research on Innovative Areas "Genome Science" (to TK), for Scientific Research (C) (#23591491; to TH).

Author details

Takeo Kubota*, Kunio Miyake and Takae Hirasawa

*Address all correspondence to: takeot@yamanashi.ac.jp

Department of Epigenetics Medicine, Interdisciplinary Graduate School of Medicine and Engineering, University of Yamanashi, Yamanashi, Shimokato, Chuo, Yamanashi, Japan

References

[1] Glenn CC, Porter KA, Jong MT, Nicholls RD, Driscoll DJ. Functional imprinting and epigenetic modification of the human SNRPN gene. Hum Mol Genet 1993:2(12): 2001-5.

[2] Kubota T, Das S, Christian SL, Baylin SB, Herman JG, Ledbetter DH. Methylation-specific PCR simplifies imprinting analysis. Nat Genet 1997;16(1):16-7.

[3] Kubota T, Wakui K, Nakamura T, Ohashi H, Watanabe Y, Yoshino M, Kida T, Okamoto N, Matsumura M, Muroya K, Ogata T, Goto Y, Fukushima Y. Proportion of the cells with functional X disomy is associated with the severity of mental retardation in mosaic ring X Turner syndrome females. Cytogenet Genome Res 2002;99(1-4):276-84.

[4] Okano M, Bell DW, Haber DA, Li E. DNA methyltransferases Dnmt3a and Dnmt3b are essential for de novo methylation and mammalian development. Cell 1999;99(3): 247-57.

[5] Shirohzu H, Kubota T, Kumazawa A, Sado T, Chijiwa T, Inagaki K, Suetake I, Tajima S, Wakui K, Miki Y, Hayashi M, Fukushima Y, Sasaki H. Three novel DNMT3B mutations in Japanese patients with ICF syndrome. Am J Med Genet 2002;112(1):31-7.

[6] Kubota T, Furuumi H, Kamoda T, Iwasaki N, Tobita N, Fujiwara N, Goto Y, Matsui A, Sasaki H, Kajii T. ICF syndrome in a girl with DNA hypomethylation but without detectable DNMT3B mutation. Am J Med Genet A 2004;129A(3):290-3.

[7] Amir RE, Van den Veyver IB, Wan M, Tran CQ, Francke U, Zoghbi HY. Rett syndrome is caused by mutations in X-linked MECP2 encoding methyl-CpG-binding protein 2. Nat Genet 1999;23(2):185-8.

[8] Chunshu Y, Endoh K, Soutome M, Kawamura R, Kubota T. A patient with classic Rett syndrome with a novel mutation in MECP2 exon 1. Clin Genet 2006;70(6):530-1.

[9] Zoghbi HY. Postnatal neurodevelopmental disorders: meeting at the synapse? Science 2003;302(5646):826-30.

[10] Persico AM, Bourgeron T. Searching for ways out of the autism maze: genetic, epigenetic and environmental clues. Trends Neurosci 2006; 29(7):349-58.

[11] Qiu J. Epigenetics: unfinished symphony. Nature 2006;441(7090):143-5.

[12] Weaver IC, Cervoni N, Champagne FA, D'Alessio AC, Sharma S, Seckl JR, Dymov S, Szyf M, Meaney MJ. Epigenetic programming by maternal behavior. Nat Neurosci 2004:7(8):847-54.

[13] Lillycrop KA, Phillips ES, Jackson AA, Hanson MA, Burdge GC. Dietary protein restriction of pregnant rats induces and folic acid supplementation prevents epigenetic modification of hepatic gene expression in the offspring. J Nutr 2005;135(6):1382-6.

[14] Lillycrop KA, Phillips ES, Torrens C, Hanson MA, Jackson AA, Burdge GC. Feeding pregnant rats a protein-restricted diet persistently alters the methylation of specific cytosines in the hepatic PPAR alpha promoter of the offspring. Br J Nutr 2008;100(2): 278-282.

[15] Fraga MF, Ballestar E, Paz MF, Ropero S, Setien F, Ballestar ML, Heine-Suñer D, Cigudosa JC, Urioste M, Benitez J, Boix-Chornet M, Sanchez-Aguilera A, Ling C, Carlsson E, Poulsen P, Vaag A, Stephan Z, Spector TD, Wu YZ, Plass C, Esteller M.Epigenetic differences arise during the lifetime of monozygotic twins. Proc Natl Acad Sci USA 2005;102(30):10604-9.

[16] Miyake K, Yang C, Minakuchi Y, Ohori K, Soutome M, Hirasawa T, Kazuki Y, Adachi N, Suzuki S, Itoh M, Goto YI, Andoh T, Kurosawa H, Oshimura M, Sasaki M, Toyoda A, Kubota T.Comparison of genomic and epigenomic expression in monozygotic twins discordant for Rett syndrome. PLoS ONE 8(6):e66729, 2013.

[17] Szabó PE, Mann JR. Biallelic expression of imprinted genes in the mouse germ line: implications for erasure, establishment, and mechanisms of genomic imprinting. Genes Dev 1995;9(15):1857-68.

[18] Sato S, Yoshimizu T, Sato E, Matsui Y. Erasure of methylation imprinting of Igf2r during mouse primordial germ-cell development. Mol Reprod Dev 2003;65(1):41-50.

[19] Weaver JR, Susiarjo M, Bartolomei MS. Imprinting and epigenetic changes in the early embryo. Mamm Genome 2009;20(9-10):532-43.

[20] Hackett JA, Sengupta R, Zylicz JJ, Murakami K, Lee C, Down TA, Surani MA. Germline DNA demethylation dynamics and imprint erasure through 5-hydroxymethylcytosine.Science. 2013;339(6118):448-52.

[21] Tsankova NM, Berton O, Renthal W, Kumar A, Neve RL, Nestler EJ. Sustained hippocampal chromatin regulation in a mouse model of depression and antidepressant action. Nat Neurosci 2006;9(4):519-25.

[22] Jessberger S, Nakashima K, Clemenson GD Jr, Mejia E, Mathews E, Ure K, Ogawa S, Sinton CM, Gage FH, Hsieh J.Epigenetic Modulation of Seizure-Induced Neurogenesis and Cognitive Decline. J Neurosci 2007;27(22):5967-75.

[23] Dong E, Nelson M, Grayson DR, Costa E, Guidotti A. Clozapine and sulpiride but not haloperidol or olanzapine activate brain DNA demethylation. Proc Natl Acad Sci USA 2008;105(36):13614-9.

[24] Dong E, Chen Y, Gavin DP, Grayson DR, Guidotti A. Valproate induces DNA demethylation in nuclear extracts from adult mouse brain. Epigenetics 2010;5(8):730-5.

[25] Wang Q, Xu X, Li J, Liu J, Gu H, Zhang R, Chen J, Kuang Y, Fei J, Jiang C, Wang P, Pei D, Ding S, Xie X. Lithium, an anti-psychotic drug, greatly enhances the generation of induced pluripotent stem cells. Cell Res 2011;21(19):1424-35.

[26] Rimland, B. Controversies in the treatment of autistic children: vitamin and drug therapy. J Child Neurol 1988;3 Suppl, S68-S72.

[27] James SJ, Cutler P, Melnyk S, Jernigan S, Janak L, Gaylor DW, Neubrander JA. Metabolic biomarkers of increased oxidative stress and impaired methylation capacity in children with autism. Am. J. Clin. Nutr. 2004;80(6):1611-7.

[28] Moretti P, Sahoo T, Hyland K, Bottiglieri T, Peters S, del Gaudio D, Roa B, Curry S, Zhu H, Finnell RH, Neul JL, Ramaekers VT, Blau N, Bacino CA, Miller G, Scaglia F. Cerebral folate deficiency with developmental delay; autism; and response to folinic acid. Neurology 2005;64(6):1088-90.

[29] Ohtsuki A, Kimura MT, Minoshima M, Suzuki T, Ikeda M, Bando T, Nagase H, Shinohara, K, Sugiyama H. Synthesis and properties of PI polyamide–SAHA conjugate. Tetrahedron Lett 2009;50:7288-92.

[30] Matsuda H, Fukuda N, Ueno T, Katakawa M, Wang X, Watanabe T, Matsui S, Aoyama T, Saito K, Bando T, Matsumoto Y, Nagase H, Matsumoto K, Sugiyama H: Transcriptional inhibition of progressive renal disease by gene silencing pyrrole-imidazole polyamide targeting of the transforming growth factor-β1 promoter. Kidney Int 2011;79(1):46-56.

[31] Franklin TB, Russig H, Weiss IC, Gräff J, Linder N, Michalon A, Vizi S, Mansuy IM. Epigenetic transmission of the impact of early stress across generations. Biol Psychiatry 2010;68(5):408-15.

[32] Inoue K, Kanai M, Tanabe Y, Kubota T, Kashork CD, Wakui K, Fukushima Y, Lupski JR, Shaffer LG. Prenatal interphase FISH diagnosis of PLP1 duplication associated with Pelizaeus-Merzbacher disease. Prenat Diagn 2001;21(13):1133-6.

[33] Reiner O, Carrozzo R, Shen Y, Wehnert M, Faustinella F, Dobyns WB, Caskey CT, Ledbetter DH. Isolation of a Miller-Dieker lissencephaly gene containing G protein beta-subunit-like repeats. Nature 1993;364(6439):717-21.

[34] Bi W, Sapir T, Shchelochkov OA, Zhang F, Withers MA, Hunter JV, Levy T, Shinder V, Peiffer DA, Gunderson KL, Nezarati MM, Shotts VA, Amato SS, Savage SK, Harris DJ, Day-Salvatore DL, Horner M, Lu XY, Sahoo T, Yanagawa Y, Beaudet AL, Cheung SW, Martinez S, Lupski JR, Reiner O. Increased LIS1 expression affects human and mouse brain development. Nat Genet 2009;41(2):168-77.

[35] Online Mendelian Inheritance in Man (OMIM): #118220 http://www ncbi nlm nih gov/entrez/

[36] Obi T, Nishioka K, Ross OA, Terada T, Yamazaki K, Sugiura A, Takanashi M, Mizoguchi K, Mori H, Mizuno Y, Hattori N. Clinicopathologic study of a SNCA gene duplication patient with Parkinson disease and dementia. Neurology 2008;70(3):238-41.

[37] Li E, Beard C, Jaenisch R. Role for DNA methylation in genomic imprinting. Nature 1993;366(6453):362-5.

[38] Takizawa T, Nakashima K, Namihira M, Ochiai W, Uemura A, Yanagisawa M, Fujita N, Nakao M, Taga T. DNA methylation is a critical cell-intrinsic determinant of astrocyte differentiation in the fetal brain. Dev Cell 2001;1(6):749-758.

[39] Sakashita K, Koike K, Kinoshita T, Shiohara M, Kamijo T, Taniguchi S, Kubota T: Dynamic DNA methylation change in the CpG island region of p15 during human myeloid development. J Clin Invest 2001;108(8):1195-204.

[40] Abel T and Zukin RS. Epigenetic targets of HDAC inhibition in neurodegenerative and psychiatric disorders. Curr Opin Pharmacol 2008;8(1):57-64.

[41] Urdinguio RG, Sanchez-Mut JV, Esteller M. Epigenetic mechanisms in neurological diseases: genes syndromes and therapies: Lancet Neurol 2009;8(11):1056-72.

[42] Wu H, Tao J, Chen PJ, Shahab A, Ge W, Hart RP, Ruan X, Ruan Y, Sun YE. Genome-wide analysis reveals methyl-CpG-binding protein 2-dependent regulation of microRNAs in a mouse model of Rett syndrome. Proc Natl Acad Sci U S A 2010;107(42): 18161-6.

[43] Xue F, Tian XC, Du F, Kubota C, Taneja M, Dinnyes A, Dai Y, Levine H, Pereira LV, Yang X. Aberrant patterns of X chromosome inactivation in bovine clones. Nat Genet 2002:31(2):216-220.

[44] Nolen LD, Gao S, Han Z, Mann MR, Gie Chung Y, Otte AP, Bartolomei MS, Latham KE. X chromosome reactivation and regulation in cloned embryos. Dev Biol 2005;279(2):525-540.

[45] Chen WG, Chang Q, Lin Y, Meissner A, West AE, Griffith EC, Jaenisch R, Greenberg MEDerepression of BDNF transcription involves calcium-dependent phosphorylation of MeCP2. Science 2003:302(5564):885-9.

[46] Martinowich K, Hattori D, Wu H, Fouse S, He F, Hu Y, Fan G, Sun YE. DNA methylation-related chromatin remodeling in activity-dependent BDNF gene regulation. Science 2003(5646):302:890-3.

[47] Itoh M, Ide S, Takashima S, Kudo S, Nomura Y, Segawa M, Kubota T, Mori H, Tanaka S, Horie H, Tanabe Y, Goto Y. Methyl CpG-binding protein 2 (a mutation of which causes Rett syndrome) directly regulates insulin-like growth factor binding protein 3 in mouse and human brains. J Neuropathol Exp Neurol 2007:66(2):117-23.

[48] Miyake K, Hirasawa T, Soutome M, Itoh M, Goto Y, Endoh K, Takahashi K, Kudo S, Nakagawa T, Yokoi S, Taira T, Inazawa, J, Kubota T. The protocadherins, PCDHB1 and PCDH7, are regulated by MeCP2 in neuronal cells and brain tissues: implication for pathogenesis of Rett syndrome. BMC Neurosci 2011;12:81.

[49] Chahrour M, Jung SY, Shaw C, Zhou X, Wong ST, Qin J, Zoghbi HY. MeCP2, a key contributor to neurological disease, activates and represses transcription. Science 2008, 320(5880):1224-1229.

[50] Kubota T, Aradhya S, Macha M, Smith AC, Surh LC, Satish J, Verp MS, Nee HL, Johnson A, Christan SL, Ledbetter DH. Analysis of parent of origin specific DNA methylation at SNRPN and PW71 in tissues: implication for prenatal diagnosis. J Med Genet. 1996 Dec;33(12):1011-4.

[51] Fombonne E. Epidemiology of pervasive developmental disorders. Pediatr Res 2009;65(6):591-8.

[52] Ma DK, Jang MH, Guo JU, Kitabatake, Y, Chang ML, Pow-Anpongkul N, et al. Neuronal Activity–Induced Gadd45b Promotes Epigenetic DNA Demethylation and Adult Neurogenesis. Science 2009;323(5917):1074-7.

[53] McGowan PO, Sasaki A, D'Alessio AC, Dymov S, Labonté B, Szyf M, Turecki G, Meaney MJ. Epigenetic regulation of the glucocorticoid receptor in human brain associates with childhood abuse. Nat Neurosci 2009;12(3):342-8.

[54] Murgatroyd C, Patchev AV, Wu Y, Micale V, Bockmühl Y, Fischer D, Holsboer F, Wotjak CT, Almeida OF, Spengler D. Dynamic DNA methylation programs persistent adverse effects of early-life stress. Nat Neurosci 2009;12(12):1559-66.

[55] Renthal W, Kumar A, Xiao G, Wilkinson M, Covington HE 3rd, Maze I, Sikder D, Robison AJ, LaPlant Q, Dietz DM, Russo SJ, Vialou V, Chakravarty S, Kodadek TJ, Stack A, Kabbaj M, Nestler EJ. Genome-wide analysis of chromatin regulation by cocaine reveals a role for sirtuins. Neuron 2009;62(3):335-48.

[56] Pascual M, Boix J, Felipo V, Guerri C. Repeated alcohol administration during adolescence causes changes in the mesolimbic dopaminergic and glutamatergic systems and promotes alcohol intake in the adult rat. J Neurochem 2009;108(4):920-31.

[57] Gluckman PD, Seng CY, Fukuoka H, Beedle AS, Hanson MA. Low birthweight and subsequent obesity in Japan. Lancet 2007;369(9567):1081-2.

[58] Painter RC, de Rooij SR, Bossuyt PM, Simmers TA, Osmond C, Barker DJ, Bleker OP, Roseboom TJ. Early onset of coronary artery disease after prenatal exposure to the Dutch famine. Am J Clin Nutr 2006;84(2):322-7.

[59] St Clair D, Xu M, Wang P, Yu Y, Fang Y, Zhang F, Zheng X, Gu N, Feng G, Sham P, He L. Rates of adult schizophrenia following prenatal exposure to the Chinese famine of 1959-1961. JAMA 2005;294(5):557-62.

[60] Silveira PP, Portella AK, Goldani MZ, Barbieri MA. Developmental origins of health and disease (DOHaD). J Pediatr (Rio J) 2007;83(6):494-504.

[61] Lillycrop KA, Phillips ES, Torrens C, Hanson MA, Jackson AA, Burdge GC: Feeding pregnant rats a protein-restricted diet persistently alters the methylation of specific cytosines in the hepatic PPAR alpha promoter of the offspring. Br J Nutr 2008;100(2): 278-82.

[62] Tobi EW, Lumey LH, Talens RP, Kremer D, Putter H, Stein AD, et al. DNA methylation differences after exposure to prenatal famine are common and timing-and sex-specific. Hum Mol Genet 2009;18(21):4046-53.

[63] Lim D, Bowdin SC, Tee L. Clinical and molecular genetic features of Beckwith-Wiedemann syndrome associated with assisted reproductive technologies. Hum Reprod 2009; 24(3):741-7.

[64] Bliek J, Alders M, Maas SM, Oostra RJ, Mackay DM, van der Lip K, et al. Lessons from BWS twins: complex maternal and paternal hypomethylation and a common source of haematopoietic stem cells. Eur J Hum Genet 2009;17(12):1625-34.

[65] Basic investigation report for handicapped children 2005 (in Japanese). http://www.mhlw.go.jp/toukei/saikin/hw/titeki/index.html (Sep 9; 2013).

[66] Yeargin-Allsopp M, Rice C, Karapurkar T, Doernberg N, Boyle C, Murphy C. Prevalence of autism in a US metropolitan area. JAMA. 2003;289(1):49-55.

[67] Holden C. Autism Now. Science 2009;323:565.

[68] Fombonne E. Epidemiology of pervasive developmental disorders. Pediatr Res 2009;65(6):591-8.

[69] Kim YS, Leventhal BL, Koh YJ, Fombonne E, Laska E, Lim EC, et al. Prevalence of autism spectrum disorders in a total population sample. Am J Psychiatry 2011;168(9): 904-12.

[70] Lord C. Epidemiology: How common is autism? Nature 2011;474(7350):166-8.

[71] Waterland RA, Jirtle RL. Transposable elements: targets for early nutritional effects on epigenetic gene regulation. Mol Cell Biol 2003;23(15):5293-300.

[72] Kucharski R, Maleszka J, Foret S, Maleszka R. Nutritional control of reproductive status in honeybees via DNA methylation. Science 2008;319(5871):1827-30.

[73] Yaoi T, Itoh K, Nakamura K, Ogi H, Fujiwara Y, Fushiki S. Genome-wide analysis of epigenomic alterations in fetal mouse forebrain after exposure to low doses of bisphenol A. Biochem Biophys Res Commun 2008;376(3):563-7.

[74] Gore AC, Walker DM, Zama AM, Armenti AE, Uzumcu M. Early life exposure to endocrine-disrupting chemicals causes lifelong molecular reprogramming of the hypothalamus and premature reproductive aging. Mol Endocrinol 2011;25(12):2157-68.

[75] Kondo M, Gray LJ, Pelka GJ, Christodoulou J, Tam PP, Hannan AJ. Environmental enrichment ameliorates a motor coordination deficit in a mouse model of Rett syndrome-Mecp2 gene dosage effects and BDNF expression. Eur J Neurosci 2008;27(12): 3342-50.

[76] Lonetti G, Angelucci A, Morando L, Boggio EM, Giustetto M, Pizzorusso T. Early environmental enrichment moderates the behavioral and synaptic phenotype of MeCP2 null mice. Biol Psychiatry 2010;67(7):657-65.

[77] Nag N, Moriuchi JM, Peitzman CG, Ward BC, Kolodny NH, Berger-Sweeney JE. Environmental enrichment alters locomotor behaviour and ventricular volume in Mecp2 1lox mice. Behav Brain Res 2009;196(1):44-8.

[78] Kerr B, Silva PA, Walz K, Young JI. Unconventional transcriptional response to environmental enrichment in a mouse model of Rett syndrome. PLoS One 2010;5(7):e11534.

[79] Luikenhuis S, Giacometti E, Beard CF, Jaenisch R. Expression of MeCP2 in postmitotic neurons rescues Rett syndrome in mice. Proc Natl Acad Sci USA 2004;101(16): 6033-8.

[80] Guy J, Gan J, Selfridge J, Cobb S, Bird A. Reversal of neurological defects in a mouse model of Rett syndrome. Science 2007;315(5815):1143-7.

[81] Lioy DT, Garg SK, Monaghan CE, Raber J, Foust KD, Kaspar BK, et al. A role for glia in the progression of Rett's syndrome. Nature 2011;475(7357):497-500.

[82] Vecsler M, Simon AJ, Amariglio N, Rechavi G, Gak E. MeCP2 deficiency downregulates specific nuclear proteins that could be partially recovered by valproic acid in vitro. Epigenetics 2010;5(1):61-7.

[83] Abel T, Zukin RS. Epigenetic targets of HDAC inhibition in neurodegenerative and psychiatric disorders. Curr Opin Pharmacol. 2008;8(1):57-64.

[84] Cassel S, Carouge D, Gensburger C, Anglard P, Burgun C, Dietrich JB, Aunis D, Zwiller J. Fluoxetine and cocaine induce the epigenetic factors MeCP2 and MBD1 in adult rat brain. Mol Pharmacol. 2006;70(2):487-92.

[85] Popp C, Dean W, Feng S, Cokus SJ, Andrews S, Pellegrini M, et al. Genome-wide erasure of DNA methylation in mouse primordial germ cells is affected by AID deficiency. Nature 2011;463(7284):1101-5.

[86] Daxinger L, Whitelaw E. Transgenerational epigenetic inheritance: more questions than answers. Genome Res 2010;20(12):1623-8.

[87] Horsthemke, B. Heritable germline epimutations in humans. Nat Genet 2007;39(5): 573-4.

[88] Chong S, Youngson NA, Whitelow E. Heritable germline epimutation is not the same as transgenerational epigenetic inheritance. Nat Genet 2007;39(5):574-5.

[89] Rakyan VK, Chong S, Champ ME, Cuthbert PC, Morgan HD, Luu KV, WhitelawE. Transgenerational inheritance of epigenetic states at the murine Axin(Fu) allele occurs after maternal and paternal transmission. Proc Natl Acad Sci USA 2003;100(5): 2538-43.

[90] Relton CL, Davey Smith G. Two-step epigenetic Mendelian randomization: a strategy for establishing the causal role of epigenetic processes in pathways to disease. Int J Epidemiol 2012;41(1):161-76.

[91] Kappeler L, Meaney MJ. Epigenetics and parental effects. Bioessays 2010;32(9): 818-27.

[92] Waterland RA, Travisano M, Tahiliani KG. Diet-induced hypermethylation at agouti viable yellow is not inherited transgenerationally through the female. FASEB J. 2007;21(12):3380-5.

[93] Anway MD, Cupp AS, Uzumcu M, Skinner MK. Epigenetic transgenerational actions of endocrine disruptors and male fertility. Science 2005;308(5727):1466-9. Erratum in: Science 2010;328(5979):690.

[94] Manikkam M, Tracey R, Guerrero-Bosagna C, Skinner MK. Plastics derived endocrine disruptors (BPA, DEHP and DBP) induce epigenetic transgenerational inheritance of obesity, reproductive disease and sperm epimutations. PLoS One 2013;8(1):e55387.

[95] Seong KH, Li D, Shimizu H, Nakamura R, Ishii S. Inheritance of Stress-Induced, ATF-2-Dependent Epigenetic Change. Cell 2011;145(7):1049-61.

[96] Champagne FA, Weaver IC, Diorio J, Dymov S, Szyf M, Meaney MJ. Maternal care associated with methylation of the estrogen receptor-alpha1b promoter and estrogen receptor-alpha expression in the medial preoptic area of female offspring. Endocrinology 2006;147(6):2909-15.

[97] Crews D, Gillette R, Scarpino SV, Manikkam M, Savenkova MI, Skinner MK. Epigenetic transgenerational inheritance of altered stress responses. Proc Natl Acad Sci USA 2012;109(23):9143-8.

[98] Becker C, Weigel D. Epigenetic variation: origin and transgenerational inheritance. Curr Opin Plant Biol 2012;15(5):562-7.

[99] Rakyan V, Whitelaw E. Transgenerational epigenetic inheritance. Curr Biol 2003;13(1):R6.

[100] Schmitz RJ, Schultz MD, Lewsey MG, O'Malley RC, Urich MA, Libiger O, Schork NJ, Ecker JR. Transgenerational epigenetic instability is a source of novel methylation variants. Science 2011;334(6054):369-73.

[101] Zocchi L, Sassone-Corsi P. Joining the dots: from chromatin remodeling to neuronal plasticity. Curr Opin Neurobiol 2010;20(4):432-40.

[102] Lister R, Mukamel EA, Nery JR, Urich M, Puddifoot CA, Johnson ND, et al. Global epigenomic reconfiguration during mammalian brain development. Science 2013;341(6146):1237905.

[103] Crews D, Gillette R, Scarpino SV, Manikkam M, Savenkova MI, Skinner MK. Epigenetic transgenerational inheritance of altered stress responses. Proc Natl Acad Sci USA 2012;109(23):9143-8.

[104] Ng SF, Lin RC, Laybutt DR, Barres R, Owens JA, Morris MJ. Chronic high-fat diet in fathers programs β-cell dysfunction in female rat offspring. Nature 2010;467(7318): 963-6.

[105] Ferguson-Smith AC, Patti ME. You are what your dad ate. Cell Metab 2011;13(2): 115-7.

[106] Law JA, Du J, Hale CJ, Feng S, Krajewski K, Palanca AM, Strahl BD, Patel DJ, Jacobsen SE. Polymerase IV occupancy at RNA-directed DNA methylation sites requires SHH1.Nature 2013;498(7454):385-9.

[107] Konermann S, Brigham MD, Trevino AE, Hsu PD, Heidenreich M, Cong L, Platt RJ, Scott DA, Church GM, Zhang F. Optical control of mammalian endogenous transcription and epigenetic states. Nature 2013;500(7463):472-6.

6

Apicomplexa and Histone Variants: What's New?

Laura Vanagas, Susana Marisol Contreras
and Sergio Oscar Angel

Abstract

Plasmodium spp. and *Toxoplasma gondii* present a conserved nucleosome composition based on canonical H3 and variants, H4, canonical H2A and variants, and H2B. One-off, the phylum has also a variant H2B, named H2B.Z, which was shown to form a double variant nucleosome H2A.Z/H2B.Z. These histones also present conserved and unique post-translational modifications (PTMs). Histone variants have shown particular genomic localization and PTMs along euchromatin and heterochromatin, including telomere-associated sequences (TAS), suggesting fine-grained chromatin structure modulation. Several other nonhistone proteins present remarkable participation in controlling chromatin state, especially at TAS. Based on that, we discuss the role of epigenetics (PTMs and histone variants) in *Plasmodium* and *Toxoplasma* gene expression, replication, and DNA repair. We also discuss TAS structures and chromatin composition and its impact on antigenic variant expression in *Plasmodium*.

Keywords: *Plasmodium*, *Toxoplasma*, epigenetics, histone variants, H2B.Z, chromatin, antigenic variation, telomere-associated region

1. Introduction

Apicomplexa is a large phylum of unicellular obligate intracellular protozoan parasites responsible for a range of human and animal diseases with considerable medical and economic impact worldwide [1]. The phylum comprises several well-known genera such as *Cryptosporidium*, *Eimeria, Babesia,* and *Theileria,* but the most studied genera are *Plasmodium* and *Toxoplasma.*

Plasmodium genus is comprised by several species of which five infect humans: *P. falciparum*, *P. ovale, P. malariae, P. vivax,* and *P. knowlesi*. The infection due to *Plasmodium* genus is known as Malaria, a mosquito-borne infectious disease endemic in the tropical and subtropical zones of Asia, Africa, South, and Central America. Malaria also constitutes a serious problem for travelers as well as for people working in endemic regions. In 2016, an infection rate of 216 million cases was reported, causing some 445,000 deaths globally. Data show a stalling in declining burden of *Plasmodium* observed over the last decade (http://apps.who.int/iris/bitstream/10665/259492/1/9789241565523-eng.pdf?ua=1). In addition, the mass drug administration program has shown a limit due to the spreading of multidrug-resistant malaria [2]. The severe disease is mainly caused by *P. falciparum,* whereas *P. vivax* causes the majority of malaria morbidity outside Africa. The clinical manifestations of malaria include fever, shivering, arthralgia (joint pain), vomiting, jaundice, hemoglobinuria, convulsions, metabolic alterations, renal failure, liver and lung dysfunctions, anemia, and cerebral malaria (coma).

Toxoplasma gondii is the only one species of the *Toxoplasma* genus, and it is able to infect birds and mammals, including human, and cause toxoplasmosis. The infection occurs worldwide and the chronic stage reaches more than 500 million people [3]. During the first few weeks of infection, toxoplasmosis is either asymptomatic or causes a mild flu-like illness. However, those with a weakened immune system, such as AIDS patients, infected fetus during gestation or newborns with a congenital infection, may become seriously ill, and occasionally die. The parasite can cause encephalitis (inflammation of the brain) and neurologic diseases, and can affect the heart, liver, inner ears, and eyes (chorioretinitis). Recent research has also linked toxoplasmosis with neuropsychiatric symptoms such as attention-deficit hyperactivity disorder, obsessive compulsive disorder, bipolar disease, and schizophrenia [4–8]. The present chemotherapy for toxoplasmosis is efficient but, sometimes, it is not well tolerated by individuals with AIDS, and it is effective against the acute or active stage, but not against the chronic/latent stage.

2. Genome and nucleus

Both *Plasmodium* protozoan parasites and *T. gondii* present a highly complex life cycle, involving several stages along the cycle (**Figure 1**). The genome sizes are 23.3 Mb for *Plasmodium* and 80 Mb for *Toxoplasma,* being haploid (1 N) almost all their life cycle but diploid during sexual replicative stages (2 N) (**Figure 1**). *Plasmodium* genus and *T. gondii* were the first apicomplexan parasites to be included in genome projects [9, 10]. Since then, several other apicomplexan parasites genome projects were taken forward and the data uploaded at EuPathDB (https://eupathdb.org/eupathdb/). From these databases, it could be observed that *T. gondii* and *P. falciparum* present about 5300 (https://protists.ensembl.org/Plasmodium_falciparum/Info/Index) and 8172 (http://protists.ensembl.org/Toxoplasma_gondii/Info/Annotation/#assembly) gene transcripts, respectively, organized as single copy genes along the chromosomes, and in general, they are not clustered by function, pathway, or stage of expression. All of these data suggest that these genes are finely regulated throughout the cell cycle and the life cycle by transcriptional regulators and chromatin. Regarding transcription factors, they are poorly represented in apicomplexan, with only one large family of transcriptional regulators, with 24 AP2 family factors in *P. falciparum* and 68 in *T. gondii* [11, 12]. In this context, epigenetic

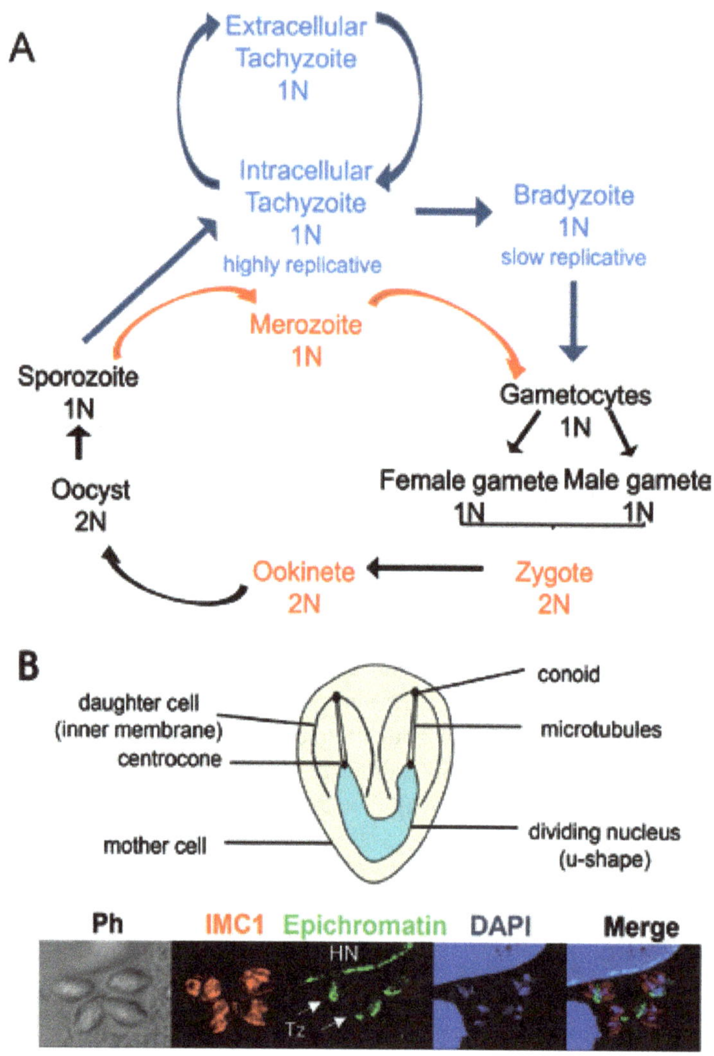

Figure 1. (A) Life cycles of T. gondii and P. falciparum. Haploid and diploid DNA content is referred to as 1 and 2 N. Black arrows and letters represent common parasite stages, blue arrows and letters represent T. gondii specific stages, and red arrows and letters represent P. falciparum-specific stages. (B) Epichromatin labeling in T. gondii. Epichromatin is a conformational epitope formed by DNA and histones H2A and H2B localized only at the exterior chromatin surface. During tachyzoite replication, the 2 N nucleus is divided, entering one genome to each budding cell, forming a typical U shape. The nuclear envelope does not disappear, and chromosomes do not present high level of condensation. Epichromatin labels predominantly one side of the nucleus, suggesting a nonhomogeneous organization of chromosomes and nuclear envelope interaction. IMC1: inner membrane complex 1.

control was proposed as a key element to facilitate parasite gene expression, DNA replication, and DNA repair [13–15].

An interesting aspect of apicomplexan parasites is that they never lose the nuclear envelope during cell division, and their chromosomes do not present the higher order level of condensation observed in metaphase chromosomes of higher eukaryotes [16]. So, the nucleus presents the same aspect along the cell cycle. However, it seems to be not homogenous: *Toxoplasma gondii* nuclear envelope and chromosomes seem to have a dynamic relocalization and/or rotation inside the nucleus during parasite budding as observed by epichromatin localization (**Figure 1B**). Epichromatin is a conformational epitope formed by DNA and histones H2A and H2B localized only at the exterior chromatin surface [17, 18]. More recently, it was observed that epichromatin forms superbead domains associated to DNA-A at the nuclear envelope [19]. A 3D analysis also shows that *P. falciparum* nucleus presents a polarization of the nuclear pore complex: in the early multinucleated schizont, it clusters in the nucleus region facing the mother plasma membrane, whereas in the late stages, when prepared for budding, it clusters toward the cytoplasm of the incipient merozoite [20].

In addition to putative polarization of the genome inside the nucleus of Apicomplexan parasites, in *T. gondii,* it was observed that the centromeres (CenH3, see below) are localized at a single spot at the apical region of the nucleus, indicating that all of them are attached to the centrocone, a structure associated to the nuclear envelope, which is traversed by microtubules coordinating the cell division [21]. Similarly, Chromo1, a *T. gondii* protein that binds to the telomere, presents a focalized localization in the nucleus, also suggesting a certain degree of chromosome organization within the parasite nucleus [22]. In *P. falciparum* prior to replication, in late ring stages and young trophozoites, CenH3 localizes to a single nuclear focus suggesting that centromeres are clustered in a single spot that most likely continues to be attached to the mitotic spindle until the end of schizogony and the intraerythrocytic developmental cycle, similar to that observed in *T. gondii* [23].

3. H3 histones: a multivariant family

H3 histone family presents canonical forms: H3, H3.1, H3.2 and variants: H3.3 and cenH3 [24]. H3.3 differs from canonical H3s in various aspects. Canonical H3s are expressed and associate to chromatin during the S-phase of cell cycle. Canonical H3s and H3.3 are highly identical differing in only four to five amino acids. The CAF-1 complex is involved in the incorporation of canonical H3s whereas CHD1/ATRX remodelers as well as HIRA chaperone complex are involved in the incorporation of H3.3 [25–30]. In addition, H3.3 is enriched in transcribed genes, enhancers, regulatory elements, and also heterochromatic repeats, including telomeres and pericentromeric regions [31–34]. In general, H3.3 is linked to gene activation or open chromatin. Moreover, it has been found to be methylated at K4, K36, and K79 and acetylated at K9 and K14, all being marks of active chromatin [32, 35]. H3.3 and H2A.Z were detected at active promoters generating nucleosomes that promote gene transcription [36–38]. Recently, it was found that H3.3 plays an essential biological role during mammal development since mice that lack H3.3 presented developmental retardation and early embryonic lethality [39]. Rather than gene expression troubles, H3.3 depletion causes genome instability due to dysfunction of heterochromatin structures at telomeres, centromeres, and pericentromeric regions of chromosomes, leading to mitotic defects.

There is little information regarding H3 histone family and the variants H3.3 in Apicomplexan parasites. The first approach is from W.J Sullivan [40] who was able to clone the entire ORFs encoding H3 and H3.3 in *Toxoplasma gondii* and also in *Plasmodium falciparum*. In this work, it was confirmed that, like in most other organisms, there is not much difference between the two variants: only four amino acids in *T. gondii* and eight between the *P. falciparum* variants. In most other species, the critical residues that differ between H3 and H3.3, resulting in different roles of these histones, are a motif, which contains SAVM in H3 canonical histone, but changes to AAIG in H3.3 [24]. However, while PfH3 has the typical SAVM motif, it changes to QAVL in PfH3.3, whereas in TgH3, the motif is SAVL and changes to QAIL in TgH3.3 [40]. Besides, there is another difference in Apicomplexa, which seems to be exclusive: KF changes for RY at position 54–55 in H3.3 [40].

In *Plasmodium*, H3.3 had a similar expression pattern to another important histone variant, H2A.Z, namely localization to active chromatin [41] (see **Figure 2**). As observed in other eukaryotic cells, it has been recently demonstrated by ChiP-seq experiments that euchromatic regions in the genome are demarcated by the presence of the H3.3 variant histone [42]. However, in *P. falciparum*, there is a particular AT versus GC content along the genome with euchromatic intergenic regions richer in AT-content compared to coding sequences with less AT content [23]. Fraschka et al. [42] have seen a particular correlation between enrichment in PfH3.3 histone variant and GC content, with this variant mainly located not only in euchromatic GC-rich sequences, but also in subtelomeric GC-rich repetitive regions. Interestingly, this correlation with the nucleotide composition is also observed with the double-variant nucleosome H2A.Z-H2B.Z (see below), but in this case, it is just the contrary: the regions with more AT content show abundance of this nucleosome [42]. However, GC-poor intergenic regions show the lowest H3.3 coverage, but the authors still argue that the incorporation of this variant to coding regions is more dependent on GC content than transcriptional activity.

It is well documented that *P. falciparum* depends on the *var* multigene family, encoding for a highly variable cytoadherence protein called *P. falciparum* erythrocyte membrane protein 1 (PfEMP1) to avoid host immunity [43–46]. This is due to the expression of only one of the ~60 *var* gene family members in any given parasite.

Regarding this important gene family, H3.3 stably occupies the promoter region and coding sequence of the active *var* gene but is evidently less incorporated into the promoter and coding sequence of silenced *var* genes [42] (see **Figure 3**). Additionally, it has been demonstrated that the PTMs affecting histone H3 are extremely important in the regulation of *var* expression. Data from fluorescence *in situ* hybridization (FISH) suggest that the *P. falciparum* SETvs (*P. falciparum variant-silencing SET* gene), which encodes an ortholog of *Drosophila melanogaster* ASH1 and controls histone H3 lysine 36 trimethylation (H3K36me3) on *var* genes, is specifically involved in *var* gene silencing, and its *knock-out* results in the transcription of virtually all *var* genes in the single parasite nuclei [47]. Besides, ChIP-qPCR analysis showed that the TSS occupancy of H3K36me3 is considerably higher in the silent *var* genes compared to the active one (see **Figure 3**) [47].

A detailed mass spectrometry study has been accomplished for *P. falciparum* histone PTMs by Trelle et al. [48], and it has been established that lysines 4, 9, 14, 18, 23, and 27 of both H3 and H3.3 are capable of being modified by acetylations and/or methylations. Also, arginine in position 17 may be mono or bimethylated. Some of these modifications had already been

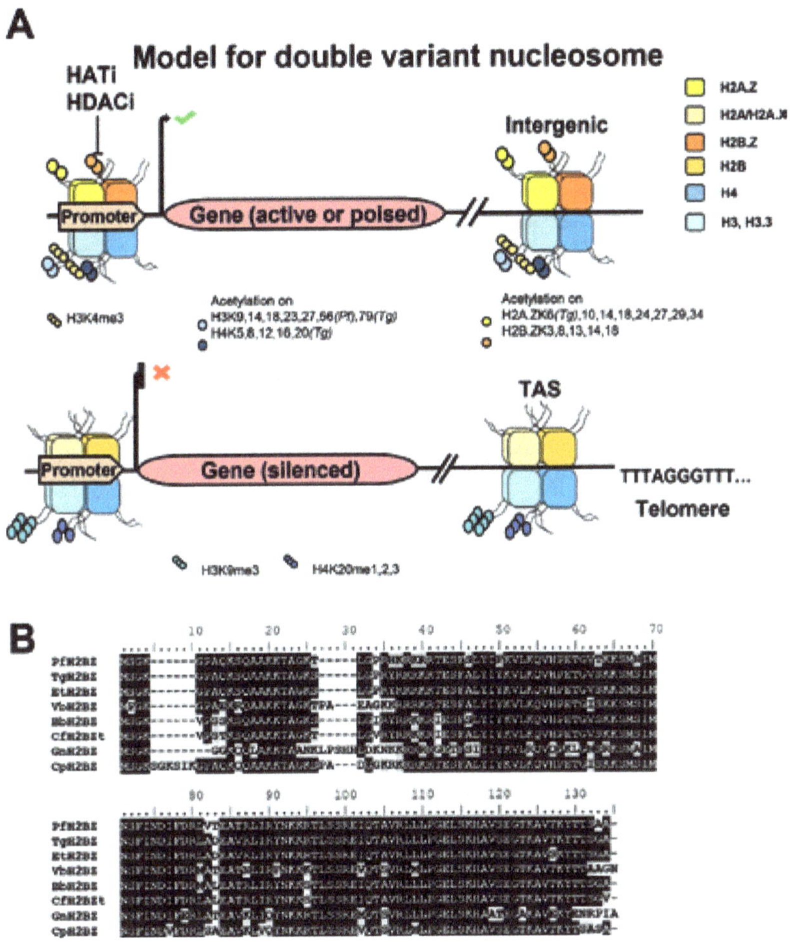

Figure 2. (A) Schematic model for double-variant nucleosome in T. gondii and P. falciparum. Hypothetical active (or poised) and silenced genes are represented with the nucleosome composition in each promoter and also downstream the genes. PTM marks are represented as well and listed below with the differences found in the literature between both the parasites. Specific HATs and HDACs are speculated to acetylate/deacetylate the unique H2B.Z histone variant. (B) Sequence alignment of histone variant H2B.Z in Apicomplexa. Pf: Plasmodium falciparum, Tg: Toxoplasma gondii, Et: Eimeria tenella, Vb: Vitrella brassicaformis, Bv: Babesia bovis, Cf: Cytauxzoon felis, Gn: Gregarina niphandrodes and Cp: Cryptosporidium parvum. All sequences can be found in EuPathDB (https://eupathdb.org/eupathdb/).

identified for H3 and H3.3 also by Miao et al. [41]. More recently, a lysine residue in the core of H3, K56, was also indicated as a site of acetylation [49, 50]. In the same way, *T. gondii* histone H3 has many lysines and also arginines capable of being modified: lysines in the positions 4, 9, 14, 23, 27 and also 36, 37, 56, 115 and 122 can be acetylated, methylated and besides some of them receive formylation, ubiquitination, or succinylation [51]. Besides, arginines 2, 17, 26, 40, and 83 can be methylated [51].

But not only acetylations and methylations are marking histones; with the development of improved acid and high-salt purification methods for *P. falciparum* histone phosphoprotein analysis, multiple phosphorylation sites have been found mostly at the N-terminal region of

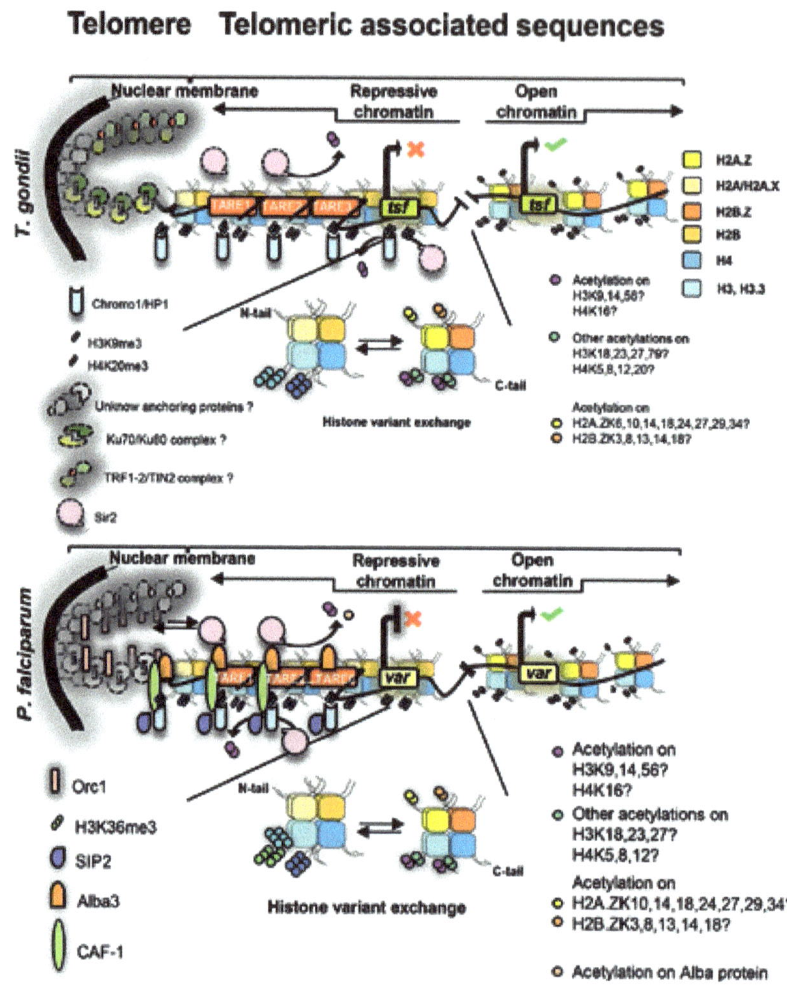

Figure 3. Hypothetical telomeric and subtelomeric structure in T. gondii (upper panel) and P. falciparum (lower panel). Here, we show the TgTAS and PfTAS composition and the possible protein interactors listed in **Table 1** and described in Section 6. In P. falciparum, we only illustrate three of the six TAREs associated. The punctuated lines define proteins described in other organisms, but some of them present an ortholog in any of those parasites. The proteins represented in continuous lines have already been described for those parasites. Proteins illustrated in grey are unknown proteins. We also show the possible histone variant exchange on silenced or active *tsf* or *var* genes. Specific PTMs on silenced or active genes are described in the figure. The questions are open because these proteins and PTMs have not been confirmed yet in these TAS regions.

most histones, including H3 and H3.3 [52]. These marks are frequently seen in combination with neighboring lysine acetylation (and methylation). In this work, they also described a Pf14-3-3 as a phosphohistone mark binding protein.

In parasites, among the most conserved modifications is histone 3 trimethylation of lysine 4 (H3K4me3), a marker of potentially active promoters. Opposed to that is H3K9 methylation, associated with silent genes and densely packed heterochromatin, although protozoan parasite histones are more highly enriched in the activation marks associated with euchromatin with lower abundance of histone modifications associated with heterochromatin [53]. However, it has been shown that the epigenome in *P. falciparum* is highly dynamic, and dependent on the stage, and, for example, H3K4me3 and H3K9ac are cycle regulated at *P. falciparum* genes [49]. This could also probably be true for *T. gondii*, where the tachyzoite to bradyzoite conversion is regulated at an epigenetic level. In this sense, it has been speculated that the H3R17me2 mark may have significance during the tachyzoite to bradyzoite differentiation process, as it was found only restricted to a subset of promoters, and taking into account the importance of arginine methylation during early development of mouse embryo [54]. In this study, using ChIP-on-chip technique, they found that H3K9ac, H4ac, and H3K4me3 modifications co-localize at focused loci in the *T. gondii* genome and correlate with significant gene expression, while the H3K4me1 and the H3K4me2 modifications were found at equal amounts in active and inactive chromatin [54].

4. Centromeric H3

CenH3, the centromere-specific H3, has been observed in animals, fungi, and plants [24] and also in Apicomplexa, including *T. gondii, Plasmodium spp.,* and *N. caninum* [55]. This fact was recently confirmed by Fraschka et al. [42] who found the centromeres depleted of PfH3.3 and PfH3, but occupied by PfCenH3. In *T. gondii*, this histone variant was characterized with the aim to understand the way in which chromosomes are delivered to the daughter cells after mitosis, a process that is still intriguing [21]. In this work, the authors labeled all the histone H3 variants, and used TgCenH3 as a marker of centromeres, to perform ChIP and microarray assays [21]. They found a particular combination of histone PTMs surrounding centromeres; this region had a huge concentration of H3K9 di- and trimethylation, marks usually associated to heterochromatin and found in subtelomeric regions in *P. falciparum* but not in *T. gondii.* In this parasite, these modifications concentrate in two peaks directly flanking the center of the centromere in each chromosome, while H3K4me3 or H3K9ac are not present [21, 52]. In contrast, H3K9me3 and heterochromatin protein 1 (HP1, chromodomain protein that binds to H3K9me3) were not associated with centromeres in *P. falciparum* [23], but rather found in islands of the genome that contain transcriptionally silent members of multigene families [56]. In this parasite, the enrichment of PfCenH3 on centromeres of all the chromosomes has also been demonstrated by genome-wide ChIP-seq analysis [23]. Besides, it has been characterized that a region within the carboxy-terminal histone fold domain, which is also named CENP-A targeting domain (CATD), is essential for mediating centromere targeting, while the N-terminus is not [57].

5. H2A.Z-H2B.Z: the double variant nucleosome

H2A family also has a canonical H2A and several variants: H2A.Z, H2A.X, both exchangeable by H2A.Z-H2B or H2A.X-H2B, allowing the modulation of gene transcription, DNA replication, and/or DNA damage repair [58, 59]. In vertebrates, the H2A family has two more variants: H2Abd and macro-H2A. When talking about H2A-H2B and the incorporation of variants into such nucleosomes, there are vast differences if we take a glance at Apicomplexan parasites compared to most other eukaryotes. One of the most surprising discoveries in these parasites was the presence of a novel H2B variant (formerly named H2Bv, but recently reclassified as H2B.Z [60]), a histone, which is known to be deficient in variants, similar to H4 [58, 61]. Variants of this histone family, though, are not only found in these parasites, but also in *Trypanosomatids* (even though they are not evolutionary related), and some rare testis-specific variants in human and other mammalian species (reviewed in [55]).

Different studies performed in *Toxoplasma* have shown a nucleosome composition in which H2A.Z, but not H2A.X, dimerizes with H2B.Z, while H2A.X dimerizes with canonical H2B (H2Ba in *T. gondii*), but never with H2B.Z [62, 63]. This fact is also seen in *P. falciparum*, although this parasite lacks H2A.X variant [41] and has driven the hypothesis of a new double variant nucleosome exclusive of parasites with particular characteristics that will be described in this section [64, 65] (**Figure 2A**). As it can be observed in the sequence alignment of H2B.Z in many Apicomplexan species, this histone variant is quite conserved (**Figure 2B**), suggesting that this histone, and likely the double variant nucleosome H2A.Z-H2B.Z, may have had an important role in the expansion of the phylum.

Since H2B.Z is not represented in yeast, insects, or mammals, almost all the current knowledge about the double-variant nucleosome relies on H2A.Z studies. H2A.Z is so widespread that has been catalogued as "universal" because of its origin before the divergence of eukaryotes [66]. The first observation that appears is the hyperacetylation of its N-terminal tail in most species [48–50, 67–69]. It is thought that this possibility gives H2A.Z the faculty of mediating responsiveness to the environmental changes, with so varied and seemingly contradictory effects as gene activation, heterochromatic silencing, transcriptional memory, and others, depending on the binding of activating or repressive complexes [66]. H2A.Z containing nucleosomes mark active and bivalent promoters as well as enhancers, correlating with open chromatin [70, 71]. However, acetylation of H2A.Z is necessary for gene induction and is most often associated with active gene transcription [67, 68, 70, 71], whereas ubiquitylation, which can occur at the C-terminal tail, is linked to transcriptional repression and polycomb silencing [72–75]. Acetylated H2A.Z composes nucleosomes flanking the nucleosome-depleted regions [76]. Regulation of gene expression by acetylation of H2A.Z histone tail may be a result of the participation of other proteins as "readers" in the histone code; for example, the SWR-C chromatin remodeling enzyme and related INO80 family are well characterized to catalyze chromatin incorporation of the histone variant from yeast to human, and the acetylation of histone H3 on lysine 56 (H3-K56Ac) was said to lead to promiscuous dimer exchange in which either H2A.Z or H2A can be exchanged from nucleosomes, although this is in discussion [77–82]. NuA4 acetylation activity, which is homologous to the TIP60/p400 complex, was found to be associated with SWR1-driven incorporation of H2A.Z into chromatin [83]. Besides, bromodomain-containing proteins are known to be implicated in "reading" the acetylation patterns of H2A.Z: acetylated lysines in histones, and other proteins are recognized by this motif, common in remodelers [77, 78, 84, 85]. In fact, for SWR1, bromodomains have been studied to recognize a pattern of acetylation (including H3K14ac), which may influence the deposition of H2A.Z-H2B variant dimers into the appropriate nucleosome [77, 78]. By using *Tetrahymena* as a model, it could be observed that these protozoa cannot survive with all acetylatable lysines replaced by arginines, indicating that H2A.Z acetylation modulates a charge patch with an essential function in chromatin regulation [69, 75]. Unlike the histone code, these changes need not to be site-specific. If this hypothesis is true, modulation of the charge at any one of a number of clustered sites could inhibit nucleosome condensation, facilitating transcription [86].

T. gondii H2A.Z, together with H2B.Z, was enriched in the promoters of active genes in tachyzoites, while repressed genes were enriched with H2A.X-H2Ba nucleosomes [63] (**Figure 2A**). In addition, H2A.Z-H2B.Z was also recruited within the coding region of silent bradyzoite-specific genes and within promoter regions but not coding regions of actively expressed genes [87]. It is tempting to speculate that the enrichment at active promoters or poised regions could be ruled by different PTM stages of these histone variants. In agreement with this, H2A.Z and H2B.Z have shown to be highly acetylated at the amino-terminal tail, in contrast to canonical H2A and H2B histones and the H2A.X variant [51]. Considering that H2A.Z has shown to be essential in regulating the changing gene expression program during differentiation [79–81, 88–90], and recently, it was observed that overexpression of mutated version of H2A.Z, where all five potential acetylatable lysines on H2A.Z-GFP (K4, 7, 11, 13, and 15) were mutated to arginines, blocked myoblast differentiation through disruption of myoD expression [91], it may be that the H2B variant is involved in the *T. gondii* cell differentiation process as part of H2A.Z-H2B.Z nucleosome. Whether through a patch charge modulation and/or histone code remains an open question, considering that *T. gondii* presents several bromodomain-containing proteins that can recognize some of the acetylated lysine [92].

As stated above, the sequence alignment of H2B.Z in many Apicomplexan species reveals a high degree of conservation for this histone variant (**Figure 2B**). Interestingly, every lysine that has been proved to be acetylated in *T. gondii* and *P. falciparum*, H2B.Z was detected in the other Apicomplexan species, which is also true for H2A.Z [50, 53]. Maybe, the double-variant nucleosome is present in the phylum with same PTMs and similar biological role.

5.1. Double-variant nucleosome in var genes

In *P. falciparum*, H2A.Z-containing nucleosomes were proposed to demarcate intergenic/regulatory regions of the genome, serving as a scaffold for stage specific as well as transcription-coupled recruitment of histone modifying enzymes [93]. H3K9ac and H3K4me3 were found preferentially placed/retained on or next to H2A.Z-containing nucleosomes [49]. However, it was observed that *P. falciparum* intergenic regions, including promoters, display a global nucleosome depletion, while telomeres harbored the highest nucleosomal occupancy, except for the *var* gene with the highest expression level, which again showed the lowest nucleosomal occupancy [94]. Apparently, the little amount of nucleosomes in these areas is composed largely of variant nucleosomes. Petter et al. [95] also showed an enrichment of PfH2A.Z in the promoter of a set of developmentally regulated genes in the euchromatin compartment, although not correlated with transcription levels nor with acetylation status. *P. falciparum* H2A.Z-H2B.Z promoter occupancy in *var* genes was found to be strongly associated with transcriptional activity, whereas silent or poised *var* genes would be depleted of double-variant nucleosome (see **Figure 3**) [65, 86]. The authors have speculated that it may function as a similar physical switch to control gene expression in response to temperature change (for example, during fever or as *P. falciparum* is transmitted between its two hosts), as a thermosensory response that was seen in *Arabidopsis thaliana* and yeast [96]. This could be due to reduced DNA wrapping of H2A.Z containing nucleosomes at higher temperatures, resulting in a relaxed chromatin structure, although this variant histone has also been associated with a tighter relationship with DNA, especially in heterotypic H2A.Z/H2A nucleosomes [97]. While heterochromatic intergenic regions showed to contain low levels of histone variant H2B.Z [64], it is interesting that double-variant nucleosomes are depleted from silent *var* gene promoters but not from silent promoters of heterochromatic invasion gene families, which have similar patterns of variegated expression [65]. Besides, this correlation between double-variant nucleosome presence and expression was only seen in *var* genes, while this nucleosome was also found enriched in intergenic regions across the genome, associated with euchromatic histone modifications and not necessarily associated with transcription [64, 65, 86]. Moreover, long promoter containing intergenic regions that maintain higher variant histone levels as compared with 3′UTR containing regions, which are considerably shorter, presents higher AT content, so this correlation could simply be due to the minimal length of the AT-rich content in these short 3′UTR regions [64]. As it was previously observed for H3.3 variant histone (see Section 3), a correlation between nucleosome occupancy and GC/AT content in the genome was observed, although contrary to H3.3 that was correlated with rich GC regions [42], here both H2B.Z and H2A.Z histone variant occupancy displayed a clear positive correlation toward genomic AT content [64]. In **Figure 2A**, a schematic representation of *P. falciparum* and *T. gondii* nucleosome occupancy is proposed.

6. Heterochromatin, telomeres, and subtelomeres

The telomere-associated sequences (TAS), also named subtelomeres, are heterochromatic regions adjacent to the telomeric-end looking toward the centromere. The telomeres and the TAS regions are the final structures at the chromosomes and integrate with the centromere the constitutive heterochromatin in the genome. These TAS regions have been described in *Plasmodium* and *Toxoplasma* with a size of 20–40 and near 30 Kpb, respectively (**Figure 3**) [98–100]. In *T. gondii*, the structure contains three tandem repeated elements (TARE), separated by noncoding DNA and flanked at one end by the telomere and at the other, downstream TARE 3, by a *Toxoplasma*-specific gene family, the *tsf* gene, of unknown function [100]. In general, there is only one *tsf* gene per TAS. Interestingly, based on predicted amino acidic sequence, TSF proteins present a high degree of conservation in the N-tail and middle regions while being highly variable at the C-terminal end. Up to now, only few studies were performed on chromatin modulation of *T. gondii* TAS.

The TAS element in *Plasmodium*, instead, has been deeply studied because of the presence of different families of genes associated to virulence and pathogenicity with a clonal pattern of expression [101, 102]. Telomeres are spatially restricted to nuclear periphery, where they form clusters of three to seven heterologous chromosome ends [103–105]. *Plasmodium* TAS is composed of six different TAREs, and the coding part of the genome is localized directly downstream TARE 6, and is characterized by members of multiple antigen gene families including *var*, *rif*, *stevor*, and *pfmc-2tm* genes [94, 95].

The telomeres and TAS regions are dynamic structures associated to a plethora of specific factors that not only give it structure, but also configures all the regions as constitutive heterochromatin that participates in an epigenetic way to regulate subtelomeric genes expression (**Figure 3**). This epigenetic mechanism is carried out by proteins that introduce, recognize, and implement a repressive state over the gene expression under normal environmental conditions. It has been reported that under nutritional or environmental stress, the repressed subtelomeric genes activate their expression in response to events promoting growth and survival [87, 106–109].

It is important to highlight that the *T. gondii* TAS regions show a nucleosome composition enriched in H2A.X and heterochromatin markers [100]. An *in silico* analysis using the *Plasmodium* and *Toxoplasma* databases reveals the presence of only some orthologs to the yeast and mammal's telomeric-subtelomeric proteins as TRF1-2, HP1, KU70/KU80, and Sir2 proteins (**Table 1**). But interestingly, the principal actor in this scenario would be the histone deacetylase type III -Sir2. This NAD+ deacetylase-dependent has also been implicated in different signaling pathways. *P. falciparum* has two Sir2 paralogues, Sir2A and B; with overlapping but distinct roles that regulate different subsets of *var* genes[110], binding reversibly with the promoter regions of silent but not active subtelomeric *var* genes [111]. PfSir2A is implicated in telomere length regulation [112]. In *T. gondii*, two deacetylases containing the Sir2-domain were identified: TgSir2A and TgSir2B, but their function has not been characterized yet. Another protein that had been described in *Plasmodium* is PfOrc1 (origin recognition complex 1), which together with Sir2 promotes the epigenetic silencing in *P. falciparum* TAS [113]. PfOrc1 has a role in DNA replication but also cooperates with Sir2 to coordinate the spreading of heterochromatin and regulation of *var* gene expression [114]. In general, Sir2 proteins act by removing acetyl groups in cytosolic targets and at the nuclear level at H3K9, K14 and K56, but it also was described to act on the histone mark H4K16 promoting the deposition of methyl groups on H4K20, H4K20me3 being a chromatin mark associated with heterochromatin [115]. Thus, Sir2 seems to play a very important role in linking signaling processes to gene expression and chromosome architecture.

Additionally, a member of the Alba protein family (PfAlba3) was demonstrated via ChIP assays to bind to telomeric and subtelomeric regions co-localizing with Sir2A in the periphery of the nucleus. PfAlba3 inhibits transcription *in vitro* by binding to DNA. PfSir2A was shown to interact with PfAlba3 deacetylating the lysine residue of N-terminal peptide of PfAlba3 specific for DNA binding [116] (**Figure 3**). In archaea, this interaction had been reported, in which Sir2 regulates silencing through deacetylation of the major archaeal chromatin protein Alba, highlighting an ancestrally conserved mechanism of gene regulation [117].

As stated above, heterochromatin protein 1 (HP1) is a very important protein that has been described to recognize the trimethylation on H3K9, a critical mark for the establishment, maintenance and silencing of centromeric and telomeric heterochromatic regions in various model organisms. In *P. falciparum*, it has been identified as PfHP1 [118] and the H3K9me3 mark was mainly associated with *var* genes at TAS regions, as said before [119]. Moreover, high levels of H3K9me3 correlate with genes localized to the nuclear periphery, implying chromosome loop formation. In addition, an association between PfSir2 and H3K9me3 was found, since the lack of the sirtuin deacetylases causes changes in H3K9me3 localization at the chromosome and generates disruption of the monoallelic transcription of *var* genes, suggesting the existence of perinuclear repressive centers associated with control of expression of malaria parasite genes involved in phenotypic variation and pathogenesis [119].

Flueck et al. [120] described the presence of an ApiAP2 family member in *P. falciparum*, designated as SIP2 that binds to TARE-2 and TARE-3 regions and the upstream regions of *var* upsB *in vivo*. Immunofluorescence and genome-wide high-resolution ChIP analyses demonstrated that *P. falciparum* SIP2 and HP1 proteins co-localize and associate with the same subtelomeric region, suggesting that both proteins participate in the assembly of telomeric heterochromatin. A recent report from Gupta et al. [121] has demonstrated that the protein CAF-1, a chaperone that loads the H3-H4 to the nucleosome assembly after DDR, co-localizes with PfHP1

Yeast	Mammals	*T. gondii* (ToxoDB number)	*P. falciparum* (PlasmoDB PF3D7 number)
Sir2 (P06700)	Sir2 (Q8IXJ6)	Sir2A (227020)	Sir2A (1328800)
		Sir2B (267360)	Sir2B (1451400)
Sir3 (P06701)	Sir3 (Q9NTG7)	ATPase, AAA family protein (283900)*	Orc1/Sir3 like activity (1203000)*
Sir4 (P11978)	Sir4 (Q9Y6E7)	NF	NF
RAP1 (P11938)	RAP1 (Q9NYB0)	NF	NF
RIF1 (P29539)	RIF1 (Q5UIP0)	NF	NF
RIF2 (Q06208)	NF	NF	NF
Ku70 (P32807)	XRCC6 (B1AHC9)	Ku70 (248160)	NF
Ku80 (Q04437)	XRCC5 (P13010)	Ku80 (312510)	NF
Taz1 (P79005)	TRF1 (P54274)	NF	NF
NF	TRF2 (Q15554)	NF	NF
NF	TIN2 (Q9BSI4)	NF	NF
NF	HP1 (Q13185)	Chromo1 (268280)	HP1 (1220900)
Stn1 (P38960)	NF	NF	NF
Ten1 (Q07921)	NF	NF	NF
Cdc13 (P32797)	NF	NF	NF
NF	TPP1 (Q96AP0)	NF	NF
NF	POT1 (Q9NUX5)	NF	NF
Pif1 (P07271)	Pif1 (Q9H611)	NF	NF

NF: Not found.*P. falciparum Orc1 complement yeast Sir3 activity [113]. T. gondii counterpart was detected by searching ToxoDB with PfOrc1 amino acidic sequence by BlastP.

Table 1. Telomeric proteins.

at the same subtelomeric localization, in the nuclear periphery, and also demonstrated its binding to TARE1-3 and co-localization with H3K56ac, a signal of completion on chromatin reassembly after DDR [122]. Interestingly, immunoprecipitation with PfCAF1 followed by LC-MS/MS analysis demonstrated that this protein would be interacting not only with PfHP1 but also with PfAlba3 among others [121].

In *T. gondii*, an HP1 protein was identified as TgChromo1, linked to the sequestration of chromosomes at the nuclear periphery and the process of cell division of the parasite [22]. TgChromo1 has shown to localize at *T. gondii* telomeres but not subtelomeres. However, by that time, subtelomeric regions had not yet been described and, in some cases, the sequences in these regions were not correctly assembled. Also, the presence of H4K20me3 and H2A.X at some TARE sequences and a region near *tsf* gene, previously named TgIRE, was observed [62, 63, 100, 123].

7. Double-strand break repair: H2A.X and chromatin

Cells are exposed to DNA lesions produced by exogenous (e.g., chemicals, UV-irradiation, and ionization) or endogenous factors (e.g., DNA replication stress, meiotic recombination). One of the most deleterious forms of DNA damage is the double-strand break (DSB) [124]. DSBs activate the signal transduction pathway to induce DNA damage checkpoints that delay cell cycle progression, which allows the cell to activate DNA repair mechanism [125]. The phosphorylation of SQE/DΦ motif (where Φ represents a hydrophobic residue) on histone H2A.X (referred to as γH2A.X) is one of the earliest responses to DSB [126, 127]. H2A.X seems to be incorporated randomly in the genome of resting cells [128], whereas γH2A.X is clearly observed forming foci, labeling the DSB and replication fork sites, spreading along the chromosome up to 2 Mb from the damaged site. In addition, chromatin is subjected to several changes at damage sites playing an important role in regulating DNA repair [129]. DSB can be produced by various events, either external as ionizing and UV radiations or internal such as collapse of replication forks and transcription-associated damage, among others [130, 131]. DSB can be repaired by two main mechanisms: nonhomologous end joining (NHEJ) and homologous recombination repair (HRR); the first is an error-prone mechanism available along the cell cycle, and the second is an error-free mechanism active at S/G2 phases of cell cycle because of the requirement of sister chromatid as template [131–134]. Both mechanisms were described in *T. gondii* [14, 135], but *Plasmodium* genus is thought to rely only on HRR [136–138].

Before the election of NHEJ or HRR mechanism, DSB triggers a cascade of events that starts with Mre11-RAD50-Nbs1/Xrs2 (MRN in mammals and MRX in yeast) complex binding to the damaged site, which recruits and activates ATM kinase (**Figure 4A**) [139]. ATM is able to phosphorylate H2A.X at SQE motif as well as other DSB repair enzymes allowing the spreading of γH2A.X and a correct DNA damage response (DDR) at DSB site (**Figure 4A**). ATM kinase is present in *T. gondii* and *P. falciparum* [14]. In *T. gondii*, the MYST family lysine acetyltransferase TgMYST-B has shown to mediate DDR induced by methyl methanesulfonate (MMS) and to stimulate the ATM expression at gene level [140]. In addition to this finding, histone acetyltransferases (HATs) have a predominant role in DDR on the basis of chromatin modulation. Chromatin responds to DSB first by increasing the compaction stage by replacing H2A/H2A.X with the H2A.Z variant and by methylating H3K9 by suv39h1 methyltransferase, which is recruited after spreading the DDR response at both sides of DSB sites (**Figure 4B**) [141, 142]. The arrival of H3K9me3 allows its interaction with the HAT Tip60 and the acetylation of H4 on K16 together with the acetylation of ATM kinase, an important PTM for the activation of autophosphorylation and subsequent activation of ATM (**Figure 4**) [143, 144]. The H3K9me3 and H4K16ac marks were identified in *T. gondii* and *P. falciparum* by mass spectrometry analysis [48–51]. However, in the case of *T. gondii,* an acetylated residue was also detected in H3K9 in a more frequent fashion than H3K9me1,2,3, suggesting that chromatin is preferentially in an open state and that this lysine PTM can be regulated [51]. As it was stated before, H3K9me2/3 is also enriched in centromeres in *T. gondii* [21]. In addition, *T. gondii* H4K16ac was one of the most abundant PTMs found in the mass spectrometry analysis [51]. In the case of *P. falciparum,* the treatment with MMS has increased the level of H4K8ac and H4K16ac and reduction of H3K9ac [145]. Both, *T. gondii* and *P. falciparum* present H3K9me1,2,3 and H3K9ac in normal conditions suggesting a conserved mechanism of chromatin modulation [51]. The role of these histone marks on Apicomplexan histones and the connections with DNA repair remain to be elucidated.

As mentioned above, γH2A.X spreading is a crucial step to initiate a correct DDR at DSB sites. In *T. gondii,* this PTM mark is accompanied by other DDR marks such as H3K9me2,3 and H4K16 in normal conditions of growth, opening the question whether DSBs are being produced during parasite replication [51, 135]. The *T. gondii* tachyzoite replicates at high rates, in a range of 5–9 hours [146]. So, a putative collapse of replication fork could be occurring in this stage. However, *T. gondii* ATM kinase could not be detected in normal conditions by Western blot, but it was detected by tachyzoites overexpressing MYST-B HAT [140].

The chromatin compaction that occurs early during DDR includes the remodeling of chromatin at DSB sites in which the H2A-H2B dimer is replaced by H2A.Z-H2B [142, 147]. This event is transient, allowing the recruitment of repressive kap-1(TRIM28)/HP1/suv39h1 complex that can be important to inhibit transcription. The presence of H2A-H2B dimer in the nucleosomal core particle produces a unique negatively charged region on the surface of the nucleosome, called the "acidic patch," which is extended in H2A.Z (**Figure 4B**) [148–150]. The acidic patch favors the binding of H4 N-tail, resulting in an increase in the interaction between nucleosomes and chromatin compaction [150]. Interestingly, this seems a necessary step to continue with a relaxed chromatin state, since this compaction and recruitment of kap-1(TRIM28)/HP1/suv39h1 complex lead to methylation of H3K9 and phosphorylation of KAP-1 by ATM kinase, which in turn promote H4K16 acetylation by Tip60 and release kap-1(TRIM28)/HP1/suv39h1 (**Figure 4B**) (see [142]). *T. gondii* and *P. falciparum* have the novel H2A.Z-H2B.Z double-variant nucleosome (see Section 5). However, *T. gondii* and *P. falciparum* H2A-H2B and variants conserve the acidic patch (**Figure 4B**). To note, *T. gondii* and *P. falciparum* do not appear to have KAP-1 protein at ToxoDB and PlasmoDB databases [151].

In higher eukaryotes, another important PTM mark associated to DDR is ubiquitination by E3 ubiquitin ligases RNF168 and RNF8 at DSB site after γH2A.X and MDC1 protein foci

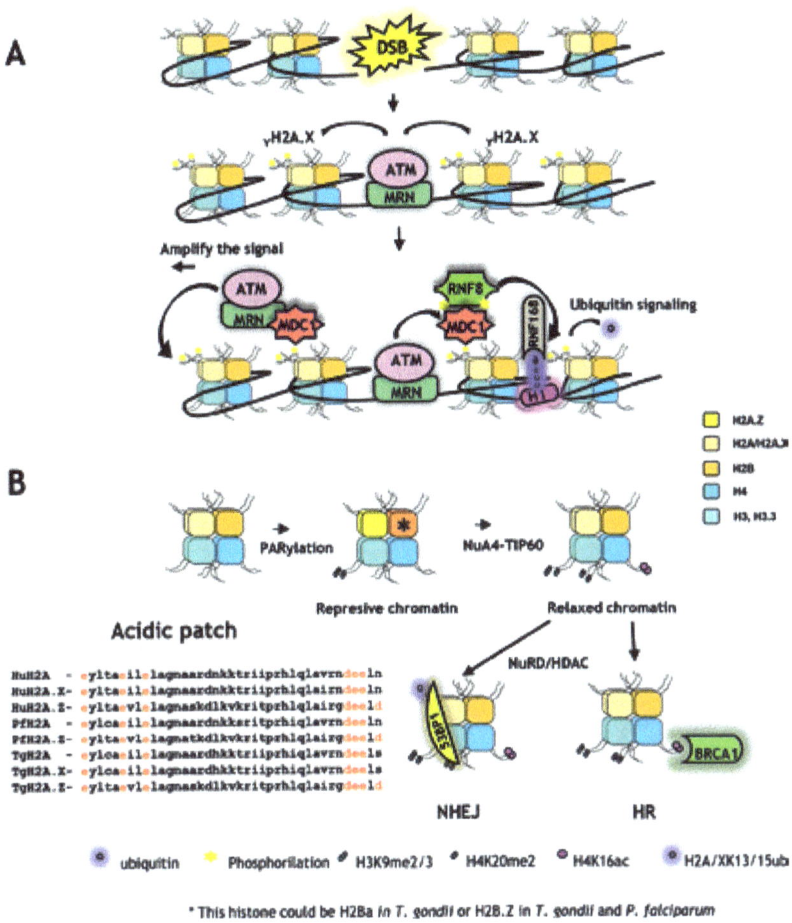

Figure 4. (A) Recognition of DSB and initial steps of DDR pathways. MRN complex and ATM kinase are recruited to a DSB. ATM phosphorylates several DDR proteins and checkpoint kinases. Phosphorylation by ATM allows the spreading of γH2A.X and DDR foci. RNF8 E3 ubiquitin ligase complexes ubiquitinate H2A and H1 histones to compact and generate histone marks, which will be read by other DDR factors such as MDC1 and E3 ubiquitin ligase RNF168. (B) Model of chromatin modulation after DSB. During PARylation, the p400 ATPase (NuA4-Tip60 complex) replaces H2A-H2B dimers by H2A.Z containing nucleosomes. Since T. gondii and P. falciparum present a double-variant nucleosome, we speculate that H2A-H2B or H2A.X-H2Ba dimers may be replaced by H2A.Z-H2B.Z dimers. This exchange might increase the interaction of the acidic patch with the N-tail of H4 increasing the chromatin compaction (see the sequence alignment: in red letters are written the acidic residues involved in generating the acidic patch). PARylation also produces an increase in H3K9me2/3 and histone deacetylation repressive marks. After a short time, the H2A.Z containing nucleosome is replaced by H2A-H2B dimer and N-tail of H4 is acetylated leading to a relaxed chromatin and recruitment of different DDR factors, among them those related to the DDR pathway choice, such as 53BP1 or BRCA1.

spreading (**Figure 4A**). MDC1 is also phosphorylated by ATM kinase allowing the recruitment of RNF168 and RNF8 [152]. Ubiquitination on H1 and H2A recruits several BRCT domain containing proteins such as BRCA1 and 53BP1 [129]. In the case of 53BP1, its binding requires the H2AK13/15ub and H4K20me2 and addresses the DDR to NHEJ pathway (**Figure 4B**). By contrast, the presence of H4K16ac impairs the 53BP1 binding to the nucleosome allowing the recruitment of BRCA, which addresses the DDR to HRR (**Figure 4B**) (see [141, 142]). As stated above, in *T. gondii* and *P. falciparum*, the mark H4K20me1,2,3 was found [48, 51, 53]. However, *T. gondii* and *P. falciparum* H2As did not contain H2AK15ub and lysine 13 ubiquitylation was not detected either [51]. In addition, *T. gondii* and *P. falciparum* did not show the presence of orthologs of BRCA1 and/or 53BP1, though *T. gondii* presents three different BRCT domain containing proteins [14].

T. gondii and *P. falciparum* conserve several histone marks present in chromatin-associated DDR to DBS, as well as histone variants—in the case of *T. gondii*, the DDR, well studied H2A.X, is present, whereas *Plasmodium* has only canonical H2A [55], involved in the recruitment of several factors that spread and choose the DDR pathway in higher eukaryotes. Although, *T. gondii* and *P. falciparum* lack some key DDR regulators such as KAP-1, 53BP1, BRCA1, MDC1, RNF168 and RNF8 [14], both parasites present the HRR mechanism of DNA repair, whereas NHEJ is present only in *T. gondii*. So, the modulation of both DDR pathways is still an intriguing issue.

8. Concluding remarks

In protozoan parasites, the modulation of chromatin seems to be a key biological process to regulate gene expression, pathogenicity and DNA repair, the latter probably associated to DNA replication, ergo, the cell cycle. In Apicomplexa, highly evident in *Plasmodium* genus, the TAS or subtelomeric regions play an important role in the control of a group of genes essential in parasite pathogenicity. This fact suggests that subtelomeres have not a trivial impact in the evolution of these organisms, and their structure can influence the features of the cell. How this genomic domain has evolved within the Apicomplexa phylum remains to be elucidated. *T. gondii*, in which to date a scenario of variant antigenicity was not detected, has shown a someway conserved structure with the presence of tandem repeated boxes and a gene family of unknown function (*tsf*). Different from *Plasmodium*, which variant antigen-associated gene is represented by hundreds of members, *T. gondii* has only one gene per TAS. However, the predicted protein sequences show conserved N-tail and middle regions, with highly variable C-terminal ends. We believe that the elucidation of the localization, role, and antigenic potential of these gene family proteins will be of high impact in our knowledge of this parasite. Also, it could be interesting to know if the members of this gene family show a regulation of gene expression similar to *Plasmodium* variable antigen gene family.

In addition to the presence of PTM marks similar to other organisms but with currently less-well characterized readers and erasers, Apicomplexa chromatin presents a double-variant nucleosome based on the new histone variant H2B.Z. If considering the partitioned knowledge in these parasites, specially *P. falciparum*, where H3.3 variant has been found in the same regions as this double-variant nucleosome, but in different studies, it would be possible that a triple-variant nucleosome exists in Apicomplexa. Since the presence of H2B.Z arose early in Apicomplexa evolution, it is expected that the double-variant nucleosome could have been important in the expansion of the phylum, maybe modulating chromatin structure during the execution of different biological processes. Interestingly, the genome-wide analyses seem to indicate that *Plasmodium* and *Toxoplasma* double-variant nucleosomes do not have the same behavior. In *T. gondii*, it is enriched in active and poised genes, whereas in *P. falciparum*, it is localized in active and silent promoters, excepting the *var* genes, in which the presence of the double-variant nucleosome is associated to active promoters. The analysis of this novel nucleosome in the different genera of the phylum can give more information to elucidate the reason of the presence of this H2B variant.

Chromatin is also important to the DDR and has an important role in determining the different pathways of DNA repair after DSB. *T. gondii* seems to have every histone variant and histone mark as well as important proteins associated to every DDR pathway to repair a DSB: NHEJ (e.g., Ku70/Ku80) and HRR (RAD51). Different from *T. gondii, Plasmodium* does not present the histone variant H2A.X, whose phosphorylation (γH2A.X) is linked to the localization of DSB on DNA. Moreover, *T. gondii* has shown a basal level of γH2A.X, even without damage. Not expected, the proteins associated to the DDR pathway choice (NHEJ or HRR), which read the chromatin, were not detected in *T. gondii* nor in *Plasmodium*. So, it is unknown if these marks are associated to other proteins (*T. gondii* has three BRCT domain containing proteins) with similar roles and/or chromatin modulates DDR in another way.

Taken all together, these differences are not only interesting at the light of evolution but also can be analyzed in the context of the identification of new parasite-specific drug targets. Gene regulation, DNA replication, pathogenicity, and DNA repair are crucial biological processes, and all of them may offer new targets to exploit as future treatments against Apicomplexan pathogens.

Acknowledgements

SO Angel (Researcher), L. Vanagas (Researcher), and S.M. Contreras (Fellow) are members of National Research Council of Argentina (CONICET). SO Angel and L. Vanagas are professors of Universidad Nacional General San Martin (UNSAM). This chapter was supported by ANPCyT PICT 2015 1288 (S.O.A.) and National Institute of Health (NIH, NIAID 1R01AI083162) grants.

Author details

Laura Vanagas, Susana Marisol Contreras and Sergio Oscar Angel*

*Address all correspondence to: sangel@intech.gov.ar

Instituto Tecnológico de Chascomús (INTECH), CONICET/UNSAM, Chascomús, Provincia de Buenos Aires, Argentina

References

[1] Black MW, Boothroyd JC. Lytic cycle of *Toxoplasma gondii*. Microbiology and Molecular Biology Reviews. 2000;**64**(3):607-623

[2] Zuber JA, Takala-Harrison S. Multidrug-resistant malaria and the impact of mass drug administration. Infection and Drug Resistance. 2018;**11**:209-336

[3] Tenter AM, Heckeroth AR, Weiss LM. *Toxoplasma gondii*: From animals to humans. International Journal for Parasitology. 2000;**30**(12-13):1217-1258

[4] Fuller Torrey E, Bartko JJ, Yolken RH. *Toxoplasma gondii* and other risk factors for schizophrenia: An update. 2012;**38**(3):642-647

[5] Fuglewicz AJ, Piotrowski P, Stodolak A. Relationship between toxoplasmosis and schizophrenia: A review. Advances in Clinical and Experimental Medicine. 2017;**26**(6):1031-1036

[6] Flegr J, Horá Ček J. Toxoplasma-infected subjects report an obsessive-compulsive disorder diagnosis more often and score higher in obsessive-compulsive inventory. European Psychiatry. 2017;**40**:82-87

[7] Sutterland AL et al. Beyond the association. *Toxoplasma gondii* in schizophrenia, bipolar disorder, and addiction: Systematic review and meta-analysis. Acta Psychiatrica Scandinavica. 2015;**132**(3):161-179

[8] Yolken R, Fuller Torrey E, Dickerson F. Evidence of increased exposure to *Toxoplasma gondii* in individuals with recent onset psychosis but not with established schizophrenia. PLoS Neglected Tropical Diseases. 2017;**6**(11):e0006040

[9] Kissinger JC, Gajria B, Li L, Paulsen IT, Roos DS. ToxoDB: Accessing the *Toxoplasma gondii* genome. Nucleic Acids Research. 2003;**31**(1):234-236

[10] Gardner MJ et al., Genome sequence of the human malaria parasite Plasmodium falciparum. Nature. 2002;**419**(6906):498-511

[11] De Silva EK et al. Specific DNA-binding by apicomplexan AP2 transcription factors. Proceedings of the National Academy of Sciences of the United States of America. 2008;**105**(16):8393-8398

[12] Behnke MS et al. Coordinated progression through two subtranscriptomes underlies the tachyzoite cycle of *Toxoplasma gondii*. PLoS One. 2010;**5**(8):e12354

[13] Dixon SE, Bhatti MM, Uversky VN, Dunker AK, Sullivan WJ. Regions of intrinsic disorder help identify a novel nuclear localization signal in *Toxoplasma gondii* histone acetyltransferase TgGCN5-B. Molecular and Biochemical Parasitology. 2011;**175**(2):192-195

[14] Fenoy IM, Bogado SS, Contreras SM, Gottifredi V, Angel SO. The knowns unknowns: Exploring the homologous recombination repair pathway in *Toxoplasma gondii*. Frontiers in Microbiology. 2016;**7**(May):1-15

[15] Batugedara G, Lu XM, Bunnik EM, Le Roch KG. The role of chromatin structure in gene regulation of the human malaria parasite. Trends in Parasitology. 2017;**33**:364-377

[16] Striepen B, Jordan CN, Reiff S, van Dooren GG. Building the perfect parasite: Cell division in apicomplexa. PLoS Pathogens. 2007;**3**(6):e78

[17] Olins AL, Ernst A, Zwerger M, Herrmann H, Olins DE. An in vitro model for Pelger-Huët anomaly. Nucleus. 2010;**1**(6):506-512

[18] Vanagas L, Dalmasso MC, Dubremetz JF, Portiansky EL, Olins DE, Angel SO. Epichromatin is conserved in *Toxoplasma gondii* and labels the exterior parasite chromatin throughout the cell cycle. Parasitology. 2013;**140**(9):1-1110

[19] Erenpreisa J, Krigerts J, Salmina K, Selga T, Sorokins H, Freivalds T. Differential staining of peripheral nuclear chromatin with Acridine orange implies an A-form epichromatin conformation of the DNA. Nucleus. 2018;**9**(1):171-181

[20] Weiner A et al. 3D nuclear architecture reveals coupled cell cycle dynamics of chromatin and nuclear pores in the malaria parasite *Plasmodium falciparum*. Cellular Microbiology. 2011;**13**(7):967-977

[21] Brooks CF, Francia ME, Gissot M, Croken MM, Kim K, Striepen B. *Toxoplasma gondii* sequesters centromeres to a specific nuclear region throughout the cell cycle. Proceedings of the National Academy of Sciences of the United States of America. 2011; **108**(9):3767-3772

[22] Gissot M, Walker R, Delhaye S, Huot L, Hot D, Tomavo S. *Toxoplasma gondii* chromodomain protein 1 binds to heterochromatin and colocalises with centromeres and telomeres at the nuclear periphery. PLoS One. 2012;**7**(3):e32671

[23] Hoeijmakers WAM et al. *Plasmodium falciparum* centromeres display a unique epigenetic makeup and cluster prior to and during schizogony. Cellular Microbiology. 2012; **14**(9):1391-1401

[24] Ahmad K, Henikoff S. Histone H3 variants specify modes of chromatin assembly. Proceedings of the National Academy of Sciences USA. 2002;**99**(Suppl 4):16477-16484

[25] Smith S, Stillman B. Purification and characterization of CAF-I, a human cell factor required for chromatin assembly during DNA replication in vitro. Cell. 1989;**58**(1):15-25

[26] Verreault A, Kaufman PD, Kobayashi R, Stillman B. Nucleosome assembly by a complex of CAF-1 and acetylated histones H3/H4. Cell. 1996;**87**(1):95-104

[27] Tagami H, Ray-Gallet D, Ve Almouzni G, Nakatani Y. Histone H3.1 and H3.3 complexes mediate nucleosome assembly pathways dependent or independent of DNA synthesis. Cell. 2004;**116**:51-61

[28] Konev AY et al. The CHD1 motor protein is required for deposition of histone variant H3.3 into chromatin in vivo Science. 2007;**317**(5841):1087-1090

[29] Drané P, Ouararhni K, Depaux A, Shuaib M, Hamiche A. The death-associated protein DAXX is a novel histone chaperone involved in the replication-independent deposition of H3.3 Genes and Development. 2010;**24**(12):1253-1265

[30] Lewis PW, Elsaesser SJ, Noh K-M, Stadler SC, Allis CD. Daxx is an H3.3-specific histone chaperone and cooperates with ATRX in replication-independent chromatin assembly at telomeres. Proceedings of the National Academy of Sciences. 2010;**107**(32):14075-14080

[31] Wirbelauer C, Bell O, Schübeler D. Variant histone H3.3 is deposited at sites of nucleosomal displacement throughout transcribed genes while active histone modifications show a promoter-proximal bias. Genes and Development. 2005;**19**(15):1761-1766

[32] Loyola A, Almouzni G. Marking histone H3 variants: How, when and why? Trends in Biochemical Sciences. 2007;**32**(9):425-433

[33] Goldberg AD et al. Distinct factors control histone variant H3.3 localization at specific genomic regions. Cell. 2010;**140**(5):678-691

[34] Szenker E, Ray-Gallet D, Almouzni G. The double face of the histone variant H3.3. Cell Research. 2011;**21**(3):421-434

[35] Mckittrick E, Gafken PR, Ahmad K, Henikoff S. Histone H3.3 is enriched in covalent modifications associated with active chromatin. Proceedings of the National Academy of Sciences USA. 2004;**101**(6):1525-1530

[36] Jin C et al. H3.3/H2A.Z double variant-containing nucleosomes mark 'nucleosome-free regions' of active promoters and other regulatory regions in the human genome. Nature Genetics. 2009;**41**(8):941-945

[37] Jin C et al. H3.3/H2A.Z double variant–containing nucleosomes mark 'nucleosome-free regions' of active promoters and other regulatory regions. Nature Genetics. 2009; **41**(8):941-945

[38] Chen PB et al. *Plasmodium falciparum* PfSET7: Enzymatic characterization and cellular localization of a novel protein methyltransferase in sporozoite, liver and erythrocytic stage parasites. Scientific Reports. 2016;**6**:21802

[39] Jang C-W, Shibata Y, Starmer J, Yee D, Magnuson T. Histone H3.3 maintains genome integrity during mammalian development. Genes & Development. 2015;**29**(13):1377-1392

[40] Sullivan WJ. Histone H3 and H3.3 variants in the protozoan pathogens *Plasmodium falciparum* and *Toxoplasma gondii*. DNA Sequence. 2003;**14**(3):227-231

[41] Miao J, Fan Q, Cui L, Li J, Cui L. The malaria parasite *Plasmodium falciparum* histones: Organization, expression, and acetylation. Gene. 2006;**369**:53-65

[42] Anne-Kristin Fraschka S, Wilhelmus Maria Henderson R, Bártfai R. H3.3 demarcates GC-rich coding and subtelomeric regions and serves as potential memory mark for virulence gene expression in *Plasmodium falciparum*. Scientific Reports. 2016;**6**:31965

[43] Scherf A, Lopez-Rubio JJ, Riviere L. Antigenic Variation in *Plasmodium falciparum*. Annual Review of Microbiology. 2008;**62**(1):445-470

[44] Baruch DI et al. Cloning the gene encoding PfEMPl, a malarial variant antigen and adherence receptor on the surface of parasitized human erythrocytes. Cell. 1995;**92**:77-97

[45] Smith JD et al. Switches in expression of *Plasmodium falciparum* var genes correlate with changes in antigenic and cytoadherent phenotypes of infected erythrocytes. Cell. 1995;**82**(1):101-110

[46] Su XZ et al. The large diverse gene family var encodes proteins involved in cytoadherence and antigenic variation of *Plasmodium falciparum*-infected erythrocytes. Cell. 1995;**82**(1):89-100

[47] Jiang L et al. PfSETvs methylation of histone H3K36 represses virulence genes in *Plasmodium falciparum*. Nature. 2013;**499**(7457):223-227

[48] Trelle MB, Salcedo-Amaya AM, Cohen AM, Stunnenberg HG, Jensen ON. Global histone analysis by mass spectrometry reveals a high content of acetylated lysine residues in the malaria parasite *Plasmodium falciparum*. Journal of Proteome Research. 2009;**8**(7):3439-3450

[49] Salcedo-Amaya AM et al. Dynamic histone H3 epigenome marking during the intra-erythrocytic cycle of *Plasmodium falciparum*. Proceedings of the National Academy of Sciences. 2009;**106**(24):9655-9660

[50] Cui L, Miao J. Chromatin-mediated epigenetic regulation in the malaria parasite *Plasmodium falciparum*. Eukaryotic Cell. 2010;**9**(8):1138-1149

[51] Nardelli SC et al. The histone code of *Toxoplasma gondii* comprises conserved and unique posttranslational modifications. MBio Journal. 2013;**4**(6):e00922-13

[52] Dastidar EG et al. Comprehensive histone phosphorylation analysis and identification of Pf14-3-3 protein as a histone H3 phosphorylation reader in malaria parasites. PLoS One. 2013;**8**(1):e53179

[53] Croken MM, Nardelli SC, Kim K. Chromatin modifications, epigenetics, and how protozoan parasites regulate their lives. Trends in Parasitology. 2012;**28**(5):202-213

[54] Gissot M, Kelly KA, Ajioka JW, Greally JM, Kim K. Epigenomic modifications predict active promoters and gene structure in *Toxoplasma gondii*. PLoS Pathogens. 2007;**3**(6):e77

[55] Dalmasso MC, Sullivan WJ, Angel SO. Canonical and variant histones of protozoan parasites. Frontiers in Bioscience (Landmark Ed.). 2011;**16**:2086-2105

[56] Fischer T et al. Diverse roles of HP1 proteins in heterochromatin assembly and functions in fission yeast. Proceedings of the National Academy of Sciences of the United States of America. 2009;**106**(22):8998-9003

[57] Verma G, Surolia N. *Plasmodium falciparum* CENH3 is able to functionally complement Cse4p and its, C-terminus is essential for centromere function. Molecular and Biochemical Parasitology. 2013;**192**(1-2):21-29

[58] Talbert PB, Henikoff S. Histone variants—Ancient wrap artists of the epigenome. Nature Reviews. Molecular Cell Biology. 2010;**11**(4):264-275

[59] Henikoff S, Smith MM. Histone variants and epigenetics. Cold Spring Harbor Perspectives in Biology. 2015;**7**(1):a019364

[60] Talbert PB et al. A unified phylogeny-based nomenclature for histone variants. Epigenetics & Chromatin. 2012;**5**:7

[61] Malik HS, Henikoff S. Phylogenomics of the nucleosome. Nature Structural Biology. 2003;**10**(11):882-891

[62] Dalmasso MC, Onyango DO, Naguleswaran A, Sullivan WJ, Angel SO. Toxoplasma H2A variants reveal novel insights into nucleosome composition and functions for this histone family. Journal of Molecular Biology. 2009;**392**:33-47

[63] Bogado SS et al. Canonical histone H2Ba and H2A.X dimerize in an opposite genomic localization to H2A.Z/H2B.Z dimers in *Toxoplasma gondii*. Molecular and Biochemical Parasitology. 2014;**197**(1-2):36-42

[64] Hoeijmakers WAM et al. H2A.Z/H2B.Z double-variant nucleosomes inhabit the AT-rich promoter regions of the *Plasmodium falciparum* genome. Molecular Microbiology. 2013; **87**(5):1061-1073

[65] Petter M et al. H2A.Z and H2B.Z double-variant nucleosomes define intergenic regions and dynamically occupy *var* gene promoters in the malaria parasite *Plasmodium falciparum*. Molecular Microbiology. 2013;**87**(6):1167-1182

[66] Talbert PB, Henikoff S. Environmental responses mediated by histone variants. Trends in Cell Biology. 2014;**24**(11):642-650

[67] Millar CB, Xu F, Zhang K, Grunstein M. Acetylation of H2AZ Lys 14 is associated with genome-wide gene activity in yeast. Genes & Development. 2006;**20**(6):711-722

[68] Bruce K et al. The replacement histone H2A.Z in a hyperacetylated form is a feature of active genes in the chicken. Nucleic Acids Research. 2005;**33**(17):5633-5639

[69] Ren Q, Gorovsky MA. Histone H2A.Z acetylation modulates an essential charge patch. Molecular Cell. 2001;**7**(6):1329-1335

[70] Hartley PD, Madhani HD. Mechanisms that specify promoter nucleosome location and identity. Cell. 2009;**137**(3):445-458

[71] Saeed S et al. Chromatin accessibility, p300, and histone acetylation define PML-RAR and AML1-ETO binding sites in acute myeloid leukemia. Blood. 2012;**120**(15):3058-3068

[72] Valdés-Mora F et al. Acetylation of H2A.Z is a key epigenetic modification associated with gene deregulation and epigenetic remodeling in cancer. Genome Research. 2012;**22**(2):307-321

[73] Valdés-Mora F et al. Acetylated histone variant H2A.Z is involved in the activation of neo-enhancers in prostate cancer. Nature Communications. 2017;**8**(1):1346

[74] Sarcinella E, Zuzarte PC, Lau PNI, Draker R, Cheung P. Monoubiquitylation of H2A.Z distinguishes its association with euchromatin or facultative heterochromatin. Molecular and Cellular Biology. 2007;**27**(18):6457-6468

[75] Draker R, Sarcinella E, Cheung P. USP10 deubiquitylates the histone variant H2A.Z and both are required for androgen receptor-mediated gene activation. Nucleic Acids Research. 2011;**39**(9):3529-3542

[76] Talbert PB, Henikoff S. Histone variants on the move: Substrates for chromatin dynamics. Nature Reviews. Molecular Cell Biology. 2017;**18**(2):115-126

[77] Clapier CR, Cairns BR. The biology of chromatin remodeling complexes. Annual Review of Biochemistry. 2009;**78**(1):273-304

[78] Van C, Williams JS, Kunkel TA, Peterson CL. Deposition of histone H2A.Z by the SWR-C remodeling enzyme prevents genome instability. DNA Repair (Amst). 2015;**25**:9-14

[79] Ruhl DD et al. Purification of a human SRCAP complex that remodels chromatin by incorporating the histone variant H2A.Z into nucleosomes. Biochemistry. 2006;**45**(17): 5671-5677

[80] Watanabe S, Radman-Livaja M, Rando OJ, Peterson CL. A histone acetylation switch regulates H2A.Z deposition by the SWR-C remodeling enzyme. Science (80-). 2013; **340**(6129):195-199

[81] Wang F, Ranjan A, Wei D, Wu C. Comment on "A histone acetylation switch regulates H2A.Z deposition by the SWR-C remodeling enzyme". Science (80-). 2016;**353**(6297): 358-358

[82] Watanabe S, Peterson CL. Response to comment on "A histone acetylation switch regulates H2A.Z deposition by the SWR-C remodeling enzyme". Science (80-). 2016; **353**(6297):358-358

[83] Altaf M et al. NuA4-dependent acetylation of nucleosomal histones H4 and H2A directly stimulates incorporation of H2A.Z by the SWR1 complex. The Journal of Biological Chemistry. 2010;**285**(21):15966-15977

[84] Perell GT, Mishra NK, Sudhamalla B, Ycas PD, Islam K, Pomerantz WCK. Specific acetylation patterns of H2A.Z form transient interactions with the BPTF bromodomain. Biochemistry. 2017;**56**(35):4607-4615

[85] Draker R, Ng MK, Sarcinella E, Ignatchenko V, Kislinger T, Cheung P. A combination of H2A.Z and H4 acetylation recruits Brd2 to chromatin during transcriptional activation. PLoS Genetics. 2012;**8**(11):e1003047

[86] Ren Q, Gorovsky MA. The nonessential H2A N-terminal tail can function as an essential charge patch on the H2A.Z variant N-terminal tail. Molecular and Cellular Biology. 2003;**23**(8):2778-2789

[87] Jeffers V, Tampaki Z, Kim K, Sullivan WJ. A latent ability to persist: Differentiation in *Toxoplasma gondii*. Cellular and Molecular Life Sciences. 2018;**75**(13):2355-2373

[88] Whittle CM et al. The genomic distribution and function of histone variant HTZ-1 during *C. elegans* embryogenesis. PLoS Genetics. 2008;**4**(9):e1000187

[89] Updike DL, Mango SE. Temporal regulation of foregut development by HTZ-1/H2A.Z and PHA-4/FoxA. PLoS Genetics. 2006;**2**(9):e161

[90] Ridgway P, Brown KD, Rangasamy D, Svensson U, Tremethick DJ. Unique residues on the H2A.Z containing nucleosome surface are important for *Xenopus laevis* development. The Journal of Biological Chemistry. 2004;**279**(42):43815-43820

[91] Law C, Cheung P. Expression of non-acetylatable H2A.Z in myoblast cells blocks myoblast differentiation through disruption of MyoD expression. The Journal of Biological Chemistry. 2015;**290**(21):13234-13249

[92] Jeffers V, Yang C, Huang S, Sullivan WJ. Bromodomains in protozoan parasites: Evolution, function, and opportunities for drug development. Microbiology and Molecular Biology Reviews. 2017;**81**(1):e00047-e00016

[93] Bártfai R et al. H2A.Z demarcates intergenic regions of the *Plasmodium falciparum* epigenome that are dynamically marked by H3K9ac and H3K4me3. PLoS Pathogens. 2010;**6**(12):e1001223

[94] Westenberger SJ, Cui L, Dharia N, Winzeler E, Cui L. Genome-wide nucleosome mapping of *Plasmodium falciparum* reveals histone-rich coding and histone-poor intergenic regions and chromatin remodeling of core and subtelomeric genes. BMC Genomics. 2009;**10**(1):610

[95] Petter M et al. Expression of *P. falciparum* var genes involves exchange of the histone variant H2A.Z at the promoter. PLoS Pathogens. 2011;**7**(2):e1001292

[96] Kumar SV, Wigge PA. H2A.Z-containing nucleosomes mediate the thermosensory response in arabidopsis. Cell. 2010;**140**(1):136-147

[97] Horikoshi N, Arimura Y, Taguchi H, Kurumizaka H. Crystal structures of heterotypic nucleosomes containing histones H2A.Z and H2A. Open Biology. 2016;**6**(6):160127

[98] Scherf A, Figueiredo LM, Freitas-junior LH. Plasmodium telomeres: A pathogen's perspective. Current Opinion in Microbiology. 2001;**4**(4):409-414

[99] Figueiredo LM, Freitas-Junior LH, Bottius E, Olivo-Marin J-C, Scherf A. A central role for *Plasmodium falciparum* subtelomeric regions in spatial positioning and telomere length regulation. The EMBO Journal. 2002;**21**(4):815-824

[100] Dalmasso MC, Carmona SJ, Angel SO, Agüero F. Characterization of *Toxoplasma gondii* subtelomeric-like regions: Identification of a long-range compositional bias that is also associated with gene-poor regions. BMC Genomics. 2014;**15**(1):21

[101] Kaviratne M, Khan SM, Jarra W, Preiser PR. Small variant STEVOR antigen is uniquely located within Maurer's clefts in *Plasmodium falciparum*-infected red blood cells. Eukaryotic Cell. 2002;**1**(6):926-935

[102] Petter M, Haeggström M, Khattab A, Fernandez V, Klinkert M-Q, Wahlgren M. Variant proteins of the *Plasmodium falciparum* RIFIN family show distinct subcellular localization and developmental expression patterns. Molecular and Biochemical Parasitology. 2007;**156**(1):51-61

[103] Freitas-Junior LH et al. Frequent ectopic recombination of virulence factor genes in telomeric chromosome clusters of *P. falciparum*. Nature. 2000;**407**(6807):1018-1022

[104] Vernick KD, McCutchan TF. A novel class of supercoil-independent nuclease hypersensitive site is comprised of alternative DNA structures that flank eukaryotic genes. Journal of Molecular Biology. 1998;**279**(4):737-751

[105] Gardner MJ et al. Genome sequence of the human malaria parasite *Plasmodium falciparum*. Nature. 2002;**419**(6906):498-511

[106] Ai W, Bertram PG, Tsang CK, Chan TF, Zheng XFS. Regulation of subtelomeric silencing during stress response. Molecular Cell. 2002;**10**(6):1295-1305

[107] Buck MJ, Lieb JD. A chromatin-mediated mechanism for specification of conditional transcription factor targets. Nature Genetics. 2006;**38**(12):6-1451

[108] Tomar RS, Zheng S, Brunke-Reese D, Wolcott HN, Reese JC. Yeast Rap1 contributes to genomic integrity by activating DNA damage repair genes. The EMBO Journal. 2008; **27**(11):1575-1584

[109] Harari Y, Romano G-H, Ungar L, Kupiec M. Nature vs nurture: Interplay between the genetic control of telomere length and environmental factors. Cell Cycle. 2013;**12**(22): 3465-3470

[110] Tonkin CJ et al. Sir2 paralogues cooperate to regulate virulence genes and antigenic variation in *Plasmodium falciparum*. PLoS Biology. 2009;**7**(4):0771-0788

[111] Freitas LH et al. Telomeric heterochromatin propagation and histone acetylation control mutually exclusive expression of antigenic variation genes in malaria parasites. Cell. 2005;**121**(1):25-36

[112] Merrick CJ et al. Functional analysis of sirtuin genes in multiple *Plasmodium falciparum* strains. PLoS One. 2015;**10**(3):e0118865

[113] Mancio-Silva L, Rojas-Meza AP, Vargas M, Scherf A, Hernandez-Rivas R. Differential association of Orc1 and Sir2 proteins to telomeric domains in *Plasmodium falciparum*. Journal of Cell Science. 2008;**121**:2046-2053

[114] Deshmukh AS et al. The role of N-terminus of *Plasmodium falciparum* ORC1 in telomeric localization and var gene silencing. Nucleic Acids Research. 2012;**40**(12):5313-5331

[115] Serrano L et al. The tumor suppressor SirT2 regulates cell cycle progression and genome stability by modulating the mitotic deposition of H4K20 methylation. Genes & Development. 2013;**27**(6):639-653

[116] Goyal M et al. Identification and molecular characterization of an Alba-family protein from human malaria parasite *Plasmodium falciparum*. Nucleic Acids Research. 2012; **40**(3):1174-1190

[117] Bell SD. The interaction of Alba, a conserved archaeal chromatin protein, with Sir2 and its regulation by acetylation. Science (80-). 2002;**296**(5565):148-151

[118] Pérez-Toledo K et al. *Plasmodium falciparum* heterochromatin protein 1 binds to trimethylated histone 3 lysine 9 and is linked to mutually exclusive expression of var genes. Nucleic Acids Research. 2009;**37**(8):2596-2606

[119] Lopez-Rubio JJ, Mancio-Silva L, Scherf A. Genome-wide analysis of heterochromatin associates clonally variant gene regulation with perinuclear repressive centers in malaria parasites. Cell Host & Microbe. 2009;**5**(2):179-190

[120] Flueck C et al. A major role for the *Plasmodium falciparum* ApiAP2 protein PfSIP2 in chromosome end biology. PLoS Pathogens. 2010;**6**(2):e1000784

[121] Gupta MK, Agarawal M, Banu K, Reddy KS, Gaur D, Dhar SK. Role of chromatin assembly factor 1 in DNA replication of *Plasmodium falciparum*. Biochemical and Biophysical Research Communications. 2018;**495**(1):1285-1291

[122] Masumoto H, Hawke D, Kobayashi R, Verreault A. A role for cell-cycle-regulated histone H3 lysine 56 acetylation in the DNA damage response. Nature. 2005;**436**(7048):294-298

[123] Echeverria PC, Rojas PA, Martin V, Guarnera EA, Pszenny V, Angel SO. Characterisation of a novel interspersed *Toxoplasma gondii* DNA repeat with potential uses for PCR diagnosis and PCR-RFLP analysis. FEMS Microbiology Letters. 2000;**184**(1):23-27

[124] Fillingham J, Keogh M-C, Krogan NJ. GammaH2AX and its role in DNA double-strand break repair. Biochemistry and Cell Biology. 2006;**84**(4):568-577

[125] Nyberg KA, Michelson RJ, Putnam CW, Weinert TA. Toward maintaining the genome: DNA damage and replication checkpoints. Annual Review of Genetics. 2002;**36**(1): 617-656

[126] Redon C, Pilch D, Rogakou E, Sedelnikova O, Newrock K, Bonner W. Histone H2A variants H2AX and H2AZ. Current Opinion in Genetics and Development. 2002;**12**(2): 162-169

[127] Turinetto V, Giachino C. Histone variants as emerging regulators of embryonic stem cell identity. Epigenetics. 2015;**10**(7):563-573

[128] Seo J et al. Genome-wide profiles of H2AX and γ-H2AX differentiate endogenous and exogenous DNA damage hotspots in human cells. Nucleic Acids Research. 2012; **40**:5965-5974

[129] Lukas J, Lukas C, Bartek J. More than just a focus: The chromatin response to DNA damage and its role in genome integrity maintenance. Nature Cell Biology. 2011; **13**(10):1161-1169

[130] Ciccia A, Elledge SJ. The DNA damage response: Making it safe to play with knives. Molecular Cell. 2010;**40**(2):179-204

[131] Jackson SP, Bartek J. The DNA-damage response in human biology and disease. Nature. 2009;**461**(7267):1071-1078

[132] Bétermier M, Bertrand P, Lopez BS. Is non-homologous end-joining really an inherently error-prone process? PLoS Genetics. 2014;**10**(1):e1004086

[133] Guirouilh-Barbat J, Lambert S, Bertrand P, Lopez BS. Is homologous recombination really an error-free process? Frontiers in Genetics. 2014;**5**:175

[134] Sancar A, Lindsey-Boltz LA, Unsal-Kacmaz K, Linn S. Molecular mechanisms of mammalian DNA repair and the DNA damage checkpoints. Annual Review of Biochemistry. 2004;**73**(1):39-85 (0066-4154 (Print) LA–eng PT–Journal Article PT–Review RN–0 (Cross–Linking Reagents) RN–9007-49-2 (DNA) SB–IM)

[135] Smolarz B, Wilczyński J, Nowakowska D. DNA repair mechanisms and *Toxoplasma gondii* infection. Archives of Microbiology. 2014;**196**(1):1-8

[136] Kelso AA, Waldvogel SM, Luthman AJ, Sehorn MG. Homologous recombination in protozoan parasites and recombinase inhibitors. Frontiers in Microbiology. 2017;**8**:1716

[137] Fidock DA, Lee AH, Symington LS, Fidock A. DNA repair mechanisms and their biological roles in the malaria parasite *Plasmodium falciparum*. Microbiology and Molecular Biology Reviews. 2014;**3**:78

[138] Calhoun SF, Reed J, Alexander N, Mason CE, Deitsch KW, Kirkman LA. Chromosome end repair and genome stability in *Plasmodium falciparum*. MBio Journal. 2017;**8**(4): e00547-e00517

[139] Paull TT. Mechanisms of ATM activation. Annual Review of Biochemistry. 2015;**84**(1): 711-738

[140] Vonlaufen N, Naguleswaran A, Coppens I, Sullivan WJ. MYST family lysine acetyltransferase facilitates ataxia telangiectasia mutated (ATM) kinase-mediated DNA damage response in *Toxoplasma gondii*. The Journal of Biological Chemistry. 2010;**285**(15): 11154-11161

[141] Agarwal P, Miller KM. The nucleosome: Orchestrating DNA damage signaling and repair within chromatin. Biochemistry and Cell Biology. 2016;**94**(5):381-395

[142] Gursoy-Yuzugullu O, House N, Price BD. Patching broken DNA: Nucleosome dynamics and the repair of DNA breaks. Journal of Molecular Biology. 2016;**428**(9):1846-1860

[143] Sun Y, Jiang X, Chen S, Fernandes N, Price BD. A role for the Tip60 histone acetyltransferase in the acetylation and activation of ATM. Proceedings of the National Academy of Sciences of the United States of America. 2005;**102**(37):13182-13187

[144] Francia ME, Striepen B. Cell division in apicomplexan parasites. Nature Reviews Microbiology. 2014;**12**(2):125-136

[145] Gupta DK, Patra AT, Zhu L, Gupta AP, Bozdech Z. DNA damage regulation and its role in drug-related phenotypes in the malaria parasites. Scientific Reports. 2016; **6**(November):1-15

[146] Radke JR, Striepen B, Guerini MN, Jerome ME, Roos DS, White MW. Defining the cell cycle for the tachyzoite stage of *Toxoplasma gondii*. Molecular and Biochemical Parasitology. 2001;**115**(2):165-175

[147] Xu Y, Ayrapetov MK, Xu C, Gursoy-Yuzugullu O, Hu Y, Price BD. Histone H2A.Z controls a critical chromatin remodeling step required for DNA double-strand break repair. Molecular Cell. 2012;**48**(5):723-733

[148] Luger K, Rechsteiner TJ, Flaus AJ, Waye MM, Richmond TJ. Characterization of nucleosome core particles containing histone proteins made in bacteria. Journal of Molecular Biology. 1997;**272**(3):301-311

[149] Luger K, Suto RK, Clarkson MJ, Tremethick DJ. Crystal structure of a nucleosome core particle containing the variant histone H2A.Z. Nature Structural Biology. 2000; **7**(12):1121-1124

[150] Park Y-J, Dyer PN, Tremethick DJ, Luger K. A new fluorescence resonance energy transfer approach demonstrates that the histone variant H2AZ stabilizes the histone octamer within the nucleosome. The Journal of Biological Chemistry. 2004;**279**(23):24274-24282

[151] Aurrecoechea C et al. EuPathDB: The eukaryotic pathogen database. Nucleic Acids Research. 2013;**41**(D1):D684-D691

[152] Jackson SP, Durocher D. Regulation of DNA damage responses by ubiquitin and SUMO.Molecular Cell. 2013;**49**(5):795-807

7

Epigenome, Cancer Prevention and Flavonoids and Curcumin

Višnja Stepanić, Renata Novak Kujundžić and
Koraljka Gall Trošelj

1. Introduction

Epigenome is a common name for heritable chemical modifications of DNA and histone molecules, of which DNA methylation and histone acetylation and methylation represent the most studied parts. Nucleosomes, the chromatin building units, are positioned in a way that is strictly dependent on the epigenome changes. Based on the presence of a specific epigenetic modification, the chromatin becomes less or more condensed. These changes in chromatin structure are inevitably related to gene activity. For example, DNA hypermethylation joined with histone hypoacetylation is frequently related to a condensed form of chromatin, marking the region of DNA that should not be active during a specific time window. This implies that genes in that specific region may become active once the aforementioned marks are removed. Indeed, epigenome represents a very powerful, extremely flexible "tool" for regulating gene activity and the major reason for the well-known phenomena of "time specific" and "tissue specific" gene expression.

In the field of cancer research, epigenome changes are considered to be among the first steps in carcinogenesis, preceding the structural changes in the DNA molecule, known generally as "gene mutations". Specifically, the most prominent change in the earliest phases of cancer is inactivation of tumor suppressor genes which are frequently silenced through DNA methylation and histone deacetylation taking place in the regions corresponding to their promoters. It is known that enzymes regulating these processes, DNA methyltransferases (DNMTs) and histone deacetylases (HDACs) are aberrantly up-regulated not only in a developed cancer, but also in the early phases of carcinogenesis (as recently shown for ductal *in situ* breast cancer [1]). Accordingly, significant effort has been given to the discovery and development of specific chemical compounds that may act as DNA demethylating agents and histone deacetylases inhibitors (HDACi). Some of these compounds are already utilized in the clinic, like DNMT inhibitors 5-azacytidine and decitabine and HDAC inhibitor vorinostat, with specific therapeutic indications [2]. In parallel with these research efforts, considerable data has been published on the role of natural compounds. The importance of these compounds has been intensely studied in the field of cancer prevention, especially in light of the influence of a specific diet on cancer prevention (as shown for the Mediterranean diet which may have a modest beneficial effect related to the incidence of colorectal carcinoma [3]). Many dietary compounds have been revealed to significantly impact gene expression through modulating the epigenome. Logically, if a specific type of diet is considered to be protective in relation to cancer, there has to be a molecular mechanism at the level of the epigenome explaining its protective effect.

These will be addressed in this book chapter, where we describe polyphenols' molecular mechanisms of action, through well-known compounds belonging to different chemical subgroups and shown in Table 1.

2. Chromatin structure

The native state of DNA, a double helix, is formed when two antiparallel strands are held together by hydrogen bonds (H-bonds) between complementary purine and pyrimidine bases. Each human diploid cell contains approximately two meters of DNA. Obviously, in order to be kept in the nucleus, which is, on average, nine micrometers in diameter, the DNA must be 10,000-20,000 folds compacted [4].

Histones are small proteins that act as chromatin "compacting units. The tight binding of DNA and histones is considerably dependent on the charge: DNA is negatively charged molecule due to presence of phosphate groups, and the strength of interaction between DNA and histones strongly depends on posttranslational modifications of histones' tails which can modify their charge. This is possible due to a specific structure of histone proteins. Histones' globular domain represents central part that is highly structured. In addition to this part, histone proteins have "tails" at both, NH_2-and COOH-ends. These tails may be modified through numerous types of posttranslational modifications of which methylation and acetylation will be discussed in detail through this chapter. These covalent modifications, by which cell regulates access to DNA, depend on enzymes often called "writers" and "erasers" [5].

2.1. Histone modifications and gene transcription

The part of the genome that contains genes that are dynamically transcribed must be shaped in an open, flexible way. Part of the chromatin that follows this rule is called euchromatin. Non-coding parts of genome, joined with those parts that contain inactive genes (e.g., in the region of centromeres and telomeres) do not need to follow significant reshape. This condensed, closed shape of chromatin is known as heterochromatin. So, how do histone modifications influence keeping these two forms of chromatin present in the cell and, also important, how do histone modifications influence "the switch" between the two forms? In other words,

Polyphenol	Plant sources
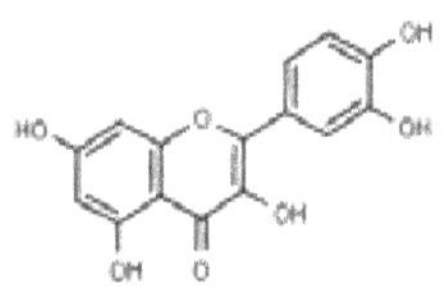 Quercetin	Apples, grapes, blackberries, cranberries, blueberries, onion, kale, capers, watercress, dill, bitter dock, red wines, black tea
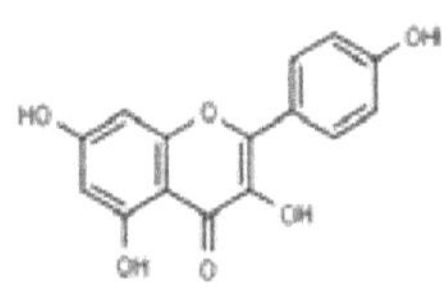 Kaempferol	Tea, kale, carrot, capers, leek, celery, apples
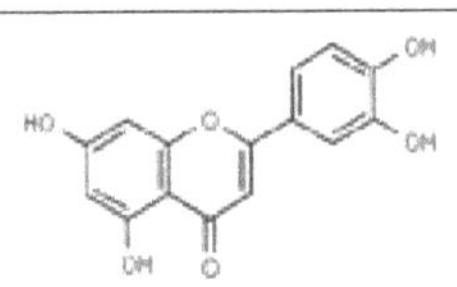 Luteolin	Sage, thyme, peppermint, carrot, broccoli, onion, chilli
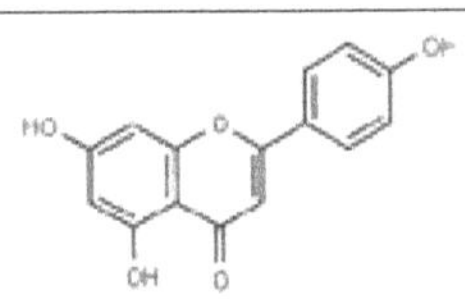 Apigenin	Chinese cabbage, parsley, papper, garlic , barley, endive, olive oil, chamomile, apples, onion
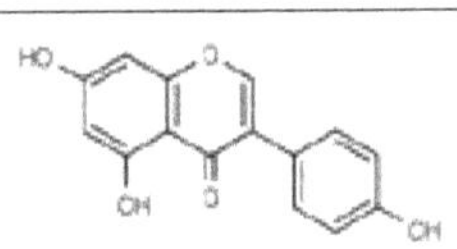 Genistein	Soy, soy food – miso, tempeh, tofu *etc.*
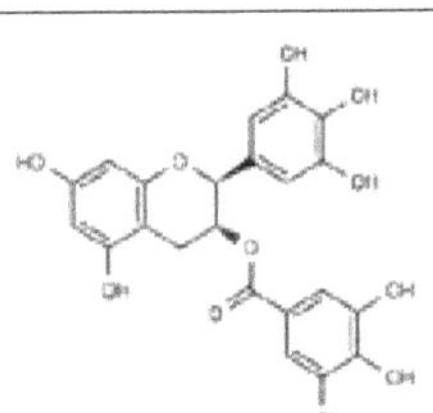 EGCG	Green tea
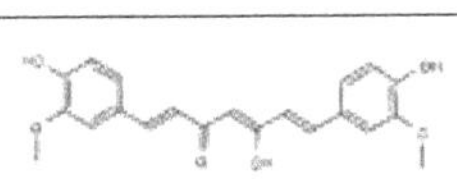 Curcumin	Turmeric (*Curcuma longa*), curry

Table 1. Structures and sources of selected polyphenols with known epigenome modifying activities.

how is the need for expression of a specific gene during very short time period regulated by histone posttranslational modifications?

There are two basic mechanisms: a) direct, influencing the overall structure of chromatin, b) indirect, through the regulation of binding of effector molecules [6]. For example, trymethylation of lysine at the position 9 of histone 3 (H3K9me3) can recruit the protein HP1 (heterochromatin protein 1). The interaction takes place in the area of heterochromatin and leads to additional compacting that physically precludes access of transcriptional machinery [7]. There is sufficient level of evidence on *cis*-interactions in chromosome-mediated gene expression. For example, H3S10 phosphorylation enhances H3K4 methylation and H3K14 acetylation, and inhibits H3K9 methylation, thus indirectly facilitating chromatin decondensation [8].

The first report on histone acetylation is 50 years old [9]. The earliest studies following this discovery, revealed association of hyperacetylated histones with gene transcription [10]. In general, keeping in mind that there is no rule that would not have an exception, hyperacetylation of histone tails induces transcriptional activation, while hypoacetylation is associated with repression of transcription. Lysine acetylation is very dynamic process, regulated by antagonistic actions of two groups of enzymes: histone acetyltransferases (HATs) and HDACs. The consequence of lysine acetylation, which occurs upon the transfer of an acetyl group to the ε-amino-group of lysine side chain, is neutralization of lysine's positive charge and hence weakening interactions between histone and DNA. Mainly as a result of cumulative charge neutralizations at multiple lysines, the chromatin takes its "open", transcriptionally active structure [11]. This process is fast and happens in only a few minutes, as measured by isotopic pulse labeling [12]. In general, HDACs have the suppressing function, they are negative regulators of gene activity. It must be told that these enzymes have also many non-histone protein substrates that are included in regulation of important cellular processes, including cell proliferation and cell death. These are but not limited to: transcription factors, hormone receptors, cytoskeletal proteins, chaperons and various signaling mediators.

Histone methylation certainly is one of the best studied histone modifications, which takes place on both lysine and arginine amino acid residues. These modifications are not only residue-dependent (K4, K9, K27, K36, K79 in histone 3 (H3)) but also status-dependent (mono-, di-and trimethylation). In most scenarios, H3K4me2/3, H3K36me1/3 and H3K79me1/2 and H4K20m1 modifications are associated with activation of transcription, while H3K9me2/3, H3K27me2/3 and H4K20me3 marks are usually associated with transcriptional repression [13]. H3K4me3 association with 5' regions of active genes strongly correlates with overall transcription rate, active RNA polymerase II occupancy and global histone acetylation (reviewed in [14]). Such outcome is a consequence of binding of different proteins that specifically interact with activators or repressors of transcription.

Histone methylation depends on activity of histone methylating (histone lysine methyltransferases, KMTs) and demethylating (histone lysine demethylases, KDMs) enzymes. Both groups of enzymes have a very important role in cancer initiation and development and their mutations have been shown to exist in different types of malignant tumors. Methylation marks on histones are highly specific, altering gene expression in a way that may be unique for particular type of normal and/or cancer cell [13]. For example, histone demethylase KDM5A contains a highly specific H3K4me3 reader domain and is probably involved in modifying nearby domains upon binding to H3K4m3. This enzyme was found to be present in regions that are enriched in H3K4me3 and are transcriptionally active. This is particularly significant in cells originating from bone marrow and peripheral blood where high expression of its target genes was also found [13]. For that reason, the ratio of various histone demethylases and histone methyltransferases, KDM/KMT, was suggested to be a sign of a specific "transcription module", trying to predict expression of specific genes, members of specific module. This fact, which should provide more specific way of acting compared to acetylation balancing enzymes, makes enzymes involved in regulation of histone methylation status good candidates for specific epigenetic interventions.

Histone lysine methylation depends on KMTs that are classified into two groups, based on the sequence and structure of their catalytic domains: SET domain containing (suppressor of variegation homologus (SUV), enhancer of zeste proteins (EZH), trithorax-group (TrxG) proteins) and non-SET domain containing (DOT1 protein family) [15].

So far, histone demethylases KDMs are grouped in two families. KDM1 family includes only two members, LSD1 (lysine-specific demethylase 1, KDM1A) and LSD2 (KDM1B). LSD1 was the first discovered histone demethylase and its discovery revealed that histone lysine methylation is reversible process [16]. LSD1 targets histone H3K4, and, when associated with androgen or estrogen receptor, it can also target histone H3K9. In addition, LSD1 has been shown to demethylate non-histone proteins, including tumor suppressor p53 and DNA methyltransferase-1 (DNMT1). The second, Jumonji C (JmjC) domain containing protein family, is numerous and includes seven subgroups with a total of 14 KDMs. There is no doubt that KDMs and KTMs must work coordinately in order to keep a precise regulation of histone methylation.

Both KDMs and KTMs are involved in cancer initiation and progression, although KDMs are much less studied. There are firm data on histone lysine methyltransferases expression change upon cell exposure to heavy metals. For example, peripheral blood mononuclear cells (PBMC) were isolated from the whole blood of healthy volunteers and exposed to varying concentration of nickel chloride (0.25, 0.5 and 1.0 mM) for 24 h and compared to untreated control samples. The transcriptome analyses (Affymetrix Human Genome U133.20 Array) combined with ChipSeq with anti-H3K4me3, have revealed that there are 1381 entities with 2-fold difference in expression upon nickel exposure. This number was reduced to 382 and 246 with more stringent cuts off - 3-fold and 5-fold, respectively. The global level of H3K4me3 was increased. This study also showed that H3K4me3 does not occupy only the promoters of genes that were transcriptionally active, but also extends into their coding regions, as previously shown for nickel-exposed human lung adenocarcinoma cell line A549 [17]. When measured in PBMC from subjects that had occupational exposure to nickel but did not have cancer, the level of H3K4me3 was significantly increased when compared with PBMC from subjects without exposure [17]. Since chronic exposure to nickel has been associated with lung and nasal carcinoma, these results, obtained on human population, clearly show that harmful exposure indeed reshapes chromatin in a direction that leads to carcinogenesis. So, if detected early, before disease onset, can these changes be reversible? Even more so, can we influence the enzymes that reshape epigenome in a procarcinogenic direction?

2.2. Interplay between DNA methylation and histone acetylation

There are several chromatin-regulating factors that recognize methylated DNA or modified histone proteins. One of them, the HP1 protein, has already been mentioned. The common characteristic of these effector molecules is that they use a range of different recognition domains such as methyl-CpG-binding domains (MBD), zinc fingers (ZnF), chromo-domain, or plant homeodomain (PHD) in order to direct establishing specific epigenomic marks and orchestrate biological events [18, 19]. However, the most of studies performed so far have been conducted using isolated DNA or histone peptides and cannot recapitulate the situation found in chromatin *in vivo*. Recently, an approach named SNAP (SILAC nucleosome affinity purification) was used for the identification of proteins that are influenced by DNA CpG methylation and histone H3 K4-, K9- or K27-methylation (or a combination thereof) in the context of a nucleosome. The approach itself seems to be very valuable in defining the chromatin "interactome" and showing that DNA methylation and histone modifications act in a concerted manner by creating a "modification landscape" that must be interpreted by proteins able to recognize large molecular assemblies [20].

This is not surprising due to the fact that there are currently 18 HDACs identified in humans, subclassified in four classes: a) class I HDACs 1, 2, 3 and 8 localized mainly in nucleus where they acetylate numerous proteins, of which p53 (cellular tumor antigen p53) and BRCA1 (breast cancer type 1 susceptibility protein) are probably the most frequently studied non-histonic substrates; b) class II with class IIa of HDAC 4, 5, 7 and 9 isoforms located in nucleus and cytoplasm and class IIb of HDACs 6 and 10 located only in the nucleus; c) class III of sirutins SIRT1-7 whose activity depends on the presence of nicotinamide adenine dinucleotide (NAD^+/NADH) and d) class IV containing only one enzyme, HDAC11 [21].

Besides actions on histone molecules, the importance of modifying "the guardian of genome" p53 represents utmost important cellular event. One of the consequences of recruitment of HDAC1 to p53, through MDM2 (E3 ubiquitin-protein ligase), is p53 deacetylation and degradation. For this very reason, there is no p53-related induction of $p21^{WAF1}$ (p21, cyclin-dependent kinase inhibitor 1) and MDM2 [22]. Luckily, p21 is not regulated only by p53, but also through many other transcription factors including Sp1 (transcription factor Sp1) for which six binding sites are present in the p53 promoter. Thus, this is only one example of multiple regulations and how complex the system has to be in keeping the balance of signals that will prevent cell from uncontrolled division, which is a hallmark of cancer.

HDACi are generally subdivided into several groups, based on their diverse chemical structures-short chain fatty acids, hydroxamates, cyclic peptides, aliphatic acids, benzamides, SIRT inhibitors, electrophilic ketones and miscellaneous compounds [23]. The member of the hydroxamate group, suberoylanilide hydroxamic acid (SAHA, vorinostat) has been approved by FDA in October of 2006 for treatment of a rare cutaneous T-lymphoma. The approval for the cyclopeptide, romidepsin (Istodax®), came in November of 2009. Although well tolerated and with manageable side effects, HDACis have not entirely fulfilled expectations that were based on well-known molecular mechanism associated with their application *in vitro*: early studies have undoubtedly shown that these HDACis upregulate p21 in p53-independent fashion leading to G2/M cell cycle arrest [24]. Only two years later it was shown that this treatment additionally increases cyclin E and decreases cyclin D1 [25].

As expected, the problem lies in insufficient selectivity of HDACis: in addition to an increase of p21 and other pro-apoptotic genes, the treatment with HDACis also induces transcription of genes that are pro-carcinogenic, like multiple isoforms of protein kinase C (PKC) and downstream regulated matrix metalloproteinases (MMPs). Among 30 cancer cell lines (12 liver, 10 lung, 5 gastric and 3 breast cancer cell lines) that were tested for cell migration (indicating metastatic potential) after being treated with HDACis belonging to different groups (including vorinostat), 43% (13/30) cell lines showed several hundred folds increase in migration potential [26]. This effect was initiated at low, non-cytotoxic sub-μM to low μM dosage of HDACis. In an *in vivo* experiment, tumor cell lines were injected into HDACi treated mice. In contrast to untreated control animals, these mice have developed metastatic disease with statistically proved significance ($p < 0.026$). However, when combined with curcumin or tamoxifen, this treatment had very promising effect both, *in vitro* and *in vivo*. Western blot analyses performed on tumor lysates obtained from mice treated with HDACi trichostatin A, combined with curcumin or tamoxifen revealed significant downregulation of PKCs and some other proteins included in tumor progression. Of importance, the high expression of p21 induced with HDACis remained unchanged.

It is well-known that dietary and other environmental factors induce epigenetic alterations. For example, smoking induces numerous harmful epigenetic alterations that can be first steps in malignant transformation. Accordingly, cellular epigenome may be protected from harmful events through a proper diet and healthy way of living.

With development of sophisticated methods applicable in all fields of molecular biology, anticancer properties have become proved for many natural compounds [27]. Their mode of action frequently influences cellular epigenome through chromatin remodeling [28]. For example, polyphenols can modulate chromatin structure through influencing expression of chromatin remodeling enzymes, HDACs and DNMTs [29]. Targeting these proteins in addition to various kinases (e.g. mitogen-activated protein kinases (MAPKs), phosphatidylinositide-3-kinase (PI3K), protein kinase B isozymes (AKT), Aurora B, Polo-like kinase 1 (PLK1)), poly(ADP-ribose) polymerase (PARP) and other epigenome modifying enzymes KDMs (LSD1, JMJD3) and HATs (p300/CBP (CREB binding protein) coactivators) [30] make them extremely powerful modifiers of cellular processes included in all aspects of cellular survival and cellular death. Besides, for all these multilevel ways of acting, affecting a large number of biochemical signaling pathways, natural polyphenols are excellent examples of polypharmacological compounds.

3. Intracellular stability and nuclear localization of polyphenols

In order to exert their effect on chromatin organization, polyphenols must be stable and able to enter cellular nucleus. There are numerous studies in the field of cancer research reporting on various changes in experiment-related pre-selected set of interesting proteins included in cellular proliferation, after adding a polyphenol to cellular medium. However, their intracellular accumulation, stability and transformation are poorly understood. This is not surprising, as there are only limited number of studies dealing with polyphenol's cellular uptake and efflux, their subcellular localization and intracellular stability [31]. These parameters are crucial for understanding their mechanism of action and biological effects.

The polyphenols are usually assumed to bind to cellular membrane and/or are in the cytosoplasm affecting membrane receptors and modulating kinases activity [32,33]. Polyphenols whose effects on chromatin are described in this review, may cross both cellular and nuclear membranes and enter nucleus. For example, quercetin has been shown to be localized mainly in the nucleus of HepG2 cells [34,35]. Flavon apigenin has been reported to localize mostly in nuclear matrix and less in cytosol, nuclear membranes and microsomes of prostate cancer cell lines DU145, LNCaP and PC-3 [36]. By using a confocal laser scanning fluorescence microscope, the autofluorescence of galangin and kaempferol appeared stronger in the nucleus than cytoplasm of mouse hepatoma Hepa-1c1c7 cells [37]. Among flavonoids, only flavonols containing the conjugated 3-OH group (Figure 1), show autofluorescence and can be detected by this approach. The highest percentage of curcumin in breast cancer cell line MCF-7 cells has been found in membrane and decreases in the following order: membrane > cytoplasm > nucleus > mitochondria [38]. The fluorescent conjugates of EGCG were localized onto the membrane as well as in the cytoplasm and nucleus of mouse fibroblasts L-929 [39], but are found on the membrane, in the cytoplasm and specifically in mitochondria of the human umbilical vein endothelial cells (HUVECs) [40]. The largest fraction of soy isoflavone genistein has been localized in cytoplasm, but it has also been registered in nuclei and mitochondria of pooled female rat liver [41]. The associated concentrations of genistein were in the nmol/g range, far below the concentrations required for most of its *in vitro* effects [41]. Concentrations of parent polyphenols within cells *in vitro* are usually in low μM to sub-μM range [42].

Namely, significant portion of a polyphenol, such as in the cases of EGCG [43] and apigenin [44], may be intracellularly transformed, depending on cell type and cell culture conditions, particularly pH of the medium [43, 45]. At the cellular level, metabolic transformations of polyphenols through phases I and II enzymes, have been well-documented, including hydroxylation by CYP450 isoforms CYP1A2, CYP3A4 [44] and CYP1B1 [46] and methylation of hydroxyl groups by catechol-O-methyl transferase (COMT) [31]. These reactions may be necessary for generation of active metabolites, as is the case with conversion of apigenin into its main metabolite, luteolin [47]. Furthermore, since polyphenols more or less readily participate in redox processes, the contribution of their oxidized quinone/quinone methide forms to their mechanisms of action may not be excluded [48], particularly when relatively high concentrations of flavonoids (high μM to mM) have been applied to cells [31].

Metabolic conjugation alters the physicochemical properties of flavonoids and it is widely assumed that this can affect their biological activity. Hence, for understanding the cellular effects of parent polyphenol compounds, the influence of their uptake, intracellular metabolism, oxidation and localization should be taken into account or *a priori* excluded [49]. This is enormously important when put in the context of cellular epigenome which is specific for each type of cell. It may not be surprising then that specific effects of metabolites are consistent with findings that polyphenols' actions are cell-type dependent.

As usual, observations presented in this review will be interpreted in terms of parent polyphenol aglycons whose structures are shown within Table 1, but one should bear in mind that they may be exerted by their metabolites and oxidized forms.

4. Dose-dependent effects of polyphenols

The cellular effects of polyphenols recorded *in vitro* are concentration- and time-dependent [49,50]. Application of quercetin and EGCG as well as other polyphenols like resveratrol, induces hormetic dose–response cellular phenomenon characterized by a low-dose stimulation and high-dose inhibition, often resulting in typical U-or J-shaped curves [50]. While showing pro-oxidant properties joined with citotoxicity at high concentrations, low doses of quercetin (1-40 μM) were shown to have antioxidant and chemopreventive properties [51]. Also, application of curcumin, even at a very low concentration (10 μM), and especially if exposure was prolonged (up to 72 h), was shown to be cytotoxic for various cancer cells, but not for fibroblasts WI-38 [52].

At the low μM doses, the polyphenols activate hormetic adaptive cellular stress response signaling pathways that include various kinases and transcription factors [50]. As a result, there is an activation of genes that encode stress resistance proteins such as antioxidant and detoxifying enzymes, protein chaperones, neurotrophic factors, and other cytoprotective proteins. Specific example of such a pathway is the Nrf2/ARE (NF-E2-related factor 2 / antioxidant response element) pathway [50]. At these concentrations, these compounds are not cytotoxic, but cytostatic. They commonly block the cell cycle in various cancer cells in S/G2 and mitotic phase, leading to cell death. They also target multiple kinases that are implicated in pathogenesis of cancer.

5. Plant polyphenols in cellular growth arrest and death

So far, all studied polyphenols have been shown to induce both, apoptosis and autophagy of cancer cells, without affecting normal cells [53,54,55]. Epicatechin and quercetin have been shown to stimulate autophagy by simultaneous promotion of cytoplasmic protein deacetylation although with different potencies and, possibly, through distinct molecular pathways [53]. Selected polyphenols can induce G0/G1 (growth arrest effect) and / or G2/S (anti-mitotic effect) phase cell cycle arrest of various human cancer cell lines [56]. The induction of autophagy and apoptosis is a very important mechanism for cancer prevention by dietary polyphenols. It represents an effective anti-cancer strategy since it is based on an effort to block or suppress the multistage process of carcinogenesis which relates to six fundamental hallmarks of cancer: self-sufficient proliferation, insensitivity to anti-proliferative signals, evasion of apoptosis, unlimited replicative potential, maintenance of vascularization, and, finally, tissue invasion and metastasis [57,58]. In addition, chemoprevention based on dietary polyphenols is not expected to be accompanied by side effects since they are selectively toxic for the cancer cells.

Mechanistically, polyphenols have been shown to induce growth arrest and increase apoptosis in cancer cells in various ways. Antiproliferative effects of dietary polyphenols are generally associated with their capacity to regulate response to oxidative stress and/or DNA damage, suppress angiogenesis, and inhibit various pro-proliferative signaling pathways. They affect all aspects of carcinogenesis at its different stages through inhibition of various survival transduction pathways related to NF-κB, PI3K, AKT and MAP kinases, as well as by stimulating expression of tumor suppressor genes (p53, BRCA1 and BRCA2) [57,58]. All polyphenols studied so far, except apigenin, are able to modify redox cellular state as potent radical scavengers [59]. They are also direct inhibitors of enzymes included in production of reactive endogenous radicals. In addition to the effect on their enzymatic activity, dietary polyphenols are also modulators of expression of proteins related to cellular antioxidant defenses and detoxification, often through regulation of transcriptional activity of Nrf2.

These multiple effects of dietary polyhenols have been reviewed many times so far. Here, we are focused on reviewing recent studies of some polyphenols' influence on alteration of gene expression through modulating epigenome by affecting DNA methylation and posttranslational modifications of histone proteins. Natural compounds seem to offer a huge source of epigenetically active compounds of which flavonoids - flavonols quercetin and kaempferol, flavones apigenin and luteolin, isoflavone genistein, catechin EGCG and curcuminoid curcumin certainly take a very important place.

6. Quercetin

Quercetin is strong natural antioxidant flavonol ubiquitously present in dietary plant sources (Table 1) [59]. Cellular sensitivity and specific response to quercetin depends on sensitivity to hydrogen peroxide, H_2O_2. For example, quercetin induces formation of 8-oxo-7,8-dihydro-2'-deoxyguanosine (8-oxodG), an indicator of oxidative DNA damage, in HL-60 cells, while in their H_2O_2-resistant clone, HP 100 cells, this effect does not occur [60]. This, again, shows that mode of action of specific nutraceuticals depends on cellular "molecular background".

In addition to its substantial redox activity, quercetin has multiple intracellular molecular targets, affecting different signaling processes that are altered in cancer cells, with limited or no toxicity against normal cells. Accordingly, quercetin inhibits carcinogenesis primarily through inhibition of pro-proliferative signaling pathways. It has been found to be a pleiotropic kinase inhibitor [61]. At 2 μM concentration, quercetin was shown to decrease the activity of 16 recombinant kinases by more than 80%, including ABL1, Aurora-A,-B,-C, CLK1, FLT3, JAK3, MET, NEK4, NEK9, PAK3, PIM1, RET, FGF-R2, PDGF-Rα and –Rß [62]. Many of these kinases are positive regulators of cell cycle. Thus, through simultaneous targeting of multiple pathways related to these kinases, quercetin may act as antiproliferative agent [61].

Part of quercetin's effects has been attributed to its ability to influence histone acetylation (Figure 1). Quercetin was reported to block the binding of different transactivators including

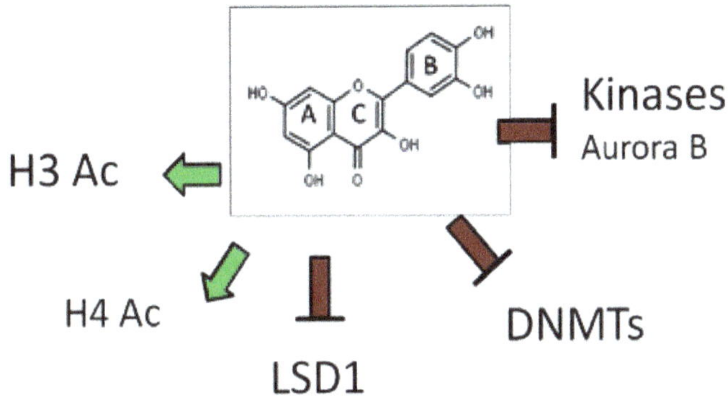

Figure 1. Epigenetic factors modulated by quercetin. Ring and atom annotations of 2-phenyl-1,4-benzopyrone scaffold.

p300, CREB2, c-Jun, C/EBPβ and NF-κB to to the promoter of proinflammatory gene, *COX2* (cyclooxygenase-2) [63]. As a consequence, there is a decrease in the level of the COX-2 protein. Generally, COX-2 decrease is considered to be a very beneficial step to a successful cancer chemoprevention [63,64]. While there is no doubt that quercetin affects numerous signaling pathways, one of these was well-explained on mouse intestinal epithelial cell line MODE-K, through its inhibitory effect on Akt phosphorylation, but without affecting cytoplasmic IKK (inhibitor of nuclear factor kappa-B (IκB) kinase) activity. Thus, in this experimental model, quercetin had no direct effect on NF-κB activation. Instead, it inhibited recruitment of the NF-κB cofactor p300/CBP to the promoters of inflammatory genes IP-10 (10 kDa interferon gamma-induced protein, C-X-C motif chemokine 10) and MIP-2 (WD repeat-containing protein 26), through modulation of histone H3 acetylation and phosphorylation [65]. At 5 μM concentration, quercetin was reported to increase acetylation of histones H3 and H4 induced by trichostatin A in A549 (expressing wild-type p53) and H1299 (a p53 null mutant) lung cancer cell lines, through p53 independent pathway [66].

Quercetin has also been found to effect activity of class III histone deacetylases SIRTs. Due to the fact that biological effects of polyphenols depend on their own chemical stability and metabolism, it is sometimes hard to predict whether *in vitro* test results may precisely predict the situation in the living organism, *in vivo*. For example, it has been observed that quercetin increases deacetylase activity of recombinant SIRT1, but at cellular level it inhibits SIRT1 activity [67]. This has been explained by metabolic transformation of quercetin. When quercetin's metabolite, quercetin-3-O-glucuronide, was taken instead of quercetin, an inhibitory function on recombinant SIRT-1 was shown. However, quercetin activates SIRT1 deacetylase activity in hypoxia-exposed or hypoxic preconditioned HepG2 cells similarly to resveratrol, resulting in hypoxic down-regulation of *c-Myc* and β-catenin [68].

Sirtuins affect the acetylation status of histones as well as other important cellular non-histone proteins like HIF-1α, c-Myc and β-catenin [68]. SIRT1-mediated histone deacetylation (H1K26, H3K9, H3K14, H4K16) is associated with the formation of heterochromatin. On the other hand, SIRT1 interacts with numerous transcription factors and, through modifying their acetylation status, modifies their function. For example, in the presence of stress stimuli, SIRT1 deacetylates p53 and FOXO3 (forkhead box protein O3) leading to inhibition of apoptosis [69]. Another mechanism for inhibition of stress-induced apoptosis is through deacetylation of repair factor Ku70 (X-ray repair cross-complementing protein 6) and consequential sequestration of the proapoptitic factor BAX (Bcl-2-associated X protein) away from mitochondria [70]. While SIRT1 is capable of protecting cells from p53-induced apoptosis, its activity augments apoptosis in response to TNF-α (tumor necrosis factor alpha) by deacetylating RelA/p65 at lysine 310 and thus supressing transcription of NF-κB regulated genes [71].

Quercetin has been found to affect other class III HDAC, SIRT6, *in vitro*. Using frontal affinity chromatographic techniques, it has been found to inhibit deacetylase activity of immobilized recombinant SIRT6 protein against H3K9 [72].

Quercetin effects have been mostly studied on blood cancers. It induces apoptosis and autophagy of human leukemia HL-60 cells through orchestrating various signaling pathways and chromatin remodeling [73]. It has been reported to induce significant histone hyperacetylation at concentrations 75 and 100 μM in human leukemia cells, indicating the possible involvement of histone hyperacetylation in its *in vitro* anticancer activity [73,74].

Quercetin has also been found to influence DNA as well as protein methylation levels. Hypermethylation of the tumor suppressor gene $p16^{INK4a}$ (p16, cyclin-dependent kinase inhibitor 2A) in human colon cancer cell line RKO was successfully reversed after 120 h of treatment with quercetin [75]. This effect was concentration dependent.

Quercetin inhibiting activity against demethylase LSD1 was shown recently [76]. LSD1, commonly upregulated in cancer, has critical role in controlling the transcription of genes involved in cell growth and differentiation [77], and its inhibition may have significant therapeutic value. LSD1 functions primarily in multiprotein complexes, which includes, for example, HDAC1/2 and SIRT1.

Quercetin, as well as other catechol polyphenols, may indirectly inhibit DNMTs and thus DNA methylation, through changing intracellular concentrations of S-adenosyl methionine (SAM) and S-adenosyl-L-homocysteine (SAH) in a manner illustrated in Figure 2 [78].

7. Kaempferol

Kaempferol is a flavonol found in various vegetables (Table 1). In comparison with quercetin, it has considerably lower antioxidant capacity due to missing catechol moiety [59]. It possesses only 4′-OH group at ring B (Figure 1). However, like quercetin, kaempferol has a wide range of pharmacological activities, including antioxidant, anti-inflammatory and anticancer activity [79]. It suppresses growth of a number of human cancer cell lines in a concentration-dependent manner, through inducing an arrest in G0/G1 or G2/M phases of cell cycle [80]. Depending on the type of the cell, kaempherol can induce apoptosis [81,82] and autophagy [80]. For example, it induces apoptosis of human breast cancer cells MCF-7, by initiation of intrinsic caspase

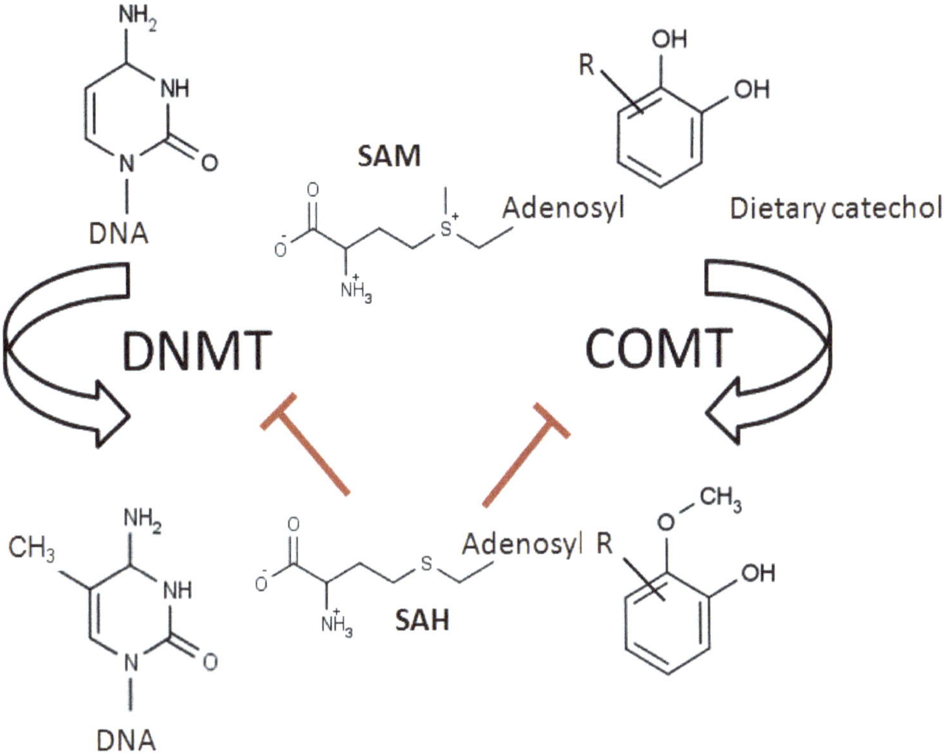

Figure 2. Indirect inhibitory effect of polyphenols with catechol (quercetin, luteolin) or galloyl (EGCG) moiety on DNMTs activity. In the O-methylation process of these polyphenols catalysed by the enzyme COMT, DNMT co-factor SAM is transformed into SAH which inhibits DNMTs and COMT.

cascade and down-regulation of the expression of nuclear kinase PLK1, an early trigger for G2/M transition and mitotic progression [83].

In human liver and colon cancer cell lines (HepG2, Hep3B, HCT-116) kaempferol (5-100 μM) was shown to induce a prominent reduction of cell viability and proliferation rate, partly mediated through induction of hyperacetylation of histone H3 complex [81]. By performing *in silico* molecular docking analysis and *in vitro* profiling on these cancer cell lines, kaempferol has been recognized as a pan-inhibitor of human HDACs of classes I, II and IV [81].

Treatment of the chronic myelogenous leukemia cell line K562 and promyelocitic human leukemia U937 with 50 μM kaempferol resulted in inhibition of PI3K and dephosphorylation of Akt at Ser473 and Thr308 as well as in an increase of the expression of deacetylase SIRT3 and its mitochondrial localization [84]. Finally, apoptotic death of these cells upon kaempferol exposure was a consequence of the induction of mitochondrial phase of the apoptotic program with an aforementioned increase of SIRT3, joined with an increase of BAX, decrease of Bcl-2, release of cytochrome c, and caspase-3 activation. Kampferol was also shown to be an inhibitor of recombinant SIRT6 activity [72].

Similar to quercetin, kaempferol has shown inhibitory effect on histone demethylase LSD1 [76]. This enzyme has been reported to inversely regulate expressions of iodothyronine deiodinases of type 2 (D2) and type 3 (D3), acting as a molecular switch that dynamically finely tunes cellular needs for active thyroid hormone during myogenesis [85]. Kaempferol has been known to interfere with many aspects of the thyroid hormones synthesis [86]. LSD1 relieves the repressive marks (H3K9me2/3) on the *DIO2* promoter and the activation marks (H3K4me2/3) on the *DIO3* promoter. This action is well-orchestrated and depends on LSD1 interaction with transcription factor FoxO3.When FoxO3 binding to DNA is abrogated, LSD1 cannot induce D2.

8. Luteolin

Luteolin is a flavone widely distributed in the plant kingdom (Table 1). In difference to quercetin, it misses conjugated 3-OH group in C-ring (Figure 1) which considerably contributes to high radical scavenging capacity of quercetin [87]. Accordingly, luteolin is less efficient radical scavenger than quercetin [59]. However, the rest of structures of luteolin and quercetin are similar and hence similar biological activities have been observed. Both flavonoids have 3′-, 4′-catechol moiety in B-ring, resorcinol-like A-ring and extended π-electron delocalisation through whole skeleton. Luteolin inhibits growth of various cancer cell lines in a concentration-dependent manner [88]. The most common effect induced with luteolin, as well as other studied polyphenols with resorcinol-like structure of A-ring, is G2/M arrest of the cell cycle [88]. However, underlying mechanisms of action vary among flavonoid family members, primarily due to different number and positions of other hydroxyl groups at a common flavone (2-phenyl-1,4-benzopyrone) backbone, leading e.g. to different antioxidant capacities and intracellular metabolic transformations. The difference in antioxidative capacity of considered flavonoids may be relevant for the observed differences in biological activities as well as molecular mechanisms of action. For example, as quercetin, luteolin induces apoptosis in HL-60 cells [60]. However, luteolin acts in non-oxidative way *via* forming a luteolin-topoisomerase II-DNA ternary complex and thus mediates DNA cleavage.

In addition to modulation of cellular redox level and inhibition of topoisomerases I and II, the underlying antiproliferative activities of luteolin relate to suppression of cell survival pathways including those related to PI3K/Akt, NF-κB and X-linked inhibitor of apoptosis protein (XIAP). It also stimulates apoptotic pathways, including those that depend on the induction of the *p53* [89, 90].

Luteolin also inhibits recombinant LSD1 *in vitro* [76]. Actually, due to the sequence homology between LSD1 and monoamine oxidases (MAO) catalytic domains, some synthetic MAO inhibitors such as *trans*-2-phenylcyclo-propylamine (TCP) and well-known natural MAO inhibitors [91,92] including luteolin, quercetin and curcumin (but not EGCG and apigenin) have been detected as potent inhibitors of LSD1 [76]. Since TCP treatment of embryonic kidney cell line HEK293 increases SIRT1 at the protein level (without recordable effect on SIRT1 mRNA level), the potent natural LSD1 inhibitors may be also expected to elevate the level of SIRT1 protein.

As measured with colorimetric HDAC Activity Assay Kit, luteolin at 50 μM inhibited total HDAC activity joined with increased acetylation of histones H3 and H4. No doubt, this finding suggests that this dietary flavonoid plays an important role in regulation of gene expression and, consequentially, has an inhibitory effect on growth of various tumor cells (LNM35, HT29, HepG2, MCF7/6 and MDA-MB231-1833) [93].

The resorcinol-like A ring was also found to be a part of flavonoid pharmacophore accounting for SIRT6 inhibition. Accordingly, luteolin inhibits deacetylase activity of recombinant SIRT 6 against H3K9 [72]. Furthermore, since luteolin is also the substrate of COMT [94], it may indirectly inhibit DNMTs by elevating endogenous SAH concentration (Figure 2) [78].

Histone H3 phosphorylation (H3S10) is a result of Aurora kinase B activity. This specific epigenetic mark is the hallmark of mitosis. Similar to quercetin [62], luteolin inhibits recombinant Aurora B enzymatic activity (equilibrium dissociation constant K_D 5.85 μM) [95]. Its inhibitory effect on endogenous Aurora B activity in different cancer cell lines was also documented [95]. The consequence of this inhibition, which was shown to be dose-dependent, is down-regulation of H3S10 phosphorylation after 24 h treatment. Inhibition of Aurora B kinase activity was also observed for fisetin and 3-hydroxyflavone [95], indicating that this effect may be related to common 2-phenyl-1,4-benzopyrone backbone (Figure 1).

In addition to inhibiting Aurora B kinase activity and hence reducing H3 phosphorylation (Figure 3), luteolin has been found to decrease the acetylation status of histone H4 at the promoter of the pro-proliferative kinase PLK-1 in PC-3 cells [88], leading to transcriptional silencing of this oncogene [83].

Luteolin is a ligand for the nuclear type II [(3)H]estradiol binding site-a binding domain on histone H4 [88]. Although, it has also been reported to stimulate c-Fos and p21 and inhibit the cell cycle pathway genes, these changes are considered to be only supportive factors in regulation of proliferation. The data obtained so far suggest that type II ligands, including luteolin, inhibit cell growth and proliferation through epigenetic control of key genes involved in cell cycle progression [88].

9. Apigenin

Apigenin is a flavone ubiquitously present in vegetables and fruits (Table 1). It induces cell cycle arrest, p53-dependent apoptosis as well as autophagy of different cancer cells. Like other polyphenols, apigenin is selectively toxic to cancer cells. However, it is much weaker radical scavenger when compared to already described flavonoids [59]. Its mechanism of action depends on cancer cell type, indicating possible existence of structural modifications caused by cellular metabolism. For example, apigenin (50 μM) blocks cellular proliferation through G2/M phase arrest of myeloid HL60 cells, leading to caspase-dependent apoptosis [96]. In contrast, it (100 μM) blocks erythroid TF1 cells in G0/G1 phase leading to autophagy. In both cell lines the JAK/STAT pathway was one of major apigenin targets.

Treatment of monocytic leukemia cells THP-1 with apigenin (50 μM) induced DNA damage mediated by kinases PKCδ and p38 [97]. The cell cycle progression at G1/S was delayed and joined with the increased number of apoptotic cells. The PKCδ-dependent phosphorylation of ataxia-telangiectasia mutated (ATM) kinase and histone γH2AX (a marker of double strand DNA breaks) upon treatment with apigenin, resulted in transcriptional down-regulation of genes involved in cell-cycle control and DNA repair. This indicates that THP-1 cells may be unable to repair DNA damage induced by apigenin, hence triggering apoptosis.

Exposure of LNCaP (hormone-dependent / p53 wild type) and PC-3 (hormone-independent / p53 mutant type) prostate cancer cells to apigenin (and also genistein, see next section) resulted in same pattern of cell cycle arrest and apoptosis, associated with p21 up-regulation and PLK1 suppression [98].

Apigenin (20-40 μM) treatment of prostate cancer cells PC-3 and 22Rv1 resulted in the inhibition of HDACs of class I, particularly HDAC1 and HDAC3, at the mRNA and protein levels [99]. Apigenin-mediated HDAC inhibition resulted in reversal of aberrant epigenetic events that promote carcinogenesis, that is, in global histone H3 and H4 acetylation, as well as localized hyperacetylation of histone H3 on the *p21* promoter. A corresponding increase in p21 and BAX mRNA and protein expressions resulted in cell cycle arrest and induction of apoptosis in both cell lines. This effect was additionally demonstrated *in vivo* by studies of PC-3 xenografts in apigenin-fed athymic nude mice.

Like already described flavonoids, arginin modulates recombinant SIRT6 deacetylase activity although more weakly than quercetin [72].

10. Genistein

Genistein is an isoflavone abundant in soybeans. Genistein represents a prototype of a phytoestrogen able to bind to nuclear hormone receptors ER-α and ER-β. It also down-regulates androgen receptor in androgen-dependent prostate cancer cell lines such as LNCaP [100]. It has been investigated as a chemopreventive agent against various cancers, particularly hormone-responsive breast and prostate malignancies. According to numerous *in vitro* experimental results accompanied with *in vivo* models, it displays pro-apoptotic, antimetastatic and antiangiogenic properties.

Genistein is only moderately strong radical scavenger [59]. However, this isoflavone exerts antioxidant effects on cellular level at low μM concentrations, which correspond to physiologically relevant concentrations in plasma. The plasma level of genistein in women consuming soy products was observed to be 0.74-6.0 μM [101]. Already at concentration of 0.5 μM, genistein increases antioxidant status of cells *via* i) interaction with estrogen receptors, ii) activation of ERK1/2 and iii) nuclear translocation of p50 subunit of NF-κB, resulting in an overexpression of MnSOD (manganese-dependent superoxide dismutase) and consequential lowering of intracellular peroxide levels [102].

Genistein can arrest cell growth and induce apoptosis in various hematological cancer cell lines [103] and cell lines of solid tumor origin (e.g. HCT-116 and SW-480 [104]). Its influence on modulation of cell cycle most commonly relates to induction of G2/M cell cycle arrest, as shown in breast, colon, malignant glioma and prostate cancer cell lines [104,105,106]. At a molecular level, this effect is commonly dependent on tumor suppressors p53, p21 and/ or p16 [106].

While genistein's anticancer effects appears similar in different cancer cell lines, the underlying molecular mechanism of its action depends on a cell type. For example, genistein was shown to have a strong inhibitory effect on cellular growth followed by apoptosis, on two different prostate cancer cell lines, LNCaP-androgen-sensitive and DuPro – androgen resistant. However, it induced G0/G1 and G2/M cell cycle arrest in LNCaP and DuPro cells, respectively [107]. In addition, cellular effects of genistein on cancer cell cycle are very dependent upon applied dose [103].

Genistein has been one of the first specific protein tyrosine kinase inhibitors which was described almost 30 years ago [108,109]. As already stated, genistein antagonizes estrogen-and androgen-mediated signaling pathways [106]. It has also been found to intervene in other cellular signal transduction pathways inhibiting carcinogenesis through inhibition of NF-κB and Akt signaling [57,109]. Significant part of genistein's action, including growth inhibition and cytotoxicity, relates to its inhibitory effect on topoisomerase II. This was very clearly shown through resistance to genistein in a model of murine transgenic cells lacking topoisomerase II beta [110,111].

Besides, genistein is also a potent modifier of epigenetic events including DNA methylation and/or histone acetylation – directly, or through steroid receptor dependent process [101]. In both aforementioned prostate cell lines, LNCaP and DuPro, genistein treatment (10-25 μM) reshaped the chromatin structure [107]. The treatment increased acetylation level of histones H3 and H4 at the transcription start sites of the two tumor suppressor genes, *p21* and *p16*. It also increased expression of transcriptional activators HATs, but did not change the global methylation status of these cells.

Genistein's effect on breast cancer cells is selective as shown recently [112]. In a dose-dependent manner genistein inhibits both precancerous (normal human mammary epithelial cells stably transfected with *SV40* and human telomerase reverse transcriptase, *hTERT)* and cancerous breast cells growth. Of importance, the apoptotic process was more prominent in precancerous than in cancerous breast cells, indicating the strong preventive potential. At the same time, there were only minor effects when applied to (commercially available) normal mammary epithelial cells [112]. *In vivo,* orthotopic breast cancer mouse model was used. The animals were orally-fed with genistein enriched diet (modified AIN-93G diet supplemented with 250 mg/kg genistein, corresponding to high-soy diet in humans). In these animals, genistein has inhibited breast cancer growth; the tumors had considerably lower wet weight and significantly less PCNA (proliferating cell nuclear antigen) positive cells, when compared with tumors that were developed in the animals fed with diet that was not supplemented with genistein. At the mRNA level, there was a strong increase in expression of tumor suppressor genes *p16* and *p21,* and dramatic decrease of oncogenes *BMI1* (polycomb complex protein BMI-1) and *c-MYC*. These changes in mRNA expression clearly point out genistein's effect on epigenome. Indeed, this was confirmed in experiments that showed that genistein induces formation of euchromatine in the region that covers promoters of *p21* and *p16*, through changing the ratio of activating and repressive histone modifications. Specifically, genistein treatment increased histone H3 acetylation and formation of H3K4me3 and, at the same time, decreased formation of suppressive chromatin marks, H3K9me3 and H3K27me3 [112]. These changes were mild in breast cancer cells, but very prominent in precancerous breast cell line, indicating, one more time, the importance of genistein in the process of cancer prevention. Based on several scientific reports, especially in the field of breast cancer, it seems that genistein significantly influences KTMs, while its effect on HDACs does not seem to be so prominent [112].

In breast cancer cell lines MCF-7 (ER-α positive) and MDA-MB 231 (ER-α negative) genistein (18.5 μM) induces decrease in trimethylated marks at H3K27, H3K9 and H3K4, at six selected genes: EZH2 (histone-lysine N-methyltransferase that adds methyl group to H3K27), BRCA1, ER-α, ER-β, SRC3 (steroid receptor coactivator protein 3, that displays HAT activity) and p300 [113]. Genistein treatment also affected histone acetylation marks in close proximity of these six selected genes recorded as an increase in H4K8ac and H3K4ac modifications.

In MDA-MB-231 cells, genistein (25 μM) restored ER-α expression by remodeling the chromatin structure in the *ER-α* promoter [112, 114,115]. This is very beneficial effect, as it increases tamoxifen-dependent anti-estrogen therapeutic sensitivity *in vitro* and *in vivo*. In addition, this effect was synergistically enhanced when combined with HDACi trichostatin A.

There are also experimental data on genistein's effect on colon cancer cells. When applied to HT29 cell line, genistein has been reported to have inhibitory effects on HDAC activity with IC_{50} value of 97 ± 18 μM [116]. Furthermore, incubation of HT29 cells with high concentration of genistein (200 μM) resulted in a significant decrease of HDAC1 protein. Similar results were obtained on human esophageal squamous cell carcinoma cells KYSE 510, in which 5 μM and 100 μM genistein inhibited 13.2% and 33% of HDAC activity, respectively [101].

Genistein was also observed to decrease expression of HDACs in other types of cells, as well. In aforementioned human breast cancer cell lines, MCF-7 and MDA-MB-231, genistein treatment (15 and 10 μM,) induced reduction (2 and ~ 4 fold, respectively) in expression of HDAC1 protein [117]. Genistein (25 μM) has been reported to significantly downregulate expression of class II HDAC6 protein in prostate cancer cells, LNCaP [100]. Since HDAC6 is a Hsp90 deacetylase, such a change leads to an increase in the acetylated form of Hsp90 and hence inhibition of its chaperone activity. The consequence of the lack of the chaperone function is ubiquitin-mediated degradation of androgen receptor protein. However, in difference to its structural isomer apigenin (Table 1), genistein does not modulate activity of recombinant SIRT6 [72].

In addition to its impact on histone acetylation and methylation, genistein was also shown to influence DNMTs *in vitro*, at the transcriptional level and also through inhibition of DNMT1 activity [117,118]. It reduces methylation specifically at promoters of tumor suppressor genes thus affecting cancer cell survival [101]. In KYSE 510 cells treated with 2–20 μM genistein, the inhibition of DNMT1 activity was associated with demethylation of the CpG islands specifically in the promoters of *p16*, *RAR-β* (retinoic acid receptor beta) and *MGMT* (O6-methylguanine methyltransferase) resulting in their consequential transcriptional reactivation [101,118]. Because genistein is a weak inhibitor of DNMTs, it does not induce global genomic hypomethylation but selective hypomethylation at hypermethyated region of genomic DNA, corresponding to aforementioned tumor suppressor genes, *p21* and *p16* [117].

Genistein can restore the expression of genes silenced by DNA hypermethylation in breast cancers not only by inhibiting enzymatic activity of DNMT1, but also through decrease of DNMT1 protein level [117]. Increased expression of DNMT1, DNMT3a, and DNMT3b is common in various cancer types, including breast cancer. Treatment of MCF-7 and MDA-MB-231 cell lines with genistein (as well as with other polyphenolic DNMT1 inhibitors, EGCG or curcumin), resulted in a significant decrease not only of HDAC1, but also of DNMT1 and MeCP2 protein levels, joined with a significant decrease in the transcript levels of all three DNMTs-DNMT1, DNMT3a, and DNMT3b [117]. The genistein effects on cell viability of these breast cancer cells were dose-dependent with IC_{50} values of 15 and 10 μM for MCF-7 and MDA-MB-231cells, respectively.

The inhibitory effects of genistein on DNMTs and HDACs may have an intrinsic synergistic effect [101]. Genistein has been observed to have additive effects on the reactivation of methylation-silenced genes in combination with other DNMT inhibitor decitabine or a HDAC inhibitor trichostatin A [101].

11. EGCG

The (-)-epigallocatechin-3-O-gallate (EGCG) is the most abundant catechin in green tea, accounting for 50-70% of green tea catechins [119]. Other green tea catechins are (−)-epigallocatechin (EGC), (−)-epicatechin-3-gallate (ECG) and (−)-epicatechin (EC).

EGCG is a strong free radical scavenger [59]. Its antioxidant activity is additionally enhanced by induction of expression of phase II detoxifying and antioxidant enzymes such as glutathione S-transferases (GST), glutathione peroxidase (GPx), glutamate cysteine ligase (GCL), heme oxygenase-1 (HO-1) and many other enzymes involved in the elimination or inactivation of reactive oxygen species (ROS) and electrophiles implicated in multi-stage carcinogenesis. EGCG acts through Nrf2/ARE dependant way *via* activated Akt and ERK1/2 signaling and / or through modifying cysteine thiols of Keap1 (Kelch-like ECH-associated protein 1), a repressor of Nrf2 [120]. EGCG can also inhibit carcinogenesis by modulating some other transduction pathways including JAK/STAT, Wnt and Notch [57,121]. EGCG-induced inhibition of EGFR (epidermal growth factor receptor) pathway is well-documented. It also negatively influences topoisomerase II [122]. In majority cancer cell lines tested so far, this catechin induces G0/G1 phase cell cycle arrest. Finally, EGCG induces apoptosis through both, p53-dependent and p53-independent pathways. These activities, joined with an inhibitory effect on NF-κB and MMPs, leads also to inhibition of angiogenesis, invansion and metastasis formation [119,121]. In addition to all these processes, chemopreventive and anticancer effects of EGCG are also based on modifications of epigenetic processes, selectively in the cancer cells. *In vitro* studies show that EGCG enters cellular nuclei and binds to both DNA and RNA [122].

As already stated, DNA methylation patterns and histone modifications significantly differ between normal and tumor cells. Accordingly, selective targeting of epigenetic marks that makes the difference between these two kinds of cells is a challenge in cancer therapy. In cancer prevention, selective "preservance" of protective epigenetic marks represents an imperative that deserves specific attention. In the field of therapy, reexpression of DNA methylation-silenced tumor suppressor genes by inhibiting the DNMTs (DNMT1, DNMT3A, and DNMT3B) has emerged as an effective strategy [123].

EGCG is a natural non-nucleoside inhibitor of DNMT1, undergoing clinical testing [124]. DNMT1 is overexpressed in the S-phase of cell cycle, particularly in highly proliferating cells, which are the basic feature of cancer. This enzyme has a high preference for hemimethylated DNA and is essential for maintaining the methylation pattern during each round of DNA replication. Strong inhibitory effect of EGCG with IC_{50} at 0.47 μM on human DNMT1-mediated DNA methylation was independent of the COMT-mediated methylation of EGCG (Figure 2) [78]. EGCG inhibits activity of the DNMT1 molecule directly by binding to its catalytic site through formation of H-bonds [78,125,126]. This binding is stabilized by Mg^{2+}ions [78]. The galloyl moiety was shown to most considerably contribute to high-affinity of EGCG for human DNMT1. Thus, DNMT1 is also directly inhibited by other polyphenols with galloyl or also pyrogallic acid (*e.g.* myricetin) moiety [78].

In breast cancer cell lines MCF-7 and MDB-MB-231 EGCG, like genistein and also curcumin, downregulates transcription of not only DNMT1, but also *de novo* DNMTs, DNMT3a, and DNMT3b. The effect extends to the proteins, lowering the level of DNMT1, HDAC1, and MeCP2, known to interact with methylated DNA CpG regions [117]. Its effects on MCF-7 and MDB-MB-231 cell viability were dose-dependent with IC_{50} of 10 and 15 μM, respectively.

Similarly to genistein, EGCG may, in physiologically attainable concentrations, reverse aberrant gene hypermethylation [101,118,126]. *In vitro* demethylation of specific promoters has been shown in various cancer cell types for many genes including *p16, MGMT, hMLH1* (human mutL homologue 1), *GSTP1* (Glutathione S-transferase Pi) and/or *RARβ* [118,126]. Epigenetic silencing of a phase II enzyme GSTP1 has been recognized as a molecular hallmark of human prostate cancer. Exposure of human prostate wild-type p53 cancer cell lines, LNCaP and MDA PCa 2b, to green tea polyphenols and EGCG alone (5-20 μM) for several days caused a concentration-and time-dependent reactivation of this enzyme, through extensive demethylation in the proximal GSTP1 promoter and regions distal to the transcription factor binding sites. This specific action of green tea polyphenols was correlated with the inhibition of both, DNMT1 expression and activity [127]. Of importance, exposure of LNCaP cells to green tea polyphenols did not result in global hypomethylation, but, instead, promoted maintenance of genomic integrity. Additionally, the exposure of LNCaP cells to EGCG reduced transcriptional activity of genes coding for HDACs 1-3 which also resulted with their decrease at the protein levels. This molecular change was joined with the increased level of acetylated histones H3 (H3K9 and H3K18) and H4.

In the context of uniqueness of cellular epigenome, in human epidermoid carcinoma cells A431 the EGCG (5-20 μM) treatment did decrease global DNA methylation level. Expectedly, it was joined with decrease of DNMT1 transcript, protein and enzymatic activity in a dose-dependent manner, although far less than upon the treatment with clinically approved demethylating drug decitabine (5 μM) [128]. In this model, EGCG treatment resulted in re-expression of the mRNA and proteins of silenced tumor suppressor genes *p16* and *p21*. There was also an increase in histones H3 (H3K9 and H3K14) and H4 (H4K5, H4K12, H4K16) acetylation and decrease in level of methylated H3K9. These phenomena were ascribed to decreased level of HDAC activity in A431 cells upon EGCG treatment [128].

In pancreatic metastatic adenocarcinoma cells AsPC-1, EGCG (10 μM) was also shown to induce Raf kinase inhibitor protein (RKIP) *via*, in part, the inhibition of HDAC activity [129]. At the same time, this treatment repressed activation of ERK and upregulated E-cadherin expression. Histone H3 expression was also increased, while Snail (zinc finger protein SNAI1) expression, NF-κB nuclear translocation and MMP-2 and-9 activities were inhibited. Of great importance, the treatment decreased metastatic potential of these cells.

Inhibition of HDAC activity and HDAC1 protein expression was recorded in a model of human colon carcinoma, HT29 [116]. EGCG at concentration 100 μM, inhibited HDAC activity by about 50%. Concomitantly, a significant decrease of the HDAC1 protein level was observed depending on EGCG concentration (significant reduction at concentrations ≥ 50 μM).

EGCG mediated, dose-and time-dependent inhibition of class I HDACs (HDAC1, 2, 3 and 8) joined with the increased acetylation of histone H3 and p53, were shown in experiments that were performed on prostate cancer cell lines LNCaP and PC-3 [130]. Acetylation of p53 resulted in its binding to the promoters of *p21* and *BAX* genes leading to increased accumulation of cells in the G0/G1 cell cycle phase and induction of apoptosis. Acetylation of p53 at Lys373 and Lys382 results in p53 accumulation due to block of its MDM-2 mediated ubiquitination [130]. Finally, EGCG was suggested to contribute also to proteasomal degradation of class I HDACs [130].

Similar to quercetin, EGCG and polyphenols with the galloyl moiety in general, stimulate the activity of recombinant SIRT1 enzyme under stabilizing antioxidant conditions (achieved by adding vitamin C or catalase) [67]. Without stabilization, recombinant SIRT1 became a target for strong inhibition by these polyphenols [49], probably due to their auto-oxidation and H_2O_2 formation [67]. These data point to the importance of testing *in vitro* stability of polyphenol aglycons and tentative effects of actual products of their (bio)chemical transformations. For example, quercetin did not show any effect on the deacetylation activity of SIRT1 in HT29 cells [67].

In addition to its influence on HDACs, EGCG has been identified as a specific inhibitor of majority of HATs [131]. In HeLa cell nuclear extract, EGCG at 100 μM concentration inhibited 90% of HAT activity while no changes in total HDAC, SIRT1 and histone methyltransferase activities were observed. The observed inhibitory action on NF-κB activation by EGCG has been ascribed to its inhibition of RelA (p65) acetylation rather than the direct inhibition of p65 phosphorylation. The mechanism was explained using HEK293 cells in which EGCG (100 μM) abrogated p300-induced p65 acetylation. Hypoacetylation of p65 increases the level of cytosolic IκBα which prevents p65 translocation into the nucleus, thus interrupting the TNFα-induced cascade of events.

EGCG (50 μM) inhibitory effect on HATs may be beneficial in hormone dependent prostate cancer due to suppression of agonist-dependent androgen receptor (AR) activation by downregulation of its acetylation. Consequentially, AR remains "locked" in the cytoplasm and cannot activate AR-related gene transcription [132]. Like p65, androgen receptor is also acetylated by p300/CBP and PCAF (HAT KAT2B)/TIP60 (HAT KAT5), supporting the hypothesis that HAT coactivators compete with HDAC corepressors for binding to promoter regions and/or protein substrates and determine the level of transcription.

12. Curcumin

Curcumin (1,7-bis(4-hydroxy-3-methoxy-phenyl)-1,6-heptadiene-3,5-dione) is a natural yellow-coloured curcumoid whose medicinal properties have long been recognized in traditional Indian Ayurvedic medicine [133]. This chemical is an important part of curry spice mix. It was brought to Western world in the 14th century.

Like other well-known polyphenols, curcumin has diverse pharmacological properties including chemopreventive activity [134]. Its proven antioxidative, anti-inflammatory, antiproliferative and antiangiogenic effects brought it in the focus for use in cancer prevention. Recently its impact on cell signal transduction pathways by regulation expression and/or activity of various proteins including NF-κB, Akt, MAPK, p53, Nrf2, Notch-1, JAK/STAT, β-catenin, and AMPK (5'-AMP-activated protein kinase) has been reviewed [135]. Curcumin induces growth arrest at G1 or G2/M phase of cell cycle leading to apoptosis of cancer cells of various types. Indeed, if one molecule has an influence on all these processes, then it has to be that it triggers basic biochemical processes in the cell.

Pharmacokinetic analyses have shown that its concentration in human plasma is far below concentrations measured in experimental cell culture systems [136]. The most likely explanation for its observed biological activity may be related to the possibility that curcumin exerts its biological activity through remodeling the epigenome network. If this kind of action indeed takes the place, one would expect that lower concentrations are required for various biological actions.

Indeed, curcumin is a strong modulator of epigenome [137]. It reduces histone acetylation mainly *via* inhibition of HAT activity [138,139]. Its first epigenome-modifying activity was shown in 2004 through its specific inhibition of acetyltransferase activity of p300/CBP in cervical cancer cells, HeLa [138]. The consequence of this event was acetylation inhibition of histones H3 and H4 with $IC_{50} \sim 25\ \mu M$. This effect was specific since the HAT activity of PCAF, histone deacetylase HDAC1 and histone methyltransferases remains unchanged. Curcumin binding to the active site of p300 also abolished p300-mediated acetylation of p53. This may be of great importance because p300/CBP directly interacts with and acetylates p53, enhances its transcriptional activation ability and, consequently, DNA repair. However, due to the fact that p53 can be target of other HATs that are not inhibited by curcumin, its acetylation status upon curcumin treatment remained in the physiological range.

Curcumin's HAT p300/CBP inhibitory activity is based on its Michael reaction acceptor functionality where its α, β unsaturated carbonyl groups in the linker (Table 1) act as reaction sites [140]. Its binding to p300/CBP induces conformational changes which result in decreased binding afinities of histones and acetyl CoA for p300 [138]. Curcumin has also been reported to promote proteasome-dependent degradation of p300 and CBP without affecting the HATs PCAF or GCN5 [140].

HAT inhibition may be a base for a variety of pharmacological effects of curcumin. HATs, have been implicated in cancer cell growth and survival, and as such, HATs represent therapeutically relevant molecular targets for anticancer drug development. HAT inhibitors also seem promising for the treatment of Alzheimer's disease and diabetes [141]. As a co-activator, p300/CBP also enhances NF-κB transcriptional activity by acetylating NF-κB/p65 as well as surrounding histones. Direct inhibition and downregulation of p300/CBP therefore contribute to the inhibition of NF-κB by curcumin. Curcumin's influence on NF-κB activity is extremely important for its chemopreventive potency [142]. Additionally, its anti-infectious activities against HIV-1 [138] and *Plasmodium falciparum* [143] can also arise from inhibition of HAT activity.

In addition, on HeLa nuclear extracts curcumin showed the potent activity as an inhibitor of HDAC [144]. At a very high concentration of 500 μM, curcumin was found to reduce ~ 50% HDAC activity and its IC_{50} was 115 μM. In the cited study, the design of the experiment did not allow for any conclusion on the mechanism of inhibition: inhibitor candidates were mixed with HeLa nuclear extract before addition of HDAC fluorometric substrate which was sensitized through deacetylation and fluorescence. Hence, only the consequence of the presence of potential inhibitor was measured. In leukemia cell lines curcumin was shown to increase expression of suppressors of cytokine signaling, SOCS1 and SOCS3, through global inhibition of HDAC activity and decreased expression of HDAC8 [145]. In curcumin (25 μM, 24 h) treated Raji cells (Epstein-Barr virus transformed lymphocyte), a decrease of HDAC8 was joined with similar levels of decrease of HDACs 1 and 3, leading to significant increase of histone H4 acetylation [146]. Curcumin was also shown to reduce HDAC activity in medulloblastoma cells and directly inhibits transcription of HDAC4 [147]. These results represent an extension of previous scientific work showing that curcumin's free binding energy and inhibition constant for HDAC8 are comparable to trichostatin A and vorinostat [144].

Like luteolin, quercetin and resveratrol, curcumin (50 μM) inhibits histone demethylase activity of recombinant LSD1 [76].

Curcumin can induce epigenetic modifications by modulating not only histone acetylation but also DNA methylation. It is considered to be a hypomethylating agent decreasing DNMT activity [137, 148]. Similarly to genistein and EGCG, curcumin (10 μM) has been demonstrated to have the potential to reverse the epigenetic changes in breast cancer cells through inducing significant decrease in protein levels of DNMT1, HDAC1 and MeCP2 as well as in the transcript levels of all three DNMTs, DNMT1, DNMT3a and DNMT3b [117]. Curcumin has been found to covalently block the catalytic thiol group within catalytic site of DNMT1 with an IC_{50} of only 3 μM after 72 h treatment, leading to reduction of DNA methylation by 15-20%, as shown in the model of AML cell line MV4-11 [148]. Curcumin treatment decreased the mRNA and protein levels of DNMT1 and downregulated its DNA methylation activity in breast cancer cells MCF-7. The downregulation of DNMT1 mRNA may well be a consequence of lack of an NF-κB/Sp1 binding to the promoter region of DNMT1 [149]. Both proteins are shown to bind to DNMT1 promoter and positively regulate DNMT1 expression. Thus, in curcumin treated cells, a decrease of NF-κB and Sp1-well known curcumin targets, may directly influence the activity of DNMT1 gene.

The most recent findings indeed confirm that curcumin decreases DNMT1 expression not only in various leukemia cell lines, but also in patient's primary AML cells treated *ex vivo* [150]. This effect was concomitant with reactivation of tumor suppressor gene *p15*^{INK4B} (p15) through hypomethylation of its promoter, G1 cell cycle arrest, and *in vitro* induction of apoptosis. This effect is, again, specific for transformed cells as it is absent in patient's healthy PBMCs treated in this way.

In contrast to non-specific global hypomethylation induced by decitabine, curcumin treatment of three colorectal cancer cell lines HCT116, HT29 and RKO, resulted in methylation changes at selected partially-methylated loci, instead of fully-methylated CpG site [151]. Curcumin has also been found to selectively induce demethylation of promoters of *NRF2* and *RARβ2* genes [152]. It also down-regulated expression of *EZH2* and thus reduced H3K27me3 methylation, as shown in in MDA-MB-435 cells [153].

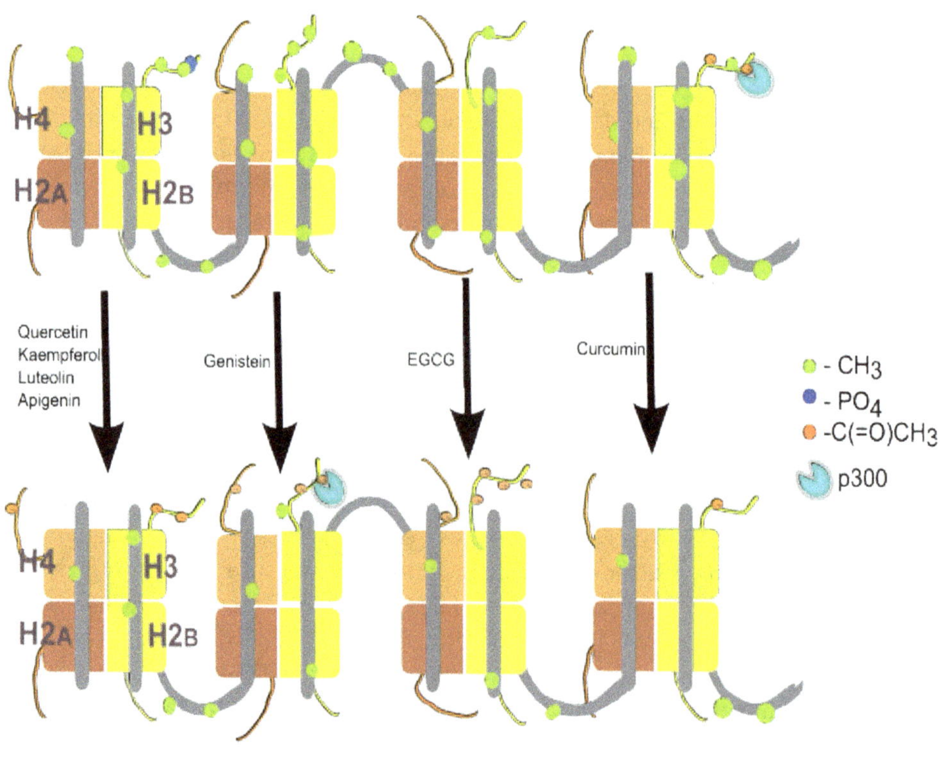

Figure 3. Epigenetic modifications induced by selected polyphenols. Molecular mechanisms of action depends upon their structures – flavonols and flavones directly inhibit histone demethylase LSD1 and indirectly DNMTs (Figure 2); genistein promotes HAT activity and DNA demethylation; EGCG is a direct DNMT inhibitor; curcumin affects many epigenome modifying enzymes.

13. Conclusion

Experimental data reported so far clearly point to dietary polyphenols as potent epigenetic modulators, able to "restore" disturbed epigenomic network which is present in premalignant and malignant cells. Polyphenols usually target more than one epigenome-modulating enzyme. In the case of curcumin the effect can be extended to enzymes with antagonistic functions. This is very interesting as it opens the question related to "epigenetic balance" and "epigenetically balanced cell". With our current knowledge, we cannot predict all possible consequences of these polyvalent modes of action.

The epigenetic effects of polyphenols are largely dependent upon compound concentration, its application time window, and, very important – on a specifically established epigenome networking which is specific for each cancer cell. As xenobiotics, natural polyphenols are substrates of various metabolic enzymes. Upon cellular uptake they can be chemically transformed by various metabolic processes that depend on both, compound concentration and the type of the cell. When studying biological effects of polyphenols, their chemical characterization has to be performed in order to detect the most probably active form.

In summary, herein considered flavonoids and curcumin represent attractive starting scaffolds for design of chemopreventive or therapeutic drugs against various cancer types. In addition, due to specific effects on epigenome, they may be useful as chemical probes that may help to understand effects of natural and synthetic molecules on epigenome and chromatin remodeling.

Acknowledgements

This work was supported by Ministry of Science, Education and Sport, Republic of Croatia.

Author details

Višnja Stepanić, Renata Novak Kujundžić and Koraljka Gall Trošelj

Laboratory for Epigenomics, Ruđer Bošković Institute, Zagreb, Croatia

References

[1] Suzuki J, Chen YY, Scott GK, Devries S, Chin K, Benz CC, Waldman FM, Hwang ES. Protein acetylation and histone deacetylase expression associated with malignant breast cancer progression. Clin Cancer Res. 2009;15(9) 3163-3171.

[2] Gall Trošelj K, Novak Kujundžić R, Grbeša I. The Importance of Aberrant DNA Methylation in Cancer. In: Tatarinova T (Ed.) DNA Methylation- From Genomics to Technology. InTech; 2012. Available from: phttp://www.intechopen.com/books/dna-methylation-from-genomics-to-technology/the-importance-of-aberrant-dna-methylation-in-cancer

[3] Bamia C, Lagiou P, Buckland G, Grioni S, Agnoli C, Taylor AJ, Dahm CC, Overvad K, Olsen A, Tjønneland A, Cottet V, Boutron-Ruault MC, Morois S, Grote V, Teucher B, Boeing H, Buijsse B, Trichopoulos D, Adarakis G, Tumino R, Naccarati A, Panico S, Palli D, Bueno-de-Mesquita HB, van Duijnhoven FJ, Peeters PH, Engeset D, Skeie G, Lund E, Sánchez MJ, Barricarte A, Huerta JM, Quirós JR, Dorronsoro M, Ljuslinder I, Palmqvist R, Drake I, Key TJ, Khaw KT, Wareham N, Romieu I, Fedirko V, Jenab M, Romaguera D, Norat T, Trichopoulou A. Mediterranean diet and colorectal cancer risk: results from a European cohort. Eur J Epidemiol. 2013;28(4) 317-328.

[4] Woodcock CL, Ghosh RP. Chromatin higher-order structure and dynamics. Cold Spring Harb Perspect Biol. 2010;2(5) a000596.

[5] Cohen I, Poreba E, Kamieniarz K, Schneider R. Histone modifiers in cancer: Friends or foes? Genes Cancer 2011;2(6) 631-647.

[6] Bannister AJ, Kouzarides T. Regulation of chromatin by histone modifications. Cell Res. 2011;21(3) 381-395.

[7] Lachner M, O'Carroll D, Rea S, Mechtler K, Jenuwein T. Methylation of histone H3 lysine 9 creates a binding site for HP1 proteins. Nature 2001;410(6824) 116-120.

[8] Baek SH. When signaling kinases meet histones and histone modifiers in the nucleus. Cell 2011;42(3) 274-284.

[9] Phillips DMP. The presence of acetyl groups in histones. Biochem J. 1963;87(2) 258-263.

[10] Allfrey V, Faulkner R, Mirsky A. Acetylation and methylation of histones and their possible role in the regulation of RNA synthesis. Proc Natl Acad Sci USA. 1964;51(5) 786–794.

[11] Zentner GE, Henikoff S. Regulation of nucleosome dynamics by histone modifications. Nat Struct Mol Biol. 2013;20(3) 259-266.

[12] Barth TK, Imhof A. Fast signals and slow marks: the dynamics of histone modifications. Trends Biochem Sci. 2010;35(11) 618-626.

[13] Islam AB, Richter WF, Lopez-Bigas N, Benevolenskaya EV. Selective targeting of histone methylation. Cell Cycle 2011;25(4) 413–424.

[14] Zhang JA, Mortazavi A, Williams BA, Wold BJ, Rothenberg EV. Dynamic transformations of genome-wide epigenetic marking and transcriptional control establish T cell identity. Cell 2012;149(2) 467-482.

[15] Dillon SC, Zhang X, Trievel RC, Cheng X. The SET-domain protein superfamily: protein lysine methyltransferases. Genome Biol. 2005;6(8) 227.

[16] Shi Y, Lan F, Matson C, Mulligan P, Whetstine JR, Cole PA, Casero RA, Shi Y. Histone demethylation mediated by the nuclear amine oxidase homolog LSD1. Cell 2004;119(7) 941–953.

[17] Arita A, Shamy MY, Chervona Y, Clancy HA, Sun H, Hall MN, Qu Q, Gamble MV, Costa M. The effect of exposure to carcinogenic metals on histone tail modifications and gene expression in human subjects. J Trace Elem Med Biol. 2012;26(2-3) 174-178.

[18] Sasai N, Defossez PA. Many paths to one goal? The proteins that recognize methylated DNA in eukaryotes. Int J Dev Biol. 2009;53(2-3) 323-334.

[19] Taverna SD, Li H, Ruthenburg AJ, Allis CD, Patel DJ. How chromatin-binding modules interpret histone modifications: lessons from professional pocket pickers. Nat Struct Mol Biol. 2007;14(11) 1025-1040.

[20] Ruthenburg AJ, Li H, Patel DJ, Allis CD. Multivalent engagement of chromatin modifications by linked binding modules. Nat Rev Mol Cell Biol. 2007;8(12) 983-994.

[21] Rajendran P, Ho E, Williams DE, Dashwood RH. Dietary phytochemicals, HDAC inhibition, and DNA damage/repair defects in cancer cells. Clin Epigenetics 2011;3(1) 4.

[22] Ito A, Kawaguchi Y, Lai CH, Kovacs JJ, Higashimoto Y, Appella E, Yao TP. MDM2-HDAC1-mediated deacetylation of p53 is required for its degradation. EMBO J. 2002;21(22) 6236-6245.

[23] Bojang P Jr, Ramos K. The promise and failures of epigenetic therapies for cancer treatment. Cancer Treat Rev. 2014;40(1) 153-169.

[24] Rajgolikar G, Chan KK, Wang HC. Effects of a novel antitumor depsipeptide, FR901228, on human breast cancer cells. Breast Cancer Res Treat. 1998;51(1) 29-38.

[25] Sandor V, Senderowicz A, Mertins S, Sackett D, Sausville E, Blagosklonny MV, Bates SE. P21-dependent G_1 arrest with downregulation of cyclin D1 and upregulation of cyclin E by the histone deacetylase inhibitor FR901228. Br J Cancer 2000;83(6) 817-825.

[26] Lin KT, Wang JW, Chen CT, Ho CM, Su WH, Jou YS. HDAC inhibitors augmented cell migration and metastasis through induction of PKCs leading to identification of low toxicity modalities for combination cancer therapy. Clin Cancer Res. 2012;18(17) 4691-4701.

[27] Orlikova B, Diederich M. Power from the garden: plant compounds as inhibitors of the hallmarks of cancer. Curr Med Chem. 2012;19(14) 2061-2087.

[28] Reuter S, Gupta SC, Park B, Goel A, Aggarwal BB. Epigenetic changes induced by curcumin and other natural compounds. Genes Nutr. 2011;6(2) 93-108.

[29] Suzuki T, Miyata N. Lysine demethylases inhibitors. J Med Chem. 2011;54(24) 8236-8250.

[30] Szarc vel Szic K, Palagani A, Hassannia B, Sabbe L, Heyninck K, Haegeman G, Berghe WV. Phytochemicals and Cancer Chemoprevention: Epigenetic Friends or Foe? In: Iraj Rasooli (Ed.), Phytochemicals - Bioactivities and Impact on Health. InTech; 2011 Available from: http://www.intechopen.com/books/phytochemicals-bioactivities-and-impact-on-health/phytochemicals-and-cancer-chemoprevention-epigenetic-friends-or-foe-

[31] Spencer JP, Abd-el-Mohsen MM, Rice-Evans C. Cellular uptake and metabolism of flavonoids and their metabolites: implications for their bioactivity. Arch Biochem Biophys. 2004;423(1) 148-161.

[32] Psahoulia FH, Drosopoulos KG, Doubravska L, Andera L, Pintzas A. Quercetin enhances TRAIL-mediated apoptosis in colon cancer cells by inducing the accumulation of death receptors in lipid rafts. Mol Cancer Ther. 2007;6(9) 2591-2599.

[33] Hironori T. Structure-dependent membrane interaction of flavonoids associated with their bioactivity. Food Chem. 2010;120(4) 1089–1096.

[34] Granado-Serrano AB, Martín MA, Bravo L, Goya L, Ramos S. Quercetin modulates Nrf2 and glutathione-related defenses in HepG2 cells: Involvement of p38. Chem Biol Interact. 2012;195(2) 154-164.

[35] Mukai R, Terao J, Shirai Y, Saito N, Ashida H. Determination of Subcellular Localization of Flavonol in Cultured Cells by Laser Scanning. In: Chau-Chang Wang (Ed.) Laser Scanning, Theory and Applications, InTech; 2011. Available from: http://www.intechopen.com/books/laser-scanning-theory-and-applications/determination-of-subcellularlocalization-of-flavonol-in-cultured-cells-by-laser-scanning

[36] Sharma H, Gupta S. Sub-cellular distribution and antioxidant potential of plant flavonoid apigenin. In: Proceedings of the 102nd Annual Meeting of the American Association for Cancer Research; 2-6 Apr 2011, Orlando, FL. Philadelphia (PA): AACR; Cancer Res. 2011;71(8 Suppl):Abstract nr 4632.

[37] Mukai R, Shirai Y, Saito N, Yoshida K, Ashida H. Subcellular localization of flavonol aglycone in hepatocytes visualized by confocal laser scanning fluorescence microscope. Cytotechnology 2009;59(3) 177-182.

[38] Kunwar A, Barik A, Mishra B, Rathinasamy K, Pandey R, Priyadarsini KI. Quantitative cellular uptake, localization and cytotoxicity of curcumin in normal and tumor cells. Biochim Biophys Acta 2008;1780(4) 673-679.

[39] Han DW, Matsumura K, Kim B, Hyon SH. Time-dependent intracellular trafficking of FITC-conjugated epigallocatechin-3-O-gallate in L-929 cells. Bioorg Med Chem. 2008;16(22) 9652–9659.

[40] Piyaviriyakul S, Shimizu K, Asakawa T, Kan T, Siripong P, Oku N. Anti-angiogenic activity and intracellular distribution of epigallocatechin-3-gallate analogs. Biol Pharm Bull. 2011;34(3) 396-400.

[41] Gu L, Laly M, Chang HC, Prior RL, Fang N, Ronis MJ, Badger TM. Isoflavone conjugates are underestimated in tissues using enzymatic hydrolysis. J Agric Food Chem. 2005;53(17) 6858-6863.

[42] Thakur VS, Gupta K, Gupta S. The chemopreventive and chemotherapeutic potentials of tea polyphenols. Curr Pharm Biotechnol. 2012;13(1) 191-199.

[43] Hong J, Lu H, Meng X, Ryu JH, Hara Y, Yang CS. Stability, cellular uptake, biotransformation, and efflux of tea polyphenol (-)-epigallocatechin-3-gallate in HT-29 human colon adenocarcinoma cells. Cancer Res. 2002;62(24) 7241-7246.

[44] Breinholt VM, Offord EA, Brouwer C, Nielsen SE, Brøsen K, Friedberg T. *In vitro* investigation of cytochrome P450-mediated metabolism of dietary flavonoids. Food Chem Toxicol. 2002;40(5) 609-616.

[45] Salucci M, Stivala LA, Maiani G, Bugianesi R, Vannini V. Flavonoids uptake and their effect on cell cycle of human colon adenocarcinoma cells (Caco2). Br J Cancer 2002;86(10) 1645-1651.

[46] Zhu Y, Chiang H, Zhou J, Xie F and Kissinger P T. *In vitro* metabolism study of resveratrol and identification and determination of its main metabolite piceatannol by LC/EC and LC/MS/MS. Asian J Drug Metab Ph. 2005;5(1) 49-54.

[47] Gradolatto A, Canivenc-Lavier MC, Basly JP, Siess MH, Teyssier C. Metabolism of apigenin by rat liver phase I and phase II enzymes and by isolated perfused rat liver. Drug Metab Dispos. 2004;32(1) 58-65.

[48] Spencer JPE, Kuhnle GG, Williams RJ, Rice-Evans C. Intracellular metabolism and bioactivity of quercetin and its *in vivo* metabolites. Biochem J. 2003;372(Pt 1) 173–181.

[49] Beekmann K, Actis-Goretta L, van Bladeren PJ, Dionisi F, Destaillats F, Rietjens IM. A state-of-the-art overview of the effect of metabolic conjugation on the biological activity of flavonoids. Food Funct. 2012;3(10) 1008-1018.

[50] Son TG, Camandola S, Mattson MP. Hormetic dietary phytochemicals. Neuromolecular Med. 2008;10(4) 236-246.

[51] Vargas AJ, Burd R. Hormesis and synergy: pathways and mechanisms of quercetin in cancer prevention and management. Nutr Rev. 2010;68(7) 418-428.

[52] Novak Kujundzić R, Grbesa I, Ivkić M, Katdare M, Gall-Troselj K. Curcumin downregulates *H19* gene transcription in tumor cells. J Cell Biochem. 2008;104(5) 1781-1792.

[53] Pietrocola F, Mariño G, Lissa D, Vacchelli E, Malik SA, Niso-Santano M, Zamzami N, Galluzzi L, Maiuri MC, Kroemer G. Pro-autophagic polyphenols reduce the acetylation of cytoplasmic proteins. Cell Cycle 2012;11(20) 3851-3860.

[54] Mukhtar E, Adhami VM, Khan N, Mukhtar H. Apoptosis and autophagy induction as mechanism of cancer prevention by naturally occurring dietary agents. Curr Drug Targets 2012;13(14) 1831-1841.

[55] Gossner G, Choi M, Tan L, Fogoros S, Griffith KA, Kuenker M, Liu JR. Genistein-induced apoptosis and autophagocytosis in ovarian cancer cells. Gynecol Oncol. 2007;105(1) 23-30.

[56] Casagrande F, Darbon JM. Effects of structurally related flavonoids on cell cycle progression of human melanoma cells: regulation of cyclin-dependent kinases CDK2 and CDK1. Biochem Pharmacol. 2001;61(10) 1205-1215.

[57] Surh YJ. (2003) Cancer chemoprevention with dietary phytochemicals. Nature Reviews Cancer 2003;3(10) 768-780.

[58] Hanahan D, Weinberg RA. Hallmarks of cancer: the next generation. Cell 2011;144(5) 646-674.

[59] Cai YZ, Mei Sun, Jie Xing, Luo Q, Corke H. Structure-radical scavenging activity relationships of phenolic compounds from traditional Chinese medicinal plants. Life Sci. 2006;78(25) 2872-2888.

[60] Yamashita N, Kawanishi S. Distinct mechanisms of DNA damage in apoptosis induced by quercetin and luteolin. Free Radic Res. 2000;33(5) 623-633.

[61] Russo GL, Russo M, Spagnuolo C, Tedesco I, Bilotto S, Iannitti R, Palumbo R. Quercetin: A pleiotropic kinase inhibitor against cancer. Cancer Treat Res. 2014;159 185-205.

[62] Boly R, Gras T, Lamkami T, Guissou P, Serteyn D, Kiss R, Dubois J. Quercetin inhibits a large panel of kinases implicated in cancer cell biology. Int J Oncol. 2011;38(3) 833-842.

[63] Xiao X, Shi D, Liu L, Wang J, Xie X, Kang T, Deng W. Quercetin suppresses cyclooxygenase-2 expression and angiogenesis through inactivation of p300 signaling. PLoS One 2011;6(8):e22934.

[64] Mutoh M, Takahashi M, Fukuda K, Matsushima-Hibiya Y, Mutoh H, Sugimura T, Wakabayashi K. Suppression of cyclooxygenase-2 promoter-dependent transcriptional activity in colon cancer cells by chemopreventive agents with a resorcin-type structure. Carcinogenesis 2000;21(5) 959-963.

[65] Ruiz PA, Braune A, Hölzlwimmer G, Quintanilla-Fend L, Haller D. Quercetin inhibits TNF-induced NF-κB transcription factor recruitment to proinflammatory gene promoters in murine intestinal epithelial cells. J Nutr. 2007;137(5) 1208-1215.

[66] Chan ST, Yang NC, Huang CS, Liao JW, Yeh SL. Quercetin enhances the antitumor activity of trichostatin A through upregulation of p53 protein expression *in vitro* and *in vivo*. PLoS One 2013;8(1):e54255.

[67] de Boer VC, de Goffau MC, Arts IC, Hollman PC, Keijer J. SIRT1 stimulation by polyphenols is affected by their stability and metabolism. Mech Ageing Dev. 2006;127(7) 618-627.

[68] Hong KS, Park JI, Kim MJ, Kim HB, Lee JW, Dao TT, Oh WK, Kang CD, Kim SH. Involvement of SIRT1 in hypoxic down-regulation of c-Myc and β-catenin and hypoxic preconditioning effect of polyphenols. Toxicol Appl Pharmacol. 2012;259(2) 210-218.

[69] Anastasiou D, Krek W. SIRT1: linking adaptive cellular responses to aging-associated changes in organismal physiology. Physiology (Bethesda) 2006;21(6) 404-410.

[70] Cohen HY, Lavu S, Bitterman KJ, Hekking B, Imahiyerobo TA, Miller C, Frye R, Ploegh H, Kessler BM, Sinclair DA. Acetylation of the C terminus of Ku70 by CBP and PCAF controls Bax-mediated apoptosis. Mol Cell 2004;13(5) 627–638.

[71] Yeung F, Hoberg JE, Ramsey CS, Keller MD, Jones DR, Frye RA, Mayo MW. Modulation of NFκB-dependent transcription and cell survival by the SIRT1 deacetylase. EMBO J. 2004;23(12) 2369–2380.

[72] Singh N, Ravichandran S, Norton DD, Fugmann SD, Moaddel R. Synthesis and characterization of a SIRT6 open tubular column: predicting deacetylation activity using frontal chromatography. Anal Biochem. 2013;436(2) 78-83.

[73] Lee WJ, Chen YR, Tseng TH. Quercetin induces FasL-related apoptosis, in part, through promotion of histone H3 acetylation in human leukemia HL-60 cells. Oncol Rep. 2011;25(2) 583-591.

[74] Jia J, Chen J. Histone hyperacetylation is involved in the quercetin-induced human leukemia cell death. Pharmazie 2008;63(5) 379-383.

[75] Tan S, Wang C, Lu C, Zhao B, Cui Y, Shi X, Ma X. Quercetin is able to demethylate the $p16^{INK4a}$ gene promoter. Chemotherapy 2009;55(1) 6–10.

[76] Abdulla A, Zhao X, Yang F. Natural polyphenols inhibit lysine-specific demethylase-1 *in vitro*. J Biochem Pharmacol Res. 2013;1(1) 56-63.

[77] Chen Y, Jie W, Yan W, Zhou K, Xiao Y. Lysine-specific histone demethylase 1 (LSD1): A potential molecular target for tumor therapy. Crit Rev Eukaryot Gene Expr. 2012;22(1) 53–59.

[78] Lee WJ, Shim JY, Zhu BT. Mechanisms for the inhibition of DNA methyltransferases by tea catechins and bioflavonoids. Mol Pharmacol. 2005;68(4) 1018-1030.

[79] Calderón-Montaño JM, Burgos-Morón E, Pérez-Guerrero C, López-Lázaro M. A review on the dietary flavonoid kaempferol. Mini Rev Med Chem. 2011;11(4) 298-344.

[80] Huang WW, Tsai SC, Peng SF, Lin MW, Chiang JH, Chiu YJ, Fushiya S, Tseng MT, Yang JS. Kaempferol induces autophagy through AMPK and AKT signaling molecules and causes G2/M arrest *via* downregulation of CDK1/cyclin B in SK-HEP-1 human hepatic cancer cells. Int J Oncol. 2013;42(6) 2069-2077.

[81] Berger A, Venturelli S, Kallnischkies M, Böcker A, Busch C, Weiland T, Noor S, Leischner C, Weiss TS, Lauer UM, Bischoff SC, Bitzer M. Kaempferol, a new nutrition-derived pan-inhibitor of human histone deacetylases. J Nutr Biochem. 2013;24(6) 977-985.

[82] Sharma V, Joseph C, Ghosh S, Agarwal A, Mishra MK, Sen E. Kaempferol induces apoptosis in glioblastoma cells through oxidative stress. Mol Cancer Ther. 2007;6(9) 2544-2553.

[83] Kang GY, Lee ER, Kim JH, Jung JW, Lim J, Kim SK, Cho SG, Kim KP. Downregulation of PLK-1 expression in kaempferol-induced apoptosis of MCF-7 cells. Eur J Pharmacol. 2009;611(1-3) 17-21.

[84] Marfe G, Tafani M, Indelicato M, Sinibaldi-Salimei P, Reali V, Pucci B, Fini M, Russo MA. Kaempferol induces apoptosis in two different cell lines *via* Akt inactivation, Bax and SIRT3 activation, and mitochondrial dysfunction. J Cell Biochem. 2009;106(4) 643-650.

[85] Ambrosio R, Damiano V, Sibilio A, De Stefano MA, Avvedimento VE, Salvatore D, Dentice M. Epigenetic control of type 2 and 3 deiodinases in myogenesis: role of lysine-specific demethylase enzyme and FoxO3. Nucleic Acids Res. 2013;41(6) 3551-3562.

[86] da-Silva WS, Harney JW, Kim BW, Li J, Bianco SD, Crescenzi A, Christoffolete MA, Huang SA, Bianco AC. The small polyphenolic molecule kaempferol increases cellular energy expenditure and thyroid hormone activation. Diabetes 2007;56(3) 767-776.

[87] Stepanić V, Gall Trošelj K, Lučić B, Marković Z, Amić D. Bond dissociation free energy as a general parameter for flavonoid radical scavenging activity. Food Chem. 2013;141(2) 1562-1570.

[88] Markaverich BM, Vijjeswarapu M. Multiple sites of type II site ligand (luteolin and BMHPC) regulation of gene expression in PC-3 cells. Int J Biomed Sci. 2012;8(4) 219-232.

[89] Lin Y, Shi R, Wang X, Shen HM. Luteolin, a flavonoid with potential for cancer prevention and therapy. Curr Cancer Drug Targets 2008;8(7) 634-646.

[90] López-Lázaro M. Distribution and biological activities of the flavonoid luteolin. Mini Rev Med Chem. 2009;9(1) 31-59.

[91] Bandaruk Y, Mukai R, Kawamura T, Nemoto H, Terao J. Evaluation of the inhibitory effects of quercetin-related flavonoids and tea catechins on the monoamine oxidase-

A reaction in mouse brain mitochondria. J Agric Food Chem. 2012 60(41) 10270-10277.

[92] Han XH, Hong SS, Hwang JS, Lee MK, Hwang BY, Ro JS. Monoamine oxidase inhibitory components from *Cayratia japonica*. Arch Pharm Res. 2007;30(1) 13-17.

[93] Attoub S, Hassan AH, Vanhoecke B, Iratni R, Takahashi T, Gaben AM, Bracke M, Awad S, John A, Kamalboor HA, Al Sultan MA, Arafat K, Gespach C, Petroianu G. Inhibition of cell survival, invasion, tumor growth and histone deacetylase activity by the dietary flavonoid luteolin in human epithelioid cancer cells. Eur J Pharmacol. 2011;651(1-3) 18-25.

[94] Chen ZJ, Dai YQ, Kong SS, Song FF, Li LP, Ye JF, Wang RW, Zeng S, Zhou H, Jiang HD. Luteolin is a rare substrate of human catechol-O-methyltransferase favoring a para-methylation. Mol Nutr Food Res. 2013;57(5) 877-885.

[95] Xie F, Lang Q, Zhou M, Zhang H, Zhang Z, Zhang Y, Wan B, Huang Q, Yu L. The dietary flavonoid luteolin inhibits Aurora B serine/threonine kinase activity and blocks proliferation of cancer cells. Eur J Pharm Sci. 2012;46(5) 388-396.

[96] Ruela-de-Sousa RR, Fuhler GM, Blom N, Ferreira CV, Aoyama H, Peppelenbosch MP. Cytotoxicity of apigenin on leukemia cell lines: implications for prevention and therapy. Cell Death Dis. 2010;1 e19.

[97] Arango D, Parihar A, Villamena FA, Wang L, Freitas MA, Grotewold E, Doseff AI. Apigenin induces DNA damage through the PKCδ-dependent activation of ATM and H2AX causing down-regulation of genes involved in cell cycle control and DNA repair. Biochem Pharmacol. 2012;84(12) 1571-1580.

[98] Seo YJ, Kim BS, Chun SY, Park YK, Kang KS, Kwon TG. Apoptotic effects of genistein, biochanin-A and apigenin on LNCaP and PC-3 cells by p21 through transcriptional inhibition of polo-like kinase-1. J Korean Med Sci. 2011;26(11) 1489-1494.

[99] Pandey M, Kaur P, Shukla S, Abbas A, Fu P, Gupta S. Plant flavone apigenin inhibits HDAC and remodels chromatin to induce growth arrest and apoptosis in human prostate cancer cells: *in vitro* and *in vivo* study. Mol Carcinog. 2012;51(12) 952-962.

[100] Basak S, Pookot D, Noonan EJ, Dahiya R. Genistein downregulates androgen receptor by modulating HDAC6-Hsp90 chaperone function. Mol Cancer Ther. 2008;7(10) 3195–3202.

[101] Fang MZ, Chen D, Sun Y, Jin Z, Christman JK, Yang CS. Reversal of hypermethylation and reactivation of $p16^{INK4a}$, *RAR-β*, and *MGMT* genes by genistein and other isoflavones from soy. Clin Cancer Res. 2005;11(19 Pt 1) 7033-7041.

[102] Borrás C, Gambini J, Gómez-Cabrera MC, Sastre J, Pallardó FV, Mann GE, Viña J. Genistein, a soy isoflavone, up-regulates expression of antioxidant genes: involvement of estrogen receptors, ERK1/2, and NFκB. FASEB J. 2006;20(12) 2136-2138.

[103] Li W, Frame LT, Hirsch S, Cobos E. Genistein and hematological malignancies. Cancer Lett. 2010;296(1) 1-8.

[104] Zhang Z, Wang CZ, Du GJ, Qi LW, Calway T, He TC, Du W, Yuan CS. Genistein induces G2/M cell cycle arrest and apoptosis *via* ATM/p53-dependent pathway in human colon cancer cells. Int J Oncol. 2013;43(1) 289-296.

[105] Schmidt F, Knobbe CB, Frank B, Wolburg H, Weller M. The topoisomerase II inhibitor, genistein, induces G2/M arrest and apoptosis in human malignant glioma cell lines. Oncol Rep. 2008;19(4) 1061-1066.

[106] Banerjee S, Li Y, Wang Z, Sarkar FH. Multi-targeted therapy of cancer by genistein. Cancer Lett. 2008;269(2) 226-242.

[107] Majid S, Kikuno N, Nelles J, Noonan E, Tanaka Y, Kawamoto K, Hirata H, Li LC, Zhao H, Okino ST, Place RF, Pookot D, Dahiya R. Genistein induces the $p21^{\mathrm{WAF1/CIP1}}$ and $p16^{\mathrm{INK4a}}$ tumor suppressor genes in prostate cancer cells by epigenetic mechanisms involving active chromatin modification. Cancer Res. 2008;68(8) 2736-2744.

[108] Akiyama T, Ishida J, Nakagawa S, Ogawara H, Watanabe S, Itoh N, Shibuya M, Fukami Y. Genistein, a specific inhibitor of tyrosine specific protein kinases. J Biol Chem. 1987;262(12) 5592-5595.

[109] Lamoral-Theys D, Pottier L, Dufrasne F, Nève J, Dubois J, Kornienko A, Kiss R, Ingrassia L. Natural polyphenols that display anticancer properties through inhibition of kinase activity. Curr Med Chem. 2010;17(9) 812-825.

[110] López-Lazaro M, Willmore E, Austin CA. Cells lacking DNA topoisomerase II beta are resistant to genistein. J Nat Prod. 2007;70(5) 763-767.

[111] Markovits J, Linassier C, Fossé P, Couprie J, Pierre J, Jacquemin-Sablon A, Saucier JM, Le Pecq JB, Larsen AK. Inhibitory effects of the tyrosine kinase inhibitor genistein on mammalian DNA topoisomerase II. Cancer Res. 1989;49(18) 5111-5117.

[112] Li Y, Chen H, Hardy TM, Tollefsbol TO. Epigenetic regulation of multiple tumor-related genes leads to suppression of breast tumorigenesis by dietary genistein. PLoS One 2013;8(1) e54369.

[113] Dagdemir A, Durif J, Ngollo M, Bignon YJ, Bernard-Gallon D. Histone lysine trimethylation or acetylation can be modulated by phytoestrogen, estrogen or anti-HDAC in breast cancer cell lines. Epigenomics 2013;5(1) 51-63.

[114] Li Y, Meeran SM, Patel SN, Chen H, Hardy TM, Tollefsbol TO. Epigenetic reactivation of estrogen receptor-α (ERα) by genistein enhances hormonal therapy sensitivity in ERα-negative breast cancer. Mol Cancer. 2013;12 9.

[115] Meeran SM, Patel SN, Li Y, Shukla S, Tollefsbol TO. Bioactive dietary supplements reactivate ER expression in ER-negative breast cancer cells by active chromatin modifications. PLoS One 2012;7(5) e37748.

[116] Groh IA, Chen C, Lüske C, Cartus AT, Esselen M. Plant polyphenols and oxidative metabolites of the herbal alkenylbenzene methyleugenol suppress histone deacetylase activity in human colon carcinoma cells. J Nutr Metab. 2013;2013 821082.

[117] Mirza S, Sharma G, Parshad R, Gupta SD, Pandya P, Ralhan R. Expression of DNA methyltransferases in breast cancer patients and to analyze the effect of natural compounds on DNA methyltransferases and associated proteins. J Breast Cancer 2013;16(1) 23-31.

[118] Fang M, Chen D, Yang CS. Dietary polyphenols may affect DNA methylation. J Nutr. 2007;137(1 Suppl) 223S-228S.

[119] Thakur VS, Gupta K, Gupta S. The chemopreventive and chemotherapeutic potentials of tea polyphenols. Curr Pharm Biotechnol. 2012;13(1) 191-199.

[120] Na HK, Surh YJ. Modulation of Nrf2-mediated antioxidant and detoxifying enzyme induction by the green tea polyphenol EGCG. Food Chem Toxicol. 2008;46(4) 1271-1278.

[121] Hou Z, Lambert JD, Chin KV, Yang CS. Effects of tea polyphenols on signal transduction pathways related to cancer chemoprevention. Mutat Res. 2004;555(1-2) 3-19.

[122] Patra SK, Rizzi F, Silva A, Rugina DO, Bettuzzi S. Molecular targets of (-)-epigallocatechin-3-gallate (EGCG): specificity and interaction with membrane lipid rafts. J Physiol Pharmacol. 2008;59(Suppl 9) 217-235.

[123] Yoo J, Medina-Franco JL. Discovery and Optimization of Inhibitors of DNA Methyltransferase as Novel Drugs for Cancer Therapy. In: Chris Rundfeldt (Ed.) Drug Development - A Case Study Based Insight into Modern Strategies. InTech; 2011. Available from: http://www.intechopen.com/books/drug-development-a-case-study-based-insight-into-modern-strategies/discovery-and-optimization-of-inhibitors-of-dna-methyltransferase-as-novel-drugs-for-cancer-therapy

[124] Schramm L. Going green: The role of the green tea component EGCG in chemoprevention. J Carcinog Mutagen. 2013;4(142) 1000142.

[125] Singh BN, Shankar S, Srivastava RK. Green tea catechin, epigallocatechin-3-gallate (EGCG): mechanisms, perspectives and clinical applications. Biochem Pharmacol. 2011;82(12) 1807-1821.

[126] Fang M, Wang Y, Ai N, Hou Z, Sun Y, Lu H, Welsh W, Yang C. Tea polyphenol (−)-epigallocatechin-3-gallate inhibits DNA methyltransferase and reactivates methylation-silenced genes in cancer cell lines. Cancer Res. 2003;63(22) 7563–7570.

[127] Pandey M, Shukla S, Gupta S. Promoter demethylation and chromatin remodeling by green tea polyphenols leads to re-expression of GSTP1 in human prostate cancer cells. Int J Cancer 2010;126(11) 2520-2533.

[128] Nandakumar V, Vaid M, Katiyar SK. (-)-Epigallocatechin-3-gallate reactivates silenced tumor suppressor genes, *Cip1/p21* and *p16*^{INK4a}, by reducing DNA methylation

and increasing histones acetylation in human skin cancer cells. Carcinogenesis 2011;32(4) 537-544.

[129] Kim SO, Kim MR. (-)-Epigallocatechin 3-gallate inhibits invasion by inducing the expression of Raf kinase inhibitor protein in AsPC-1 human pancreatic adenocarcinoma cells through the modulation of histone deacetylase activity. Int J Oncol. 2013;42(1) 349-358.

[130] Thakur VS, Gupta K, Gupta S.Green tea polyphenols increase p53 transcriptional activity and acetylation by suppressing class I histone deacetylases. Int J Oncol. 2012;41(1) 353-361.

[131] Choi KC, Jung MG, Lee YH, Yoon JC, Kwon SH, Kang HB, Kim MJ, Cha JH, Kim YJ, Jun WJ, Lee JM, Yoon HG. Epigallocatechin-3-gallate, a histone acetyltransferase inhibitor, inhibits EBV-induced B lymphocyte transformation *via* suppression of RelA acetylation. Cancer Res. 2009 69(2) 583-92.

[132] Lee YH, Kwak J, Choi HK, Choi KC, Kim S, Lee J, Jun W, Park HJ, Yoon HG. EGCG suppresses prostate cancer cell growth modulating acetylation of androgen receptor by anti-histone acetyltransferase activity. Int J Mol Med. 2012;30(1) 69-74.

[133] Krishnaswamy K. Traditional Indian spices and their health significance. Asia Pac J Clin Nutr. 2008;17(S1) 265-268.

[134] Kunnumakkara AB, Anand P, Aggarwal BB. Curcumin inhibits proliferation, invasion, angiogenesis and metastasis of different cancers through interaction with multiple cell signaling proteins. Cancer Lett. 2008;69(2) 199–225.

[135] Shehzad A, Lee YS. Molecular mechanisms of curcumin action: signal transduction. Biofactors 2013;39(1) 27-36.

[136] Fu S, Kurzrock R. Development of curcumin as an epigenetic agent. Cancer 2010;116(20) 4670-4676.

[137] Dicato M, Diederich M. Curcumin as a regulator of epigenetic events. Mol Nutr Food Res. 2013;57(9) 1619-1629.

[138] Balasubramanyam K, Varier RA, Altaf M, Swaminathan V, Siddappa NB, Ranga U, Kundu TK. Curcumin, a novel p300/CREB-binding protein-specific inhibitor of acetyltransferase, represses the acetylation of histone/nonhistone proteins and histone acetyltransferase-dependent chromatin transcription. J Biol Chem. 2004;279(4) 51163-51171.

[139] Kang J, Chen J, Shi Y, Jia J, Zhang Y. Curcumin induced histone hypoacetylation: the role of reactive oxygen species. Biochem Pharmacol. 2005;69(8) 1205-1213.

[140] Marcu MG, Jung YJ, Lee S, Chung EJ, Lee MJ, Trepel J, Neckers L. Curcumin is an inhibitor of p300 histone acetylatransferase. Med Chem. 2006;2(2) 169-174.

[141] Manzo F, Tambaro FP, Mai A, Altucci L. Histone acetyltransferase inhibitors and preclinical studies. Expert Opin Ther Pat. 2009;19(6) 761-774.

[142] Chen Lf, Fischle W, Verdin E, Greene WC. Duration of nuclear NF-κB action regulated by reversible acetylation. Science 2001;293(5535) 1653-1657.

[143] Cui L, Miao J, Cui L. Cytotoxic effect of curcumin on malaria parasite Plasmodium falciparum: inhibition of histone acetylation and generation of reactive oxygen species. Antimicrob Agents Chemother. 2007;51(2) 488-494.

[144] Bora-Tatar G, Dayangaç-Erden D, Demir AS, Dalkara S, Yelekçi K, Erdem-Yurter H. Molecular modifications on carboxylic acid derivatives as potent histone deacetylase inhibitors: Activity and docking studies. Bioorg Med Chem. 2009;17(14) 5219-5228.

[145] Chen CQ, Yu K, Yan QX, Xing CY, Chen Y, Yan Z, Shi YF, Zhao KW, Gao SM. Pure curcumin increases the expression of SOCS1 and SOCS3 in myeloproliferative neoplasms through suppressing class I histone deacetylases. Carcinogenesis 2013;34(7) 1442-1449.

[146] Liu HL, Chen Y, Cui GH, Zhou JF. Curcumin, a potent anti-tumor reagent, is a novel histone deacetylase inhibitor regulating B-NHL cell line Raji proliferation. Acta Pharmacol Sin. 2005;26(5) 603-609.

[147] Lee SJ, Krauthauser C, Maduskuie V, Fawcett PT, Olson JM, Rajasekaran SA. Curcumin-induced HDAC inhibition and attenuation of medulloblastoma growth *in vitro* and *in vivo*. BMC Cancer 2011;11 144.

[148] Liu Z, Xie Z, Jones W, Pavlovicz RE, Liu S, Yu J, Li PK, Lin J, Fuchs JR, Marcucci G, Li C, Chan KK. Curcumin is a potent DNA hypomethylation agent. Bioorg Med Chem Lett. 2009;19(3) 706-709.

[149] Du L, Xie Z, Wu LC, Chiu M, Lin J, Chan KK, Liu S, Liu Z. Reactivation of RASSF1A in breast cancer cells by curcumin. Nutr Cancer 2012;64(8) 1228-1235.

[150] Yu J, Peng Y, Wu LC, Xie Z, Deng Y, Hughes T, He S, Mo X, Chiu M, Wang QE, He X, Liu S, Grever MR, Chan KK, Liu Z. Curcumin down-regulates DNA methyltransferase 1 and plays an anti-leukemic role in acute myeloid leukemia. PLoS One 2013;8(2) e55934.

[151] Link A, Balaguer F, Shen Y, Lozano JJ, Leung HC, Boland CR, Goel A. Curcumin modulates DNA methylation in colorectal cancer cells. PLoS One 2013;8(2) e57709.

[152] Gerhauser C. Cancer chemoprevention and nutriepigenetics: state of the art and future challenges. Top Curr Chem. 2013;329 73-132.

[153] Hua WF, Fu YS, Liao YJ, Xia WJ, Chen YC, Zeng YX, Kung HF, Xie D. Curcumin induces down-regulation of EZH2 expression through the MAPK pathway in MDA-MB-435 human breast cancer cells. Eur J Pharmacol. 2010;637(1–3) 16–21.

8

Epigenetics, Protein Kinases and Heart Failure

Richard M. Millis, M. Sadegh Asadi,
Vernon Bond, Jr. and Georges E. Haddad

1. Introduction

During the past century, the diagnosis and treatment of heart failure has changed substantially. Heart failure, once viewed primarily as resulting from rheumatic valvular heart disease, presents currently as the main complications of diabetes, viral cardiomyopathy, coronary artery disease, myocardial infarction and hypertension. Although the etiologies are diverse, virtually all instances of heart failure can be characterized by a sequence of specific molecular changes in the myocardium. These molecular changes result in decrements in cardiac myocyte contractility (negative inotropy), the hallmark of heart failure. In the normal heart, contractility is mainly regulated and, therefore, maintained by G protein-coupled receptor (GPCR) signaling (Huang et al., 2011). GPCR signaling is stimulated when neurotransmitters, hormones and drugs possessing positive inotropic activity bind to β-adrenergic receptors (Leone et al., 2002). One of the main signaling problems in heart failure is that the GPCR β-adrenoceptor kinases -2 and -5 (GRK2 and GRK5) phosphorylate the GPCRs and make them insensitive to positive inotropic β-adrenoceptor ligands (Hata et al., 2004). As such, phosphorylation of the GPCRs functionally uncouples them from their G-proteins, thereby downregulating the cardiomyocyte intracellular signaling cascades which support myocardial contractility. GRK2 is the most abundant cardiac GRK and GRK2 activity is increased in several cardiovascular diseases involving impaired cardiac function and heart failure (Petrofski and Koch, 2003). GRK2 regulates myocardial signaling and heart development and the targeting of GRK activity by small molecule inhibitors of GRK2 is thought to have the potential to become an effective strategy for treatment of heart failure (Iaccarino and Koch, 2003).

1.1. Protein kinases and molecular mechanisms of negative inotropy and heart failure

Increased synthesis and release of endogenous β-adrenoceptor ligands such as norepinephrine, epinephrine and dopamine (catecholamines), mediated by sympathetic neural activity, is an attempt to drive the heart pump to compensate for heart failure. Another compensation attempts to drive the cardiac pump by upregulating the protein kinases known as cAMP-dependent protein kinase (PKA), protein kinases activated by the same signal transduction pathways as phospholipase C (PKC), phosphoinositide-3 kinases (PI3K) and mitogen-activated protein kinases (MAPK). These protein kinases phosphorylate intracellular enzymes that are functionally coupled to the signaling pathways which produce positive inotropic effects. Another compensation attempts to drive the pump by amplifying effects of the thyroid hormones on ion-channel and pump activities; however, upregulation of the thyroid hormones tri-iodothyronine (T3) and tetra-iodothyronine (T4) is also known to produce negative inotropic effects which are thought to be mediated by a T4 metabolite, 3-iodothyronamine (Axelband et al., 2011). The amplification of the effects of T3and T4 results in protein kinase mediated phosphorylation of proteins which promote calcium ion influx via L-type calcium channels and calcium removal by sarcoplasmic reticular Ca^{2+} (SERCA) pumping. Calcium influx increases contractility and results in positive inotropic effects whereas removal prevents calcium overload and, thereby, limits negative inotropy. In addition, thyroid hormones increase protein kinase-mediated phosphorylation of the sarcoplasmic reticular protein phospholemman. Phosphorylation of phospholemman is reported to stimulate sarcolemmal sodium-potassium pumping, (Na^+/K^+ ATPase) activity. Na^+/K^+ ATPase activity limits excessive depolarization associated with increases in intracellular Na^+ and may thereby prevent the arrhythmias likely to be associated with depolarization (Bers et al., 2009). Adenylyl cyclase regulates cAMP mediated signaling and the cAMP in cardiomyocytes stimulates PKA mediated phosphorylation of proteins which produces positive inotropic effects (Movsesian, 2003). Desensitization of cardiac adenylyl cyclase signaling is known to occur in heart failure. Whereas such desensitization may protect against adrenergic overstimulation, it also limits positive inotropy by downregulating β-adrenoceptors and by upregulating both the β-adrenoceptor GRKs and the inhibitory alpha subunit of G-proteins (Gi). In turn, upregulation of β-adrenoceptor GRKs decreases cardiomyocyte cAMP and the downstream positive inotropic signaling effects of PKA (El-Armouche et al., 2003). Hence, β-adrenergic antagonists are very effective treatments for heart failures; however, it remains unclear whether β-adrenoceptor blockers resensitize the β-adrenergic receptor system (Lohse et al., 2003).

1.2. Hormonal and immunologic mediators of negative inotropy and heart failure

Angiotensin II (Ang II) is also an important modulator of myocardial inotropy and the inotropic effects of Ang II are mediated by a balance of positive and negative inotropic signaling mechanisms. Heart failure is characterized by chronic exposure to high circulating levels of Ang II wherein the inotropic balance favors negative inotropy linked to activation of p38- mitogen-activated protein kinase which is activated by environmental stressors such as pro-inflammatory cytokine (p38 MAPK) signaling. Ang II also plays a role in cardiac remodeling involving hypertrophy and apoptosis mediated by Ca^{2+}/calmodulin dependent protein kinase II (CaMKII) (Palomeque et al., 2009). The sarcoplasmic reticular ryanodine receptor-2 Ca^{2+} release channel (RyR2) can be phosphorylated by several protein kinases such as PKA and CaMKII (Currie, 2009). Abnormal phosphorylation of RyR2 is also reported to contribute to the negative inotropy associated with heart failure. Although phosphorylation of RyR2 by CaMKII can produce positive inotropic effects, upregulated CaMKII activity may increase Ca^{2+} release from the sarcoplasmic reticulum, resulting in negative inotropy and cardiac arrhythmias (Currie, 2006). Negative inotropy and β-adrenergic receptor insensitivity may also result from production and release of the inducible isoform of nitric oxide synthase (iNOS) (Deswal et al., 2001). In addition, pro-inflammatory cytokines such as TNF-α appear to have the capacity to produce negative inotropy and cardiac remodeling whereby TNF-α (Levine et al., 1990) IL-6 (Kell et al., 2002) and IL-8 (Damas et al., 2000) are reported to induce apoptosis of cardiac myocytes. High circulating levels of IL-6 are associated with low cardiac muscle contractility and high levels of TNF-α have been found to be negatively correlated with a favorable clinical outcome of heart failure patients. The negative inotropy, remodeling (hypertrophy) and apoptosis associated with exposures to TNF-α seem to be mediated by activation of TNF receptor-1 (TNFR1) and inhibited by stimulation of TNF receptor-2 (TNFR2). Activity of both TNFR1 and TNFR2 are reported to be upregulated in heart failures (Chrysohoou e tal., 2009; Hamid et al., 2009). Stimulation of TNFR1 is shown to have the capacity to downregulate the rapid delayed-rectifier K^+ current (I_{Kr}) and, thereby, to delay cardiac repolarization, increasing the duration of the cardiac action potential in cardiomyocytes (Wang et al., 2004). Increased duration of the ventricular action potential is thought to be an attempt to maintain cardiac muscle contractility and limit the negative inotropy associated with heart failure. We have reported insensitivity to an agonist and to an antagonist of K_{ATP} channels, which would serve to limit the aforementioned increased duration of the ventricular action potential, in cardiomyocytes undergoing eccentric hypertrophic remodeling after volume overloading such as that which could occur during the development of heart failure associated with aortic valve regurgitation (Alvin et al., 2011). However, this increased duration of action potential also increases susceptibility to cardiac arrhythmia in hypertrophy-induced heart failure. Increased duration of the cardiac action potential is also observed in the TNF1.6 mouse model in which heart failure is produced by overexpression of TNF-α. Therefore, it seems that TNF-α induced increments in duration of the cardiac action potential and insensitivity to mechanisms that could limit the increased action potential duration may be important features of the hypertrophic remodeling associated with heart failures. Another mechanism for TNF-α induced negative inotropy is thought to result from overexpression of collagen and underexpression of the gap junction protein connexin-43 (Janczewski et al., 2004).

1.3. Intracellular transduction molecules, negative inotropy and heart failure

Myocardial infarction in mice together with estrogen receptor-β knockout is reported to increase the cardiomyocyte MAPK activities of the c-Jun, N-terminal kinase (JNK) activator protein-1 (AP-1) transcription factor component. These signaling molecules are activated by environmental stressors such as pro-inflammatory cytokines in females and the MAPK extracellular signal-related kinases (ERK1 and ERK2 also known as MAPK3 and MAPK1, respectively), cell-proliferation, growth-promoting signaling pathway in males. Estrogen protection of the myocardium associated with upregulated PI3K and the original mouse-strain Ak, thymic lymphoma transforming (Akt) cell proliferation and anti-apoptosis signaling activities in female mice suggests deficiencies of ER-β and PI3K/Akt mediated anti-apoptosis signaling in such infarction induced heart failures (Wang et al., 2009). Cardiomyocyte protection by adrenomedullin, a vasoactive peptide discovered in pheochromacytomas, also appears to involve upregulated PI3K/Akt and MAPK/ERK signaling pathways (Yanagawa and Nagaya, 2007). The myocardial protection reported with ginseng and related ginsenoside treatments are likely to decrease negative inotropy and the duration of cardiac action potentials, arrhythmias, remodeling and apoptosis by interactions with these protein kinases (Maslov and Konkovskaia, 2009). We have reported that MAPK ERK and PI3K/Akt signaling molecules play important roles in eccentrically-hypertrophied rat hearts subjected to volume overload (Teos et al., 2008; Zhao et al., 2010; Alvin et al., 2011). Substantial evidence is, therefore, emerging that the protein kinases in cardiomyocytes are invaluable biomarkers for heart failure, as well as for the effectiveness of cardiac protection by novel heart failure treatments.

2. Epigenetics, chromatin condensation for transcription and protein kinases

Chromatin participating in the transcription of DNA to mRNA is represented in the nucleus of eukaryotic cells by euchromatin, a lightly staining, unfolded structure which facilitates binding to the DNA of various gene regulatory proteins and RNA polymerases which induce transcription. The euchromatin that is not transcribed is transformed into more tightly and intensely staining heterochromatin which appears to protect the genes while they are not being actively transcribed. According to the "accessibility hypothesis," the cell uses transformation from euchromatin to heterochromatin as a method of regulating the expression and replication of genes (Yancopoulos et al., 1986). Constitutive euchromatin is the portion that is always being actively transcribed, thereby representing "housekeeping genes" which encode proteins supporting the cell survival functions (*International Human Genome Sequencing Consortium*, 2004). The condensation of chromatin for transcription is regulated by epigenetic modifications made to DNA, histones and to other regulatory proteins (Martin and Cardoso, 2010).

Epigenetics at work in the normal heart is demonstrated by the regulation of cyclic AMP-dependent protein kinase (protein kinase A, PKA), a positive-inotropic agent in cardiac myocytes and related heart tissue cells. PKA induces relaxation of the histone-3 and histone-5 (H3 and H5) associated DNA segments which condense the chromatin for transcription of the structural and functional proteins supporting normal cardiomyocyte contractility (Marion et al., 1985).

2.1. Epigenetic marks for monitoring cardiovascular disease progression

A potential use of epigenetic modifications on histones and related DNA segments is to provide a code sensitive to the progression of diseases that are impacted by environment-gene interaction. An example of this usage of epigenetic marks has been demonstrated in patients with end-stage heart failure. Heart failure in these patients appears to be correlated with differential methylation of the DNA and histones at lysine residue 36 (H3K36me3) in their cardiomyocytes. (Movassagh et al., 2011). Another example of how epigenetic marks can be useful is reported in cardiac hypertrophy wherein mRNA expression of multiple cardiomyopathy-related genes was found to be associated with a unique, specific pattern of acetylation and methylation of histone H3 in the cardiomyocytes (Gaikwad et al., 2010).

3. Histone acetylation/methylation and cardiomyopathy

3.1. Repressor element-1 silencing transcription factor (REST) and cardiomyocyte hypertrophy

Cardiomyocyte hypertrophy is a compensatory response to maintain contractility and heart function. Inhibition of expression of the gene for repressor element-1 silencing transcription factor (REST), a fetal gene transcription repressor in adult ventricular myocytes (Schoenherr and Anderson, 1995), has been linked to cardiomyocyte hypertrophy (Bingham et al., 2007). Endothelin-1 is an endogenous vasoconstrictor molecule known to be a stimulator of cardiomyocyte hypertrophy (Harada et al., 1997; Drawnel et al., 2013). Treatment of cardiomyoblast (H9C2) cells with endothelin-1 is shown to inhibit REST and the amount of hypertrophy seems to be positively correlated with acetylation of histone H4 and methylation of histone H3 lysine 4 (H3K4) (Bingham et al., 2007). Endothelin-1 also appears to employ REST to increase expression of the genes for brain and atrial natriuretic peptides, hormones that help compensate for heart failure by decreasing the circulating blood volume (Bingham et al., 2007).

3.2. Histone deacetylase GATAD1 and cardiomyopathy

Autosomal-recessive dilated cardiomyopathy in a human family has been shown to be associated with abnormal expression and subcellular localization of GATAD1 (Theis et al., 2011). GATAD1 is a gene product that is highly expressed during embryonic development of the mouse eye (Kim et al., 2010) and is a regulator of gene expression in cardiomyocytes. GATAD1 appears to function as a histone deacetylase, evidenced by its binding to a histone modification site (Theis et al., 2011). Interestingly, dilated cardiomyopathy has been produced in mice following inhibition of histone deacetylases (Theis et al., 2011). Deletion of histone deacetylase-3 (HDAC3) in embryonic cardiomyocytes is associated with a nonlethal cardiac hypertrophy and cardiomyopathy induced while animals are fed a normal diet. However, more severe hypertrophy, cardiomyopathy and heart failure occurs when these animals are fed a high-fat diet, associated with downregulation of several genes which regulate lipid metabolism (Sun et al., 2011).

3.3. DNMT inhibition, gene methylation, cardiomyocyte differentiation and cardiomyopathy

Decreased availability of β-catenin is expected to decrease developmental Wnt pathway transcription, an effect shown to be associated with inhibition of cardiomyocyte hypertrophy and left ventricular remodeling in animal models of heart failure (Bergmann, 2010). DNA methyltransferases (DNMT) are epigenetic regulators of cell differentiation and metabolism and treatment of mesenchymal stem cells with the DNMT inhibitor and demethylating agent 5-aza-2′-deoxycytidine (5-Aza) is shown to induce expression of the cardiac tissue-specific genes Nkx2.5 and α-MHC. 5-Aza treatment also upregulates glycogen synthase kinase-β (GSK3β) and downregulates the cell adhesion protein β-catenin, whereas it increases expression of GSK3α. This upregulation of GSK3β also stimulates cardiomyocyte differentiation (Cho et al., 2009). That GSK3 inhibitors (e.g., lithium) were found to be effective at blocking this 5-Aza induced upregulation implies that GSK3 is required for cardiomyocyte differentiation. That downregulation of β-catenin is closely associated with GSK3β-stimulated cardiomyocyte differentiation (Cho et al., 2009) suggests an unclear relationship between β-catenin and GSK3β and a significant difference between the 5-Aza induced mechanisms for differentiation of mesenchymal stem cells and the DNMT-dependent mechanism for inhibiting cardiomyocyte hypertrophy, ventricular remodeling and heart failure.

3.4. Methylation of PKCε and heart failure

Epidemiological studies have suggested correlations between prenatal exposure to adverse intrauterine conditions and risk for ischemic heart disease, a primary cause of heart failure, in adulthood. Hypoxia is a fetal stress known to decrease expression of the PKCε gene and increased susceptibility to myocardial ischemia and reperfusion injury in adult rat offspring (Xue and Zhang, 2009). This predilection for myocardial ischemia is associated with increased methylation of the PKCε promoter at two fetal transcription factor specific protein-1 (Sp1) binding sites. Hypoxia seems to affect the binding of Sp1 only to methylated, and not to unmethylated, sites. However, methylation of both Sp1 sites seems to decrease PKCε binding to Sp1 in both fetal and adult cardiomyocytes (Xiong et al., 2012). The DNMT inhibitor 5-Aza has been shown to block the hypoxia-induced increase in methylation of both Sp1 binding sites and to restore PKCε mRNA and protein levels to normal. These effects appear to be greater in male than in female fetal hearts. Decreased expression of PKCε mRNA was found only in the male hearts, with interactions between both estrogen receptor proteins and the Sp1 binding site (Patterson et al., 2010). Moreover, activation of PKCε is reported to cause return of high susceptibility of adult rat hearts to ischemic injury following prenatal exposure to hypoxia (Patterson et al., 2010). PKCε is also an activator of ATP-activated potassium (K_{ATP}) channels, a metabolic energy conservation measure associated with reduced energy supply stress in cardiomyocytes (Kim et al., 2006). PKCε induced K_{ATP} activation is reported to shorten the cardiomyocyte action potential and limit calcium ion influx and overload in cardiac myocyte sarcolemmal and mitochondrial membranes (Inagaki et al., 2006). PKCε also seems to mediate ischemic preconditioning, a cardioprotective countermeasure against myocardial ischemia/infarction (Inagaki et al., 2006).

Epigenetically-induced decrements in expression of PKCε, associated with aberrant methylation patterns, are also reported in relation to heart failure following experimental exposures to cocaine and nicotine (Barik, 2007). Prenatal exposure to cocaine is reported to downregulate PKCε expression in hearts, effects which persist into adulthood and increase susceptibility to myocardial ischemia and infarction and reperfusion injury (Zhang et al., 2007). Cocaine treatment of the fetal rat heart for as little as 48 h produces significant decrements in PKCε protein and mRNA expression, associated with increases in CpG methylation at two binding sites of the Sp1 in the PKCε promoter region, confirmed by the use of the DNMT inhibitor 5-Aza or procainamide to inhibit this methylation (Meyer et al., 2009). Moreover, cocaine administered to pregnant rats during gestational days 15-20 produced offspring whose fetal hearts had significantly decreased expression of PKCε mRNA and protein. We have shown that IGF-1 antagonizes the positive-inotropic effect of Ang II in atrial myocytes of aging male rats and that prenatal exposure to cocaine abolishes this response (Haddad et al., 2005), an effect that could also be mediated by decreased expression of PKCε. In addition, methylation of CpGs at the binding sites for activator protein-1 (Ap1), a human protein transcription factor, was decreased in these fetal hearts and was increased significantly by prenatal exposure to cocaine (Zhang et al., 2007). The CpG dinucleotides at Bhlhb2, Pparg, E2f, and Egr1 binding sites of the PKCε gene promoter are reported to be densely methylated in both male and female adult rats and prenatal exposure to cocaine appears to decrease methylation of the CpG dinucleotides at the two Sp1 binding sites and this binding was increased significantly by cocaine exposure, but only in the male offspring (Zhang et al., 2009).

Interestingly, prenatal exposure to nicotine, which increases release of norepinephrine, is also associated with inhibition of PKCε gene expression in the fetal rat heart, an effect which, like cocaine, persists into adulthood (Lawrence et al., 2008). This finding appears to link maternal smoking to heart failure in the offspring. Nicotine treatment of pregnant rats starting at day 4 of gestation is shown to increase methylation of the Egr-1 binding site at the PKCε gene promoter and decrease PKCε protein and mRNA expression in fetal hearts (Lawrence et al., 2011). Moreover, methylation of the Egr-1 binding site decreases Egr-1 binding to the PKCε promoter and cardiomyocyte deletion of the Egr-1 binding site decreases PKCε promoter activity and treatment of isolated fetal hearts with norepinephrine produces similar effects including increased Egr-1 binding site methylation and inhibition of PKCε gene expression. The DNMT inhibitor 5-Aza inhibited the norepinephrine-induced increase in methylation of the Egr-1 binding site and restored both Egr-1 binding and PKCε gene expression, implicating sympathetic neural overactivity in this nicotine-induced heart failure (Lawrence et al., 2011).

3.5. TNF-α methylates SERCA genes and inhibits cardiac relaxation

The aforementioned epigenetic mechanisms for heart failure are relevant mainly to the negative inotropy associated with heart failure resulting from systolic dysfunction and the majority of current treatments at increasing contractility to counteract systolic dysfunction. However, heart failure associated with diastolic dysfunction may be more common and most heart failure is, therefore, resistant to current treatments and may contribute to ethnicity-related predilections for heart failure in specific populations such as African-Americans (Khan et al., 2012). The focus of diastolic dysfunctional heart failure is an inability of cardiomyocytes to relax, a function critical to ventricular filling and, according to Starling's law of the heart, maintenance of contractility and stroke volume. In that regard, treatment with the pro-apoptotic cytokine tumor necrosis factor-α (TNF-α) is reported to methylate and decrease the cardiomyocyte sarcoplasmic reticulum calcium pump (SERCA-2A) gene activity, mRNA expression and protein transcription, thereby providing an epigenetic mechanism for diastolic heart failure (Kao et al., 2010). The promoter region of the SERCA-2A gene has a high content of CpG islands and treatment with the antihypertensive, smooth muscle relaxer apresoline, commonly used in cases of human heart failure, is reported to improve cardiac function in rat hearts by the mechanism of demethylating and increasing SERCA-2A gene expression of mRNA and protein and, thereby, improving cardiac relaxation, a key factor in heart failure associated with diastolic dysfunction (Kao et al., 2011).

3.6. Methylation patterns, cardiomyocyte apoptosis and cardiomyopathy

Aberrant methylation patterns also appear to play roles in myotonic dystrophy, a group of multisystemic diseases characterized by cardiac conduction abnormalities and CTG expansions. These CTG expansions are found to be substantially larger in cardiomyocytes than in cells of other affected tissues. The expanded repeat is reported to be a genetic biomarker for methylation wherein the CpG-free expanded CTG repeat appears to maintain a distinct pattern of CpG methylation at the myotonic dystrophy (DM1) locus, which varies markedly with age and tissue-specificity (López Castel et al., 2011). Promoter DNA methylation and Sp1 binding are also reported to be regulators of expression of human myotonic dystrophy kinase-related Cdc42 binding kinases (MRCKs) and family members of human myotonic dystrophy kinase (DMPK), RhoA-binding kinase(ROK), and citron kinase (Ng et al., 2004). These findings demonstrate an important interaction between epigenetic methylation marks (CpG-free expanded CTG repeats) and a genetic skeletal muscle disease that often produces cardiac anomalies.

Epigenetic mechanisms are also apparent in diabetic cardiomyopathy, another common cause of heart failure. Tumor suppressor protein p53-induced expression of the cyclin dependent kinasae inhibitor p21(WAF1/CIP1) is a mediator of cell cycle arrest at the G1 phase (Harper et al., 1993). When cardiomyocytes from diabetic patients and rats are subjected to oxidative stress, the change in methylation pattern and overexpression of p21(WAF1/CIP1) appears to contribute to cardiomyopathy by inducing cardiomyocyte apoptosis (Mönkemann et al., 2002).

Methylation of the insulin receptor IGF-1 and IGF-1 receptor genes at their promoter regions in cardiomyocytes of diabetic (db/db) mice is reported to be substantial and may, therefore, function as epigenetic markers for the development of diabetic cardiomyopathy. Unfortunately, their methylation patterns seem to be inadequate for differentiating db/db diabetic cardiomyocytes from those of normal control animals (Nikoshkov et al., 2011). On the other hand, the methylation patterns of three angiogenesis-related genes (angiomotin-like-2, Rho GTPase activating protein-24 and platelet/endothelial cell adhesion molecule-1) is reported to be able to differentiate left ventricular cardiomyocytes of normal control subjects from those of patients diagnosed with idiopathic end-stage cardiomyopathy (Movassagh et al., 2010).

3.7. Acetylation, cardiomyocyte survival and stress-apoptosis signaling

Stress and cardiomyocyte hypertrophy are associated with lysine acetylation of many different proteins, including histones. Lysine 53 of p38 mitogen-activated protein kinase (MAPK) appears to be acetylated and activated by histone deacetylase-3 (HDAC3) which increases the affinity of p38 MAPK for ATP, in parallel with decreased intracellular ATP concentrations in cardiomyocytes undergoing stress and hypertrophy (Pillai et al., 2011). In hypertrophied cardiomyocytes, phosphorylation of HDACs, specifically those shuttled between nucleus and cytoplasm by HDAC kinases, is associated with disinhibition of various transcription factors such as nuclear factor of activated T-cells and myocyte enhancer factor-2 (MEF2). On the other hand, the antioxidant thioredoxin 1 (Trx1) is shown to inhibit cardiomyocyte hypertrophy by decreasing cysteine residues in HDACs (Oka et al., 2009), thereby demonstrating a putative HDAC-dependent epigenetic mechanism for oxidative stress in cardiac hypertrophy and associated heart failure.

3.8. Lysine acetylation, shear stress and endothelial cell apoptosis

Blood vessel wall stress appears to be a potent epigenetic activator of sarcomeric protein transcription in vascular smooth muscle cells, a likely environment-gene interaction contributor to hypertension, the hallmark of cardiovascular disease and an important precursor to heart failure. In that regard, blood vessel wall shear stress is shown to enhance the lysine acetylation of histone H3 at position 14 (K14), as well as serine phosphorylation at position 10 (S10) and lysine methylation at position 79 (K79), and cooperated with trichostatin (TSA), an antifungal agent that is also an HDAC inhibitor, inducing acetylation of histone H4 and phosphoacetylation of S10 and K14 of histone H3. In addition, endothelial stem cells exposed to shear stress appear to strongly activate transcription from the vascular endothelial growth factor (VEGF) receptor 2 promoter. This effect was paralleled by an early induction of smooth muscle actin, smooth muscle protein 22-alpha, platelet-endothelial cell adhesion molecule-1, VEGF receptor-2, myocyte enhancer factor-2C (MEF2C), and α-actin. Moreover, the transcription factors MEF2C and Sma/MAD homolog protein 4 were isolated from shear stress-treated embryonic stem cells complexed with the cAMP response element-binding protein acetyltransferase (Illi et al., 2005). HDAC3 is known to play a crucial role in the differentiation of endothelial cells (Spallotta et al., 2010). In mature endothelial cells, HDAC3 appears to be a pro-survival molecule by activating the Akt intracellular signal transduction pathway (Zampetaki et al., 2010) and when HDAC3 is downregulated in apolipoprotein E-knockout mice, atherosclerosis and rupture is found in the isografted vessels (Zeng et al., 2006). However, at aortic bifurcations, where the endothelial cells are highly susceptible to atherosclerosis, HDAC3 expression is increased with phosphorylation of HDAC3 at serine/threonine. HDAC3 appears to bind to Akt and upregulates HDAC3 to increase phosphorylation of Akt in these endothelial cells. Increased Akt kinase activity combined with knockdown of HDAC3 could, therefore, promote both atherosclerosis and endothelial cell apoptosis by epigenetic mechanisms (Zampetaki et al., 2010). Such epigenetic mechanisms for endothelial dysfunction appear to be important, yet poorly understood, contributors to cardiovascular disease which is found to be correlated with ethnicity and may, therefore, help explain health and disease disparities such as the predilections for hypertension and heart failure in African-Americans (Khan et al., 2012).

A number of studies, during the past decade or so, have shown that HDAC inhibitors may be effective as inhibitors of cardiomyocyte hypertrophy. Class I HDACs are shown to inhibit cardiomyocyte hypertrophy associated with inhibition of the gene encoding dual-specificity phosphatase 5 (DUSP5) DUSP5, a nuclear phosphatase that downregulates hypertrophic signaling by ERK1/2 (Ferguson et al., 2013). Expression of DUSP5 in cardiomyocytes produces inhibition of hypertrophy resulting from administering prohypertrophic factors (Ferguson et al., 2013). Inhibition of DUSP5 by class I HDACs requires activity of both ERK and MAPK, that has been characterized as a self-reinforcing mechanism for promotion of cardiac ERK signaling (Ferguson et al., 2013). Moreover, in cardiomyocytes treated with highly selective class I HDAC inhibitors, nuclear ERK1/2 signaling is suppressed in a manner that is shown to be dependent on DUSP5. Research on HDAC inhibitors as therapeutic agents for heart failure has focused on the left ventricle. However, there is also research demonstrating that HDAC inhibitors may also be able to treat right heart failure by mechanisms that decrease pulmonary arterial smooth muscle contractility. A specific benzamide class I HDAC inhibitor, MGCD0103 is shown to decrease pulmonary arterial pressure more dramatically than the type 5 cGMP phosphodiesterase inhibitor and vasodilator tadalafil, a standard-of-care therapy for human pulmonary hypertension (Cavasin et al., 2012). Although this class I HDAC inhibitor only modestly reduced right ventricular hypertrophy, it had multiple beneficial effects on the right ventricle, which included suppression of pathological gene expression, inhibition of proapoptotic caspase activity, and repression of proinflammatory protein expression (Cavasin et al., 2012).

4. Therapeutic potential of HDAC inhibitors

Although the findings that cardiomyocytes expressing an HDAC mutation lack phosphorylation sites and are refractory to the development of hypertrophy (Zhang et al., 2002), mutant mice lacking the class II HDAC HDAC9 do exhibit stress-induced cardiomyocyte hypertrophy (Antos et al., 2003). These findings, although somewhat confounding, at least, suggest that modulating specific kinase activities could be key to elucidating the mechanisms of cardiac hypertrophy, as well as to developing novel heart failure treatments. Class II HDACs are known to inhibit the activity of myocyte enhancer factor-2, a mediator of responsiveness to environmental stressors and cardiac hypertrophy by binding to a stress-responsive kinase that is specific for conserved serines. (Zhang et al., 2002). The antiepileptic drug valproic acid is a class II HDAC inhibitor shown to inhibit the catalytic activity of HDAC6 (Lemon et al., 2011). Both HDAC6 and HDAC8 are apparently upregulated in experimental animal models of salt (DOCA)-sensitive hypertension and valproic acid is also shown to be an inhibitor of cardiac hypertrophy in hypertensive rats (Kee et al., 2013). PKC signaling is shown to support nuclear export of class II HDAC5 in cardiomyocytes and inhibition of PKC prevents shuttling of HDAC5 from nucleus to cytosol by a chromosome region maintenance protein (CRM1, also known as transportin-1) in response to a number of agents that promote cardiomyocyte hypertrophy (Vega et al., 2004). An HDAC5 mutant that cannot be phosphorylated is also refractory to PKC signaling and inhibits cardiomyocyte hypertrophy mediated by PKC agonists. These findings are consistent with those that demonstrate protein kinase D (PKD) phosphorylation and enhancement of HDAC5 nuclear export because PKD is a downstream effector of PKC (Vega et al., 2004). HDAC5 is only one of several transcriptional regulators of pathological cardiac hypertrophy the activities of which are regulated by subcellular distribution. For example, transcription factors belonging to the nuclear factor of activated T cells (NFAT) and GATA families of transcription factors that specifically bind to the GATA sequences of DNA are subject to CRM1-dependent nuclear export (Harrison et al., 2004). These pro-hypertrophic proteins are rapidly relocalized to the nucleus in response to pro-hypertrophic growth signaling (Harrison et al., 2004). CRM1 activity is, apparently, not required for the normal cardiomyocyte gene activation mediated by thyroid hormones (T3, T4) and IGF-1, agonists that fail to trigger the nuclear export of HDAC5. These results suggest a selective role for CRM1 in disinhibition of pathological cardiac hypertrophy and that targeting CRM1-dependent nuclear export in cardiomyocytes may ameliorate stress induced cardiomyocyte hypertrophy and provide novel therapeutic strategies for heart failure (Harrison et al., 2004).

5. Summary and conclusions

Heart failure is the result of complex environment-gene interactions between regulators of intracellular transduction molecules, intracellular/extracellular receptors and endocrine/ paracrine/ autocrine hormone-like signaling molecules. Figure 1 summarizes the main epigenetic mechanisms of cardiomyocyte hypertrophy, negative inotropy and heart failure. β-adrenoceptor activation of PKA is shown to interact directly with histones and related DNA segments at promoter regions of genes for mRNA transcription to support normal cardiac contractility. Prenatal exposures to hypoxia, cocaine or nicotine produces predilections for heart failure shown to persist into adulthood, associated with increased methylation and decreased expression of PKCε. Norepinephrine is also shown to decrease expression of PKCε, thereby implicating sympathetic overactivity in an epigenetic mechanism for cardiomyocyte hypertrophy and heart failure. Inhibition of a cardiomyocyte differentiation signaling molecule REST by endothelin-1 is shown to contribute to cardiomyocyte hypertrophy. An autosomal-recessive dilated cardiomyopathy is associated with HDAC inhibition produced by upregulation of another differentiation signaler, GATAD1. Hypermethylation of SERCA-2A gene by the pro-inflammatory cytokine TNF-α is shown to produce diastolic dysfunction, a common cause of heart failure in African-Americans and particularly resistant to current treatments. Lithium-induced inhibition of DNMTs appears to induce hypomethylation which upregulates GS3Kβ, associated with downregulation of β-catenin and inhibition of Wnt pathway signaling for differentiation, providing a mechanism for inhibiting cardiac hypertrophy and heart failure. HDAC-dependent mechanisms for stimulating stress-apoptosis pathway signaling and inducing cardiac hypertrophy have been demonstrated in cardiomyoctes, endothelial cells and vascular smooth muscle cells. These findings demonstrate multiple roles of histone and related DNA acetylations and methylations for regulating cardiomyocyte contractility. These epigenetic mechanisms provide insights that could be translated to novel clinical interventions for the prevention and treatment of heart failure.

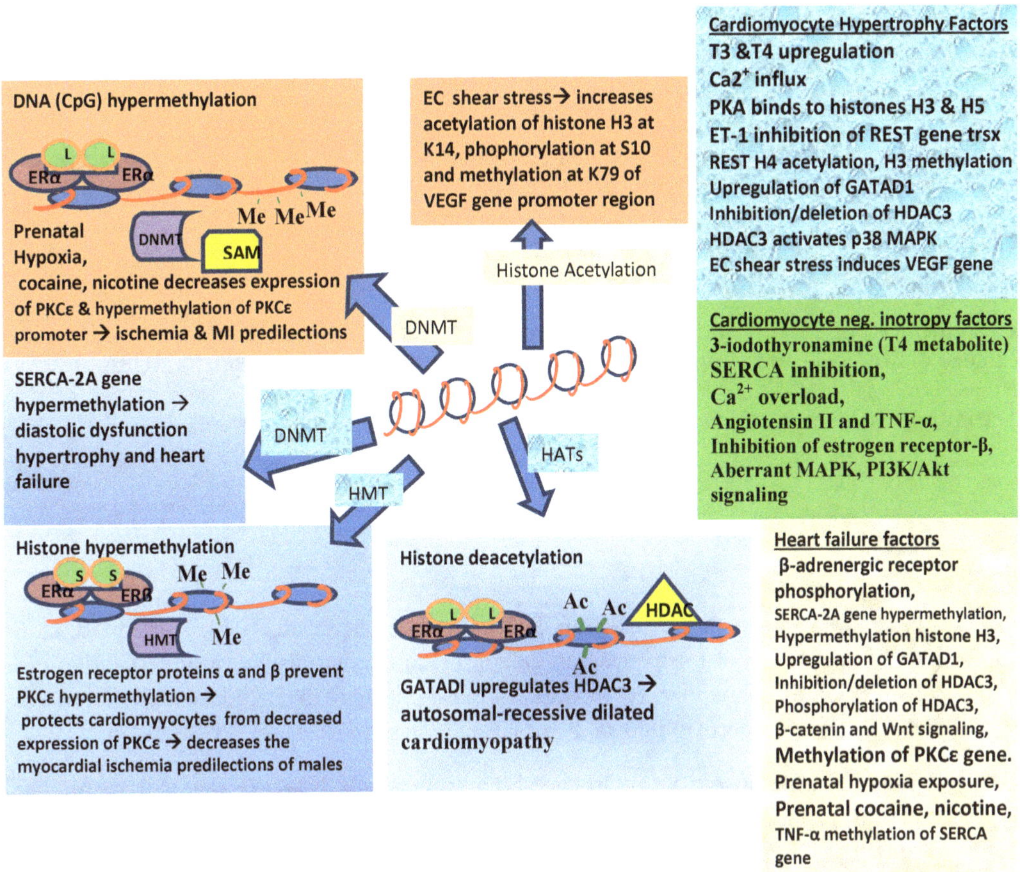

Figure 1. Main mechanisms for epigenetic alterations in heart failure. Each alteration involves many enzymes but the main players to cause methylation or acetylation are shown by arrows. These are not separate mechanisms and the enzymes do not act alone. Several enzymes act at a promoter simultaneously. 1) DNA methylatrasferase (DNMT) upregulation with S-adenosyl methionine (SAM) methylates the CpG islands at the PKCε promoter region which increases susceptibility of neonatal and adult cardiomyocytes to ischemia after prenatal exposure to hypoxia, cocaine or nicotine. 2) Upregulation of DNMTs is also associated with SERCA-2A gene hypermethylation which increases diastolic dysfunction and susceptilibity to heart failure. 3) Estrogen receptor binding to Sp1 fetal transcription factor binding sites (S) upregulates histone methyltransferases (HMTs) which protects cardiomyocytes from downregulation of PKCε expression. 4) Histone deacetylase-3 (HDAC3) upregulation is associated with expression of GATAD1, a fetal transcription factor, associated with autosomal-recessive dilated cardiomyopathy in humans and in animal models of cardiomyopathy and heart failure. 5) Histone acetylases (HACs) and histone methyltransferases (HMTs) are upregulated at a vascular endothelial growth factor (VEGF) promoter region by exposure of adult endothelial cell (EC) and embryonic stem cells to shear stress. Cardiomyocyte pro-hypertrophy factors include thyroid hormones (T3, T4), Ca2+ overload, protein kinase A (PKA) binding to histones, endothlein-1 (ET-1) inhibition of the gene for repressor element-1 silencing transcription factor (REST-1), REST gene acetylation at histone H4 and methylation at histone H3, upregulation of fetal transcription factor GATAD1, inhibition of HDAC3 and activation of p38 MAPK.

Acknowledgements

This research supported in part by NIH/NCRR/RCMI Grant 2G12RR003048 to Howard University.

Author details

Richard M. Millis[1], M. Sadegh Asadi[2], Vernon Bond, Jr.[3] and Georges E. Haddad[1]

1 Department of Physiology & Biophysics, Howard University College of Medicine and Graduate School of Arts & Sciences, Washington, DC, USA

2 Department of Neurology, Howard University College of Medicine and Graduate School of Arts & Sciences, Washington, DC, USA

3 Department of Health and Human Performance & Leisure Studies Howard University College of Medicine and Graduate School of Arts & Sciences, Washington, DC, USA

The authors have no conflicts of interest, financial or otherwise, to disclose.

References

[1] Alvin, Z, Laurence, G. G, Coleman, B. R, Zhao, A, Hajj-moussa, M, & Haddad, G. E. (2011). Regulation of L-type inward calcium channel activity by captopril and angiotensin II via the phosphatidyl inositol 3-kinase pathway in cardiomyocytes from volume-overload hypertrophied rat hearts. *Can J Physiol Pharmacol.*, 89, 206-215.

[2] Antos, C. L, Mckinsey, T. A, Dreitz, M, Hollingsworth, L. M, Zhang, C. L, Schreiber, K, Rindt, H, Gorczynski, R. J, & Olson, E. N. (2003). Dose-dependent blockade to cardiomyocyte hypertrophy by histone deacetylase inhibitors. *J Biol Chem.* , 278, 28930-28937.

[3] Axelband, F, Dias, J, Ferrão, F. M, & Einicker-lamas, M. (2011). Nongenomic signaling pathways triggered by thyroid hormones and their metabolite 3-iodothyronamine on the cardiovascular system. *J Cell Physiol.*, 226, 21-28.

[4] Barik, S. (2007). The thrill can kill: murder by methylation. *Mol Pharmacol.* , 71, 1203-1205.

[5] Bergmann, M. W. (2010). WNT signaling in adult cardiac hypertrophy and remodeling: lessons learned from cardiac development. *Circ Res.*, 107, 1198-1208.

[6] Bers, D. M, & Despa, S. (2009). Na/K-ATPase-an integral player in the adrenergic fight-or-flight response. *Trends Cardiovasc Med.*, 19, 111-118.

[7] Bingham, A. J, Ooi, L, Kozera, L, White, E, & Wood, I. C. (2007). REST regulates heart-specific gene expression using multiple chromatin-modifying complexes. *Mol Cell Biol.*, 27, 4082-4092.

[8] Cavasin, M. A, Demos-davies, K, Horn, T. R, Walker, L. A, Lemon, D. D, Birdsey, N, Weiser-evans, M. C, Harral, J, Irwin, D. C, Anwar, A, Yeager, M. E, Li, M, Watson, P.

A, Nemenoff, R. A, Buttrick, P. M, Stenmark, K. R, & Mckinsey, T. A. (2012). Selective class I histone deacetylase inhibition suppresses hypoxia-induced cardiopulmonary remodeling through an antiproliferative mechanism. *Circ Res.* , 110, 739-748.

[9] Cho, J, Rameshwar, P, & Sadoshima, J. (2009). Distinct roles of glycogen synthase kinase (GSK)-3alpha and GSK-3beta in mediating cardiomyocyte differentiation in murine bone marrow-derived mesenchymal stem cells. *J Biol Chem.* , 284, 36647-36658.

[10] Chrysohoou, C, Pitsavos, C, Barbetseas, J, et al. (2009). Chronic systemic inflammation accompanies impaired ventricular diastolic function, detected by Doppler imaging, in patients with newly diagnosed systolic heart failure (Hellenic Heart Failure Study). *Heart Vessels.* , 24, 22-26.

[11] Currie, S. (2009). Cardiac ryanodine receptor phosphorylation by CaM Kinase II: keeping the balance right. *Front Biosci.* , 14, 5134-5156.

[12] Damås, J. K, Gullestad, L, Ueland, T, et al. (2000). CXC-chemokines, a new group of cytokines in congestive heart failure-possible role of platelets and monocytes. *Cardiovasc Res.* , 45, 428-436.

[13] Deswal, A, Petersen, N. J, Feldman, A. M, Young, J. B, White, B. G, & Mann, D. L. (2001). Cytokines and cytokine receptors in advanced heart failure: an analysis of the cytokine database from the Vesnarinone trial (VEST). *Circulation.* , 103, 2055-2059.

[14] Drawnel, F. M, Archer, C. R, & Roderick, H. L. (2013). The role of the paracrine/autocrine mediator endothelin-1 in regulation of cardiac contractility and growth. *Br J Pharmacol.* , 168, 296-317.

[15] El-Armouche, A, Zolk, O, Rau, T, & Eschenhagen, T. and their role in desensitization of the adenylyl cyclase pathway in heart failure. *Cardiovasc Res.* , 60, 478-487.

[16] Ferguson, B. S, Harrison, B. C, Jeong, M. Y, Reid, B. G, Wempe, M. F, Wagner, F. F, Holson, E. B, & Mckinsey, T. A. (2013). Signal-dependent repression of DUSP5 by class I HDACs controls nuclear ERK activity and cardiomyocyte hypertrophy. *Proc Natl Acad Sci U S A.* , 110, 9806-9811.

[17] Gaikwad, A. B, Sayyed, S. G, Lichtnekert, J, Tikoo, K, & Anders, H. J. (2010). Renal failure increases cardiac myocyte histone H3 acetylation, dimethylation, and phosphorylation and the induction of cardiomyopathy-related genes in type 2 diabetes. *Am J Pathol.* , 176, 1079-1083.

[18] Haddad, G. E, Scheer, A, & Zhao, A. Clarke Jr., E., Arguinzoni, J.K., and Sobrian, S.K ((2005). Prenatal cocaine alone and combined with nicotine alter Ang II and IGF-1 induced left atrial contractions in aging male offspring. *Can J Physiol Pharmacol.* , 83, 957-965.

[19] Hamid, T, Gu, Y, Ortines, R. V, et al. (2009). Divergent tumor necrosis factor receptor-related remodeling responses in heart failure: role of nuclear factor-kappaB and inflammatory activation. *Circulation.* , 119, 1386-1397.

[20] Harada, M, Itoh, H, Nakagawa, O, Ogawa, Y, Miyamoto, Y, Kuwahara, K, Ogawa, E, Igaki, T, Yamashita, J, Masuda, I, Yoshimasa, T, Tanaka, I, Saito, Y, & Nakao, K. (1997). Significance of ventricular myocytes and nonmyocytes interaction during cardiocyte hypertrophy: evidence for endothelin-1 as a paracrine hypertrophic factor from cardiac nonmyocytes. *Circulation.*, 96, 3737-3744.

[21] Harper, J. W, Adami, G. R, Wei, N, Keyomarsi, K, & Elledge, S. J. cdk-interacting protein Cip1 is a potent inhibitor of G1 cyclin-dependent kinases. *Cell.*, 75, 805-816.

[22] Harrison, B. C, Roberts, C. R, Hood, D. B, Sweeney, M, Gould, J. M, Bush, E. W, & Mckinsey, T. A. (2004). The CRM1 nuclear export receptor controls pathological cardiac gene expression. *Mol Cell Biol.*, 24, 10636-10649.

[23] Hata, J. A, Williams, M. L, & Koch, W. J. (2004). Genetic manipulation of myocardial beta-adrenergic receptor activation and desensitization. *J Mol Cell Cardiol.*, 37, 11-21.

[24] Haudek, S. B, Taffet, G. E, Schneider, M. D, & Mann, D. L. (2007). TNF provokes cardiomyocyte apoptosis and cardiac remodeling through activation of multiple cell death pathways. *J Clin Invest.*, 117, 2692-2701.

[25] Huang, Z. M, Gold, J. I, & Koch, W. J. receptor kinases in normal and failing myocardium. *Front Biosci.*, 17, 3047-3060.

[26] Iaccarino, G, & Koch, W. J. (2003). Transgenic mice targeting the heart unveil G protein-coupled receptor kinases as therapeutic targets. *Assay Drug Dev Technol.* , 1, 347-355.

[27] Illi, B, Scopece, A, Nanni, S, Farsetti, A, Morgante, L, Biglioli, P, Capogrossi, M. C, & Gaetano, C. (2005). Epigenetic histone modification and cardiovascular lineage pro gramming in mouse embryonic stem cells exposed to laminar shear stress. *Circ Res.*, 96, 501-508.

[28] Inagaki, K, Churchill, E, & Mochly-rosen, D. (2006). Epsilon protein kinase C as a potential therapeutic target for the ischemic heart. *Cardiovasc Res.*, 70, 222-230.

[29] *International Human Genome Sequencing Consortium* ((2004). Finishing the euchromatic sequence of the human genome. *Nature.*, 431, 931-945.

[30] Janczewski, A. M, Zahid, M, Lemster, B. H, Frye, C. S, Gibson, G, Higuchi, Y, Kranias, E. G, Feldman, A. M, & Mctiernan, C. F. (2004). Phospholamban gene ablation improves calcium transients but not cardiac function in a heart failure model. *Cardiovasc Res.*, 62, 468-480.

[31] Kao, Y. H, Chen, Y. C, Cheng, C. C, Lee, T. I, Chen, Y. J, & Chen, S. A. (2010). Tumor necrosis factor-alpha decreases sarcoplasmic reticulum Ca^{2+}-ATPase expressions via the promoter methylation in cardiomyocytes. *Crit Care Med.*, 38, 217-222.

[32] Kao, Y. H, Cheng, C. C, Chen, Y. C, Chung, C. C, Lee, T. I, Chen, S. A, & Chen, Y. J. (2011). Hydralazine-induced promoter demethylation enhances sarcoplasmic reticulum Ca^{2+}-ATPase and calcium homeostasis in cardiac myocytes. *Lab Invest.* , 91, 1291-1297.

[33] Kee, H. J, Bae, E. H, Park, S, Lee, K. E, Suh, S. H, Kim, S. W, & Jeong, M. H. (2013). HDAC inhibition suppresses cardiac hypertrophy and fibrosis in DOCA-salt hypertensive rats via regulation of HDAC6/HDAC8 enzyme activity. *Kidney Blood Press Res.*, 37, 229-239.

[34] Kell, R, Haunstetter, A, Dengler, T. J, Zugck, C, Kübler, W, & Haass, M. (2002). Do cytokines enable risk stratification to be improved in NYHA functional class III patients? Comparison with other potential predictors of prognosis. *Eur Heart J.*, 23, 70-78.

[35] Khan, B. V, Rahman, S. T, Haque, T, Merchant, N, Bhaheetharan, S, & Harris, J. rd, Umar, K., Wahi, J., and Ferdinand, K.C ((2012). Vascular effects of nebivolol added to hydrochlorothiazide in African Americans with hypertension and echocardiographic evidence of diastolic dysfunction: the NASAA study. *J Cardiovasc Pharmacol Ther.*, 17, 291-297.

[36] Kim, B. S, Uhm, T. G, Lee, S. K, Lee, S. H, Kang, J. H, Park, C. S, & Chung, I. Y. (2010). The crucial role of GATA-1 in CCR3 gene transcription: modulated balance by multiple GATA elements in the CCR3 regulatory region. *J Immunol.*, 185, 6866-6875.

[37] Kim, M. Y, Kim, M. J, Yoon, I. S, Ahn, J. H, Lee, S. H, Baik, E. J, Moon, C. H, & Jung, Y. S. (2006). Diazoxide acts more as a PKC-epsilon activator, and indirectly activates the mitochondrial K(ATP) channel conferring cardioprotection against hypoxic injury. *Br J Pharmacol.*, 149, 1059-1070.

[38] Lawrence, J, Chen, M, Xiong, F, Xiao, D, Zhang, H, Buchholz, J. N, & Zhang, L. (2011). Foetal nicotine exposure causes PKCε gene repression by promoter methylation in rat hearts. *Cardiovasc Res.*, 89, 89-97.

[39] Lawrence, J, Xiao, D, Xue, Q, Rejali, M, Yang, S, & Zhang, L. (2008). Prenatal nicotine exposure increases heart susceptibility to ischemia/reperfusion injury in adult offspring. *J Pharmacol Exp Ther.*, 324, 331-341.

[40] Lemon, D. D, Horn, T. R, Cavasin, M. A, Jeong, M. Y, Haubold, K. W, Long, C. S, Irwin, D. C, Mccune, S. A, Chung, E, Leinwand, L. A, & Mckinsey, T. A. (2011). Cardiac HDAC6 catalytic activity is induced in response to chronic hypertension. *J Mol Cell Cardiol.*, 51, 41-50.

[41] Leone, M, Albanèse, J, & Martin, C. (2002). Positive inotropic stimulation. *Curr Opin Crit Care.*, 8, 395-403.

[42] Levine, B, Kalman, J, Mayer, L, Fillit, H. M, & Packer, M. (1990). Elevated circulating levels of tumor necrosis factor in severe chronicheart failure. *N Engl J Med.*, 323, 236-241.

[43] Lohse, M. J, Engelhardt, S, & Eschenhagen, T. (2003). What is the role of beta-adrenergic signaling in heart failure? *Circ Res.*, 93, 896-906.

[44] López CastelA., Nakamori, M., Tomé, S., Chitayat, D., Gourdon, G., Thornton, C.A., and Pearson, C.E ((2011). Expanded CTG repeat demarcates a boundary for abnormal CpG methylation in myotonic dystrophy patient tissues. *Hum Mol Genet.* , 20, 1-15.

[45] Marion, C, Martinage, A, Tirard, A, Roux, B, Daune, M, & Mazen, A. (1985). Histone phosphorylation in birefringence. *J Mol Biol.* , 186, 367-379.

[46] Martin, R. M, & Cardoso, M. C. (2010). Chromatin condensation modulates access and binding of nuclear proteins. *FASEB J.* , 24, 1066-1072.

[47] Maslov, L. N, & Konkovskaia, I. N. (2009). Inotropic, cardioprotective and antiarrhythmic effects of ginseng preparations. *Eksp Klin Farmakol.* , 72, 52-60.

[48] Meyer, K, Zhang, H, & Zhang, L. (2009). Direct effect of cocaine on epigenetic regulation of PKCepsilon gene repression in the fetal rat heart. *J Mol Cell Cardiol.* , 47, 504-511.

[49] Mönkemann, H, De Vriese, A. S, Blom, H. J, Kluijtmans, L. A, Heil, S. G, Schild, H. H, & Golubnitschaja, O. (2002). Early molecular events in the development of the diabetic cardiomyopathy. *Amino Acids.* , 23, 331-336.

[50] Movassagh, M, Choy, M. K, Goddard, M, Bennett, M. R, Down, T. A, & Foo, R. S. (2010). Differential DNA methylation correlates with differential expression of angiogenic factors in human heart failure. *PLoS One.* 5, e8564.

[51] Movassagh, M, Choy, M. K, Knowles, D. A, Cordeddu, L, Haider, S, Down, T, Siggens, L, Vujic, A, Simeoni, I, Penkett, C, Goddard, M, Lio, P, Bennett, M. R, & Foo, R. S. (2011). Distinct epigenomic features in end-stage failing human hearts. *Circulation.* , 124, 2411-2422.

[52] Movsesian, M. A. (2003). PDE3 inhibition in dilated cardiomyopathy: reasons to reconsider. *J Card Fail.* , 9, 475-480.

[53] Ng, Y, Tan, I, Lim, L, & Leung, T. (2004). Expression of the human myotonic dystrophy kinase-related Cdc42-binding kinase gamma is regulated by promoter DNA methylation and Sp1 binding. *J Biol Chem.* , 279, 34156-34164.

[54] Nikoshkov, A, Sunkari, V, Savu, O, Forsberg, E, Catrina, S. B, & Brismar, K. (2011). Epigenetic DNA methylation in the promoters of the Igf1 receptor and insulin receptor genes in db/db mice. *Epigenetics.* , 6, 405-409.

[55] Oka, S, Ago, T, Kitazono, T, Zablocki, D, & Sadoshima, J. (2009). The role of redox modulation of class II histone deacetylases in mediating pathological cardiac hypertrophy. *J Mol Med (Berl).* , 87, 785-791.

[56] Palomeque, J, Delbridge, L, & Petroff, M. V. a regulator of cardiomyocyte function and survival. *Front Biosci.* , 14, 5118-5133.

[57] Patterson, A. J, Chen, M, Xue, Q, Xiao, D, & Zhang, L. (2010). Chronic prenatal hypoxia induces epigenetic programming of PKC{epsilon} gene repression in rat hearts. *Circ Res.*, 107, 365-373.

[58] Petrofski, J. A, & Koch, W. J. (2003). The beta-adrenergic receptor kinase in heart failure. *J Mol Cell Cardiol.*, 35, 1167-1174.

[59] Pillai, V. B, Sundaresan, N. R, Samant, S. A, Wolfgeher, D, Trivedi, C. M, & Gupta, M. P. (2011). Acetylation of a conserved lysine residue in the ATP binding pocket of augments its kinase activity during hypertrophy of cardiomyocytes. *Mol Cell Biol.* 31, 2349-2363., 38.

[60] Schoenherr, C. J, & Anderson, D. J. (1995). The neuron-restrictive silencer factor (NRSF): a coordinate repressor of multiple neuron-specific genes. *Science.267,* 1360-1363.

[61] Spallotta, F, Rosati, J, Straino, S, Nanni, S, Grasselli, A, Ambrosino, V, Rotili, D, Valente, S, Farsetti, A, Mai, A, Capogrossi, M. C, Gaetano, C, & Illi, B. (2010). Nitric oxide determines mesodermic differentiation of mouse embryonic stem cells by activating class IIa histone deacetylases: potential therapeutic implications in a mouse model of hindlimb ischemia. *Stem Cells.*, 28, 431-442.

[62] Sun, Z, Singh, N, Mullican, S. E, Everett, L. J, Li, L, Yuan, L, Liu, X, Epstein, J. A, & Lazar, M. A. (2011). Diet-induced lethality due to deletion of the Hdac3 gene in heart and skeletal muscle. *J Biol Chem.*, 286, 33301-33309.

[63] Teos, L. Y, Zhao, A, Alvin, Z, Laurence, G. G, Li, C, & Haddad, G. E. (2008). Basal and IGF-I-dependent regulation of potassium channels by MAP kinases and PIkinase during eccentric cardiac hypertrophy. *Am J Physiol Heart Circ Physiol.* 295, H1834-H1845., 3.

[64] Theis, J. L, Sharpe, K. M, Matsumoto, M. E, Chai, H. S, Nair, A. A, Theis, J. D, De Andrade, M, Wieben, E. D, Michels, V. V, & Olson, T. M. (2011). Homozygosity mapping and exome sequencing reveal GATAD1 mutation in autosomal recessive dilated cardiomyopathy. *Circ Cardiovasc Genet.*, 4, 585-594.

[65] Vega, R. B, Harrison, B. C, Meadows, E, Roberts, C. R, Papst, P. J, Olson, E. N, & Mckinsey, T. A. (2004). Protein kinases C and D mediate agonist-dependent cardiac hypertrophy through nuclear export of histone deacetylase 5. *Mol Cell Biol.* , 24, 8374-8385.

[66] Wang, J, Wang, H, Zhang, Y, Gao, H, Nattel, S, & Wang, Z. (2004). Impairment of HERG K(+) channel function by tumor necrosis factor-alpha: role of reactive oxygen species as a mediator. *J Biol Chem.*, 279, 13289-13292.

[67] Wang, M, Wang, Y, Weil, B, Abarbanell, A, Herrmann, J, Tan, J, Kelly, M, & Meldrum, D. R. (2009). Estrogen receptor beta mediates increased activation of PI3K/Akt signaling and improved myocardial function in female hearts following acute ischemia. *Am J Physiol Regul Integr Comp Physiol.* 296, RR978., 972.

[68] Xiong, F, Xiao, D, & Zhang, L. (2012). Norepinephrine causes epigenetic repression of PKCε gene in rodent hearts by activating Nox1-dependent reactive oxygen species production. *FASEB J.*, 26, 2753-2763.

[69] Xue, Q, & Zhang, L. (2009). Prenatal hypoxia causes a sex-dependent increase in heart susceptibility to ischemia and reperfusion injury in adult male offspring: role of protein kinase C epsilon. *J Pharmacol Exp Ther.*, 330, 624-632.

[70] Yanagawa, B, & Nagaya, N. (2007). Adrenomedullin: molecular mechanisms and its role in cardiac disease. *Amino Acids.*, 32, 157-164.

[71] Yancopoulos, G. D, & Alt, F. W. (1986). Regulation of the assembly and expression of variable-region agenes. *Annu Rev Immunol.*, 4, 339-368.

[72] Zampetaki, A, Zeng, L, Margariti, A, Xiao, Q, Li, H, Zhang, Z, Pepe, A. E, Wang, G, Habi, O, Defalco, E, Cockerill, G, Mason, J. C, Hu, Y, & Xu, Q. (2010). Histone deacetylase 3 is critical in endothelial survival and atherosclerosis development in response to disturbed flow. *Circulation.*, 121, 132-142.

[73] Zhang, C. L, Mckinsey, T. A, Chang, S, Antos, C. L, Hill, J. A, & Olson, E. N. (2002). Class II histone deacetylases act as signal-responsive repressors of cardiac hypertrophy. *Cell.*, 110, 479-488.

[74] Zhang, H, Darwanto, A, Linkhart, T. A, Sowers, L. C, & Zhang, L. (2007). Maternal cocaine administration causes an epigenetic modification of protein kinase Cepsilon gene expression in fetal rat heart. *Mol Pharmacol.*, 71, 1319-1328.

[75] Zhang, H, Meyer, K. D, & Zhang, L. (2009). Fetal exposure to cocaine causes programming of Prkce gene repression in the left ventricle of adult rat offspring. *Biol Reprod.*, 80, 440-448.

[76] Zhao, A, Alvin, Z, Laurence, G, Li, C, & Haddad, G. E. (2010). Cross-talk between MAPKs and PI-3K pathways alters the functional density of I(K) channels in hypertrophied hearts. *Ethn Dis.* 20 Suppl 1, SS224., 219.

Permissions

All chapters in this book were first published in EE, by InTech Open; hereby published with permission under the Creative Commons Attribution License or equivalent. Every chapter published in this book has been scrutinized by our experts. Their significance has been extensively debated. The topics covered herein carry significant findings which will fuel the growth of the discipline. They may even be implemented as practical applications or may be referred to as a beginning point for another development.

The contributors of this book come from diverse backgrounds, making this book a truly international effort. This book will bring forth new frontiers with its revolutionizing research information and detailed analysis of the nascent developments around the world.

We would like to thank all the contributing authors for lending their expertise to make the book truly unique. They have played a crucial role in the development of this book. Without their invaluable contributions this book wouldn't have been possible. They have made vital efforts to compile up to date information on the varied aspects of this subject to make this book a valuable addition to the collection of many professionals and students.

This book was conceptualized with the vision of imparting up-to-date information and advanced data in this field. To ensure the same, a matchless editorial board was set up. Every individual on the board went through rigorous rounds of assessment to prove their worth. After which they invested a large part of their time researching and compiling the most relevant data for our readers.

The editorial board has been involved in producing this book since its inception. They have spent rigorous hours researching and exploring the diverse topics which have resulted in the successful publishing of this book. They have passed on their knowledge of decades through this book. To expedite this challenging task, the publisher supported the team at every step. A small team of assistant editors was also appointed to further simplify the editing procedure and attain best results for the readers.

Apart from the editorial board, the designing team has also invested a significant amount of their time in understanding the subject and creating the most relevant covers. They scrutinized every image to scout for the most suitable representation of the subject and create an appropriate cover for the book.

The publishing team has been an ardent support to the editorial, designing and production team. Their endless efforts to recruit the best for this project, has resulted in the accomplishment of this book. They are a veteran in the field of academics and their pool of knowledge is as vast as their experience in printing. Their expertise and guidance has proved useful at every step. Their uncompromising quality standards have made this book an exceptional effort. Their encouragement from time to time has been an inspiration for everyone.

The publisher and the editorial board hope that this book will prove to be a valuable piece of knowledge for researchers, students, practitioners and scholars across the globe.

List of Contributors

I.N. Lebedev
Institute of Medical Genetics, Tomsk, Russia

Tafari Mbadiwe and Richard M. Millis
Department of Physiology & Biophysics Howard University College of Medicine Washington,
DC, USA

Alexandra A. Majerski and Anthony C. Quinton
The Keenan Research Centre and Li Ka Shing Knowledge Institute, St. Michael's Hospital, Toronto, Canada

Philip A. Marsden
The Keenan Research Centre and Li Ka Shing Knowledge Institute, St. Michael's Hospital, Toronto, Canada
Department of Laboratory Medicine and Pathobiology, University of Toronto, Toronto, Canada

Minghua Wu
Cancer Research Institute, Central South University, Changsha, Hunan, China
Disease genome Research Center, Central South University, Changsha, Hunan, China
Key Laboratory of Carcinogenesis and Cancer Invasion, Ministry of Education; Key Laboratory of Carcinogenesis, Ministry of Health; The Center for Skull Base Surgery and Neurooncology, Hunan Province, China

Takeo Kubota, Kunio Miyake and Takae Hirasawa
Department of Epigenetics Medicine, Interdisciplinary Graduate School of Medicine and Engineering, University of Yamanashi, Yamanashi, Shimokato, Chuo, Yamanashi, Japan

Laura Vanagas, Susana Marisol Contreras and Sergio Oscar Angel
Instituto Tecnológico de Chascomús (INTECH), CONICET/UNSAM, Chascomús, Provincia de Buenos Aires, Argentina

Višnja Stepanić, Renata Novak Kujundžić and Koraljka Gall Trošelj
Laboratory for Epigenomics, Ruđer Bošković Institute, Zagreb, Croatia

Richard M. Millis and Georges E. Haddad
Department of Physiology & Biophysics, Howard University College of Medicine and Graduate School of Arts & Sciences, Washington, DC, USA

M. Sadegh Asadi
Department of Neurology, Howard University College of Medicine and Graduate School of Arts & Sciences, Washington, DC, USA

Vernon Bond, Jr.
Department of Health and Human Performance & Leisure Studies Howard University College of Medicine and Graduate School of Arts & Sciences, Washington, DC, USA

Index